MYELODYSPLASTIC SYNDROMES & SECONDARY ACUTE MYELOGENOUS LEUKEMIA

Cancer Treatment and Research
Steven T. Rosen, M.D., *Series Editor*

Goldstein, L.J., Ozols, R. F. (eds.): *Anticancer Drug Resistance. Advances in Molecular and Clinical Research.* 1994. ISBN 0-7923-2836-1.
Hong, W.K., Weber, R.S. (eds.): *Head and Neck Cancer. Basic and Clinical Aspects.* 1994. ISBN 0-7923-3015-3.
Thall, P.F. (ed): *Recent Advances in Clinical Trial Design and Analysis.* 1995. ISBN 0-7923-3235-0.
Buckner, C. D. (ed): *Technical and Biological Components of Marrow Transplantation.* 1995. ISBN 7923-3394-2.
Winter, J.N. (ed.): *Blood Stem Cell Transplantation.* 1997. ISBN 0-7923-4260-7.
Muggia, F.M. (ed): *Concepts, Mechanisms, and New Targets for Chemotherapy.* 1995. ISBN 0-7923-3525-2.
Klastersky, J. (ed): *Infectious Complications of Cancer.* 1995. ISBN 0-7923-3598-8.
Kurzrock, R., Talpaz, M. (eds): *Cytokines: Interleukins and Their Receptors.* 1995. ISBN 0-7923-363
Sugarbaker, P. (ed): *Peritoneal Carcinomatosis: Drugs and Diseases.* 1995. ISBN 0-7923-3726-3.
Sugarbaker, P. (ed): *Peritoneal Carcinomatosis: Principles of Management.* 1995. ISBN 0-7923-3727-1.
Dickson, R.B., Lippman, M.E. (eds.): *Mammary Tumor Cell Cycle, Differentiation and Metastasis.* 1995. ISBN 0-7923-3905-3.
Freireich, E.J, Kantarjian, H. (eds.): *Molecular Genetics and Therapy of Leukemia.* 1995. ISBN 0-7923-3912-6.
Cabanillas, F., Rodriguez, M.A. (eds.): *Advances in Lymphoma Research.* 1996. ISBN 0-7923-3929-
Miller, A.B. (ed.): *Advances in Cancer Screening.* 1996. ISBN 0-7923-4019-1.
Hait , W.N. (ed.): *Drug Resistance.* 1996. ISBN 0-7923-4022-1.
Pienta, K.J. (ed.): *Diagnosis and Treatment of Genitourinary Malignancies.* 1996. ISBN 0-7923-4164
Arnold, A.J. (ed.): *Endocrine Neoplasms.* 1997. ISBN 0-7923-4354-9.
Pollock, R.E. (ed.): *Surgical Oncology.* 1997. ISBN 0-7923-9900-5.
Verweij, J., Pinedo, H.M., Suit, H.D. (eds.): *Soft Tissue Sarcomas: Present Achievements and Future Prospects.* 1997. ISBN 0-7923-9913-7.
Walterhouse, D.O., Cohn, S. L. (eds.): *Diagnostic and Therapeutic Advances in Pediatric Oncology.* 1997. ISBN 0-7923-9978-1.
Mittal, B.B., Purdy, J.A., Ang, K.K. (eds.): *Radiation Therapy.* 1998. ISBN 0-7923-9981-1.
Foon, K.A., Muss, H.B. (eds.): *Biological and Hormonal Therapies of Cancer.* 1998. ISBN 0-7923-99
Ozols, R.F. (ed.): *Gynecologic Oncology.* 1998. ISBN 0-7923-8070-3.
Noskin, G. A. (ed.): *Management of Infectious Complications in Cancer Patients.* 1998. ISBN 0-7923-8150-5
Bennett, C. L. (ed.): *Cancer Policy.* 1998. ISBN 0-7923-8203-X
Benson, A. B. (ed.): *Gastrointestinal Oncology.* 1998. ISBN 0-7923-8205-6
Tallman, M.S. , Gordon, L.I. (eds.): *Diagnostic and Therapeutic Advances in Hematologic Malignanc* 1998. ISBN 0-7923-8206-4
von Gunten, C.F. (ed.): *Palliative Care and Rehabilitation of Cancer Patients.* 1999. ISBN 0-7923-852
Burt, R.K., Brush, M.M. (eds): *Advances in Allogeneic Hematopoietic Stem Cell Transplantation.* 199 ISBN 0-7923-7714-1
Angelos, P. (ed): *Ethical Issues in Cancer Patient Care* 2000. ISBN 0-7923-7726-5
Gradishar, W.J., Wood, W.C. (eds): *Advances in Breast Cancer Management.* 2000. ISBN 0-7923-78
Sparano, Joseph A. (ed.): *HIV & HTLV-I Associated Malignancies.* 2001. ISBN 0-7923-7220-4.
Ettinger, David S. (ed.): *Thoracic Oncology.* 2001. ISBN 0-7923-7248-4.
Bergan, Raymond C. (ed.): *Cancer Chemoprevention.* 2001. ISBN 0-7923-7259-X.
Leong, S.P.L. (ed.): *Atlas of Selective Sentinel Lymph Node Dissection for Melanoma, Breast Cancer ar Colon Cancer.* 2001. ISBN 0-7923-7385-5.
Raza, A., Mundle, S.D. (eds): *Myelodysplastic Syndromes & Secondary Acute Myelogenous Leukemia; Directions for the new Millennium.* 2001. ISBN 0-7923-7396-0.

MYELODYSPLASTIC SYNDROMES & SECONDARY ACUTE MYELOGENOUS LEUKEMIA:

Directions for the New Millennium

Edited by:

Azra Raza, MD

Director, MDS Center and Section of Myeloid Diseases

Suneel D. Mundle, Ph.D.

Assistant Professor of Medicine & Biochemistry, MDS Center and Section of Myeloid Diseases

RUSH CANCER INSTITUTE
RUSH PRESBYTERIAN ST. LUKE'S MEDICAL CENTER
RUSH UNIVERSITY
CHICAGO, USA

KLUWER ACADEMIC PUBLISHERS
Boston / Dordrecht / London

Distributors for North, Central and South America:
Kluwer Academic Publishers
101 Philip Drive
Assinippi Park
Norwell, Massachusetts 02061 USA

Distributors for all other countries:
Kluwer Academic Publishers Group
Distribution Centre
Post Office Box 322
3300 AH Dordrecht, THE NETHERLANDS

Library of Congress Cataloging-in-Publication Data

Printed on acid-free paper.

Printed in the United States of America

The Publisher offers discounts on this book for bulk purchases. For further information, send email to [laura.walsh@wkap.com]

****

For my mother, Zaheer Fatima, and my father, Syed Ali Raza,
the most inspiring role models in my life.
For Harvey and Sheherzad who are my two biggest strengths &
paradoxically, my two biggest weaknesses
-Azra Raza

****

****

For my Guru Dr. Nandini Sheth
-Suneel D. Mundle

****

"Surely, you have been made to see if (only) you care to see;
surely, you have been guided if (only) you care to take guidance;
& surely, you have been made to hear if (only) you care to lend your ears"
-- Ali Ibn Abu Talib
"Nahjul Balagha"

"Power Rests on Knowledge"
--Thomas Sprat

CONTENTS

LIST OF CONTRIBUTORS

Krishnan Allampallam, Ph.D., MDS Center and Section of Myeloid Diseases, Department of Medicine, Rush University, 2242 West Harrison Street, Suite 108, Chicago, IL 60612, U.S.A.

Sairah Alvi, Ph.D., MDS Center and Section of Myeloid Diseases, Department of Medicine, Rush University, 2242 West Harrison Street, Suite 108, Chicago, IL 60612, U.S.A.

M. William Audeh, M.D., Associate Clinical Professor of Medicine, Clinical Co-Chief, Division of Hematology/Oncology, Cedars-Sinai Medical Center, 8700 Beverly Boulevard, Los Angeles, CA 90048, U.S.A.

Gianluigi Castoldi, M.D., Professor of Hematology, Hematology Section, University of Ferrara, 44100 Ferrara, Italy

H. Joachim Deeg, M.D., Professor of Medicine, University of Washington School of Medicine, Fred Hutchinson Cancer Research Center, 1100 Fairview Avenue N., D1-100, Seattle, WA 98109, U.S.A.

Theo M. de Witte, M.D., Ph.D., Professor and Head, Department of Hematology, University Medical Center Nijmegen, Geert Grooteplein 8, 6500 HB Nijmegen, The Netherlands

Athanasios B.-T. Fassas, M.D., Assistant Professor, Myeloma and Transplantation Research Center, University of Arkansas for Medical Sciences, 4301 W. Markham, Slot 776, Little Rock, AR 72205

Ivana Gojo, M.D., Hematology Oncology, University of Maryland School of Medicine, Marlene and Stewart Greenebaum Cancer Center, 22 South Greene Street, Baltimore, MD 21201, U.S.A.

Judith E. Karp, M.D., Professor of Medicine and Oncology, University of Maryland School of Medicine, Marlene and Stewart Greenebaum Cancer Center, 22 South Greene Street, Baltimore, MD 21201, U.S.A.

Hans-George Klingemann, M.D., Ph.D., Coleman Professor of Medicine, Director, Section of Bone Marrow Transplant and Cell Therapy, Rush Cancer Institute, Rush University, 630 Hermitage Street, Kidston Building, Suite 404, Chicago, IL 60612, U.S.A.

Angela McGlynn, **Ph.D.,** Research Officer, Cancer and Ageing Research Group, School of Biomedical Sciences, University of Ulster at Coleraine, BT52 1SA, U.K.
Hugh McGlynn, **Ph.D.,** Senior Lecturer, Cancer and Ageing Research Group, School of Biomedical Sciences, University of Ulster at Coleraine, BT52 1SA, U.K.
Sharon Manson, RN, M.S., ACNP, Rush Cancer Institute, 1725 West Harrison Street, Suite 809, Chicago, IL 60612, U.S.A.
Hector Mayani, Ph.D., Head, Oncology Research Unit, Oncology Hospital, National Medical Center, Av. Cuauhtemoc 330, Col. Doctores, Mexico City, D.F. 06720, Mexico
Suneel D. Mundle, Ph.D., Assistant Professor of Medicine and Biochemistry, MDS Center and Section of Myeloid Diseases, Department of Medicine, Rush University, 2242 West Harrison Street, Suite 108, Chicago, IL 60612, U.S.A.
Rose Ann Padua, Ph.D., Reader, Hematology Department, University of Wales College of Medicine, Heath Park, Cardiff, CF14 4XN, U.K.
Harvey D. Preisler, M.D., Professor of Medicine, Director, Rush Cancer Institute, Chief, Hematology Oncology, Rush University, 1725 West Harrison Street, Suite 809, Chicago, IL 60612, U.S.A.
Azra Raza , M.D., Professor of Medicine, Director, MDS Center and Section of Myeloid Diseases, Department of Medicine, Rush University, 2242 West Harrison Street, Suite 108, Chicago, IL 60612, U.S.A.
Gian Matteo Rigolin, M.D., Ph.D., Assistant Professor of Hematology, Hematology Section, University of Ferrara, 44100 Ferrara, Italy
Lambert F.R. Span, M.D., Department of Hematology, University Medical Center Nijmegen, Geert Grooteplein 8, 6500 HB Nijmegen, The Netherlands
Vilasini T. Shetty, Ph.D., Assistant Professor of Medicine, MDS Center and Section of Myeloid Diseases, Department of Medicine, Rush University, 2242 West Harrison Street, Suite 108, Chicago, IL 60612, U.S.A.
Guido Tricot, M.D., Ph.D., Professor of Medicine, Director, Myeloma and Transplantation Research Center, University of Arkansas for Medical Sciences, 4301 W. Markham, Slot 776, Little Rock, AR 72205
Parameswaran Venugopal, M.D., Assistant Professor of Medicine, Rush Cancer Institute, Rush University, 1725 West Harrison Street, Suite 809, Chicago, IL 60612, U.S.A.

PREFACE

Cytopenias in older individuals are becoming almost like what prostate cancer is in older men; if you live long enough, you have a high likelihood of experiencing it. Clonality studies in disease free women have already demonstrated an age-matched increase in the incidence of monoclonal hemopoiesis. More recently, dysplastic features in the marrows of otherwise healthy older individuals without cytopenias have been identified as well. Taken together, these two findings would suggest that as the absolute number of hematopoietic stem cells decrease with increasing age, and the marrow becomes oligoclonal, the likelihood of dysplastic morphology increases. How this translates into the pernicious and potentially lethal disease called *myelodysplastic syndromes* (MDS) is a challenge requiring our immediate attention since the incidence of MDS appears to be on the rise. Limited advances in the treatment of both MDS and secondary acute myeloid leukemia (sAML) in the last two decades also add urgency to improving our understanding of the stepwise pathology involved in the evolution of these diseases. Given the enormous scope of our subject and the page limitations imposed by our publishers, this book is not meant to be the comprehensive last word on MDS and sAML. Rather, by focusing upon recent developments in intramedullary proliferation and apoptosis of hematopoietic cells, role of cytokines in the production of ineffective hematopoiesis, reasons for the poor in vitro colony growth of MDS cells, non-random cytogenetic abnormalities and sequential accumulation of molecular events leading to eventual leukemic transformation, as well as newer hypotheses regarding the etiology of MDS, we hope to provide thought-provoking suggestions to researchers in the field in this latest book on MDS and sAML.

A good example is the unique and interesting suggestion made by Dr. Harvey Preisler in the chapter on the evolution of secondary hematologic disorders. In order to dissect the sequence of events involved in the evolution of de novo MDS and/or AML in previously healthy subjects, one would have to follow thousands of individuals for years. Dr. Preisler suggests that one should be able to access an already established tissue bank maintained by the Women's Health Initiative where >100,000 women have been clinically followed for >10 years. Their blood and tissue samples have been stored at regular intervals. One can selectively examine serial blood samples for clonality studies/genetic mutations in women who were completely well at the time of enrollment on the study, but who during the course of periodic follow-up were found to have MDS and/or AML. Age-matched control samples from unaffected women would also be available in such a cohort. This study population would be different than those examined previously and composed of patients heavily pre-treated for a prior malignancy. Undeniably, access to such samples will require an extra-ordinary level of cooperation amongst investigators belonging to various disciplines, but the dividends will be far greater also.

In many ways, the pre-leukemic disorders pose a greater biologic challenge than AML. The bone marrow contains a very heterogeneous population of cells in MDS, all of which are the descendants of a transformed parent, as opposed to a monotonous population of blasts in AML. No satisfactory animal model for MDS exists, and since the hallmark of the disease is excessive intramedullary apoptosis of hematopoietic cells, immortalized tissue culture cell lines can only be considered as being partially representative of the actual pathology. But, like President Kennedy once said, America should go into space not because it is easy, but because it is hard. When one is faced with a particularly difficult challenge, paradoxically, one brings to bear both intellectual and emotional faculties.

The good news is that there appears to be a surge of interest in MDS recently. Rather than being considered an appendage of AML worth no more than a sentence or two as an aside, MDS has finally acquired the credentials and status of a full-fledged, unique disease demanding the undivided attention of its students, with a dramatic increase in the number of researchers. Several Societies and Working Groups have appeared in the last decade and International symposia solely devoted to MDS are being regularly organized. No reputable hematologic oncology meeting is considered complete without a discussion of MDS nowadays, and an unprecedented proliferation in the number of publications entirely dedicated to the study and treatment of MDS is noted. Minds, once catechized with dogmatic nonsense are beginning to dispute established tenets, weighing in with contrary views to re-think and re-examine some cherished ideas. We hope that this timely publication will add to the lively, burgeoning, rapidly expanding field by precisely locating areas ripe for translational research so that our patients can finally benefit tangibly. We apologize to those colleagues in advance who feel that their works have either not received sufficient attention in this book, or whose ideas have been challenged. It is purely the result of focusing on selected aspects of highly complex diseases, and with malice towards none. Finally we hope to invigorate our colleagues by challenging them to reconsider some of their deep-seated beliefs. Remember what the author Frank Burgess said; If in the last few years, you have not discarded a major opinion or acquired a new one, check your pulse.

Azra Raza, M.D.
Suneel D. Mundle, PhD.

March 6th, 2001

1

EVOLVING CONCEPTS IN MYELODYSPLASTIC SYNDROMES

Azra Raza,
MDS Center and Section of Myeloid Diseases, Department of Medicine
Rush University, Chicago, IL.

INTRODUCTION

Increasingly in the United States, older individuals between 60 to 75 years of age are discovered as having a variable cytopenia, most commonly detected during a routine visit to the doctor. The clinician's instinctive sense that such low-grade abnormalities would passively loiter coupled with limited therapeutic options led to the non-interventional practice of following these patients with no more than periodic blood counts. In the last two decades, this habit has been replaced by bolder attempts at more precise definitions with the result that the vast majority of such individuals are winding up with a diagnosis of Myelodysplastic Syndrome or MDS. The best proof of this statement is provided by the fact that only 143 patients were recorded as having MDS until 1973 (Saarni & Linman, 1973), while as many as 10,000 cases are being documented annually at the present time in the United States alone. This dramatic increase in incidence is the result of a combination of factors including an increase in the number of older individuals, aggressive attempts towards a specific diagnosis and probably an increase in the actual incidence of MDS due to toxic and chemical exposure. The exigent imperative for an accurate diagnosis comes first and foremost from an appreciation that MDS is not always a harmless pastiche of benign, poorly defined malaise in hematopoietic cells, but rather can be a deadly, exceedingly pernicious disease capable of killing swiftly. Rigorous classification and precise prognostication separate patients with insidious disease who can simply be followed with regular blood counts versus those requiring immediate intervention, most of which at this time remains experimental.

Unfortunately, a substantial number of individuals presenting with cytopenias continue to defy rules of classification and consequently, prognostication. The physician is then left with the unenviable task of providing reassurances to patients while attempting to explain to them the tenebrous ambiguities of the ill-defined, heterogeneous nature of their disease. The onus is more acutely felt when the patient is advised to accept treatment with drugs which themselves have been found to be the cause of MDS. At least one caveat in this context is to avoid referring rather presumptuously to MDS as a pre-leukemic disorder since that suggests a misplaced prescience. The reality in fact, is that less than a third of MDS patients overall, and less than a handful of those without excess of blasts ever evolve to a frank leukemia. For the most part, gradual, cumulative damage inflicted by the deepening profundity of persistent cytopenias eventually takes its toll in the form of resistance to transfusions and an overall deterioration in the already decrepit, weakened immune system. The terminal event usually comes in the form of a lethal bleeding episode or an intractable infection (Jandl, 1996).

THE BIOLOGY OF MYELODYSPLASTIC SYNDROMES

The paradox of pancytopenia in the presence of a hypercellular marrow

Trilineage dysplasia is the prevalent classical bone marrow abnormality in MDS, however the dysplastic features can range from minimal to bizarre, making hematopoietic precursors appear unrecognizably grotesque. Peripheral blood may show agranular, pelgeroid granulocytes, giant platelets and megaloblastic red cells (Jandl, 1996). The clonal nature of these insidious bone marrow syndromes has been repeatedly demonstrated (Janssen et al., 1989; Kamp et al., 1992; Busque & Gilliland, 1993; Anan et al., 1995; Abruzzese et al., 1996; Hotta, 1997; Schmetzer et al., 1997). Not only myeloid, erythroid and megakaryocytic cells, but also the B-lymphocytes and monocytes may all be descended from the transformed parent cell, implying disease initiation in an early progenitor cell. Greater than 90% patients with MDS demonstrate significant defects in colony forming activity in vitro affecting erythroid, monocyte-granulocytic cells, supporting the stem cell nature of the disease (Greenberg, 1992). The paradoxical finding of pancytopenia in the presence of a hypercellular marrow has recently been shown to result from increased intramedullary apoptotic death of hematopoietic cells in the majority of MDS patients (Clark & Lampert, 1990; Raza et al., 1995). While details of apoptosis in MDS are discussed elsewhere in this book, a few peculiar features need to be summarized here.

Distinctive features of apoptosis unique to MDS

Parenchymal cells belonging to all three lineages and at every stage of maturation are found to be apoptotic in MDS marrows (Raza et al., 1995a and b). S-phase cells can simultaneously undergo apoptosis in MDS and this "signal antonymy" (Hibner & Coutinho, 1994) is not demonstrable in several other malignancies using the same technique (Mundle et al., 1996a). Another interesting association is found between signal antonymy and an alteration in E2F1 transcript size versus BM cellularity. MDS patients with a hypercellular BM had low signal antonymy and a normal sized E2F1 transcript size while those with hypocellular BM had a high level of signal antonymy and a shorter E2F1 mRNA exclusively or in addition to a normal sized one (Mundle et al., 2000).

There also exists a peculiar discrepancy in the number of apoptotic cells found in different hematopoietic compartments even though all the cells are descended from the same MDS progenitor. Up to 75% cells in BM biopsies may be apoptotic, yet the matched aspirate may only show 1-5% apoptotic cells, and even that frequently needs unmasking following short-term cultures in vitro (Raza et al. 1995a and b). Peripheral blood from MDS patients actually has been shown to contain granulocytes that are more resistant to apoptosis than normal peripheral blood granulocytes (Horikawa et al., 1997). Such compartment dependency suggests the existence of cells with a wide spectrum of sensitivity to apoptosis, the most sensitive ones residing in the biopsy and the most resistant being released into the blood. This finding can be explained by one of two possibilities. Either the signal for apoptosis is extra-cellular and highly concentrated in the biopsy compartment; a site rich in accessory and stromal cells that may be the primary source of these cytokines. Or, premature apoptosis is an inherent property of the transformed stem cell that is not equally parceled out to its daughters, resulting in the production of committed CD34+ progenitors with varying degrees of sensitivity to undergo death by apoptosis. This would explain the existence of differential sensitivity to apoptosis within equally mature cells like granulocytes as they may be descended from different CD34+ progenitors despite ultimately being monoclonal. Following the rules of replicative homoplasmy, a greater uniformity is probably achieved ultimately with the marrow becoming populated by the daughters of either a dominant apoptosis sensitive stem cell (in which case, the disease progresses through ever worsening cytopenias), or apoptosis resistant stem cell (where transformation is the rule).

All this further underscores the pressing need to determine the status of apoptosis-sensitivity in CD34+ progenitors in MDS marrows. Unfortunately, the jury is out on this topic as the reports have been inconsistent so far. Some investigators have found increased apoptosis in MDS CD34+ cells (Rajapaksa et al., 1996), while others showed that blasts were clearly non-apoptotic (Raza et al., 1995a). Furthermore, when isolated CD34+ cells are examined, there is little if any increase in apoptosis, suggesting that the pro-apoptotic activity originates in $CD34^-$ cells (Anzai et al., 1997; Mundle et al., 1999). One major obstacle in addressing this question definitively and with alacrity relates to the difficulty of isolating large numbers of CD34+ cells from MDS marrows. When patients with refractory anemia (RA) are studied, the absolute number of CD34+ cells is too low for detailed, meaningful studies. When RA patients with excess of blasts (RAEB) are studied on the other hand, the CD34+ cell number may be high, but then those cells may only represent a derivative sub-population whose properties do not necessarily reflect the properties of the true MDS progenitor. While such mechanical and physical vicissitudes may eventually be negotiated, the more important question to be asked is whether these data would be of academic interest alone, or would actually have practical and immediate clinical significance. Even as anti-apoptotic agents have improved the cytopenias in at least a subset of MDS patients, no one is under the illusion that these therapies will be curative. The only cures follow consummate elimination of the MDS clone, thus far achievable only via a stem cell transplant.

Source of apoptotic signals or the role of pro-apoptotic cytokines

The cytokine milieu in MDS marrows is disconcertingly confounding. A major source of confusion is the presence of increased amounts of both pro-apoptotic and trophic factors. Finding an increase in both apoptotic and growth promoting cytokines simultaneously should not come as a surprise since both activities are enormously upregulated in MDS marrows. Increased levels of tumor necrosis factor alpha (TNF-α), transforming growth factor beta (TGF-β), interleukin-1 beta (IL-1β), IL-6, macrophage colony stimulating factor (M-CSF), as well as stem cell factor (SCF), granulocyte-CSF (G-CSF), GM-CSF and vascular endothelial growth factor (VEGF) have been demonstrated in different hematopoietic compartments of MDS patients (Zoumbos et al., 1991; Freedman et al., 1992; Verhoef et al., 1992; Koike et al., 1995; Mundle et al., 1996b; Raza et al., 1996a and b; Shetty et al., 1996;

Peddie et al., 1997; Gersuk et al., 1998; Kitagawa et al., 1998; Allampallam et al. 1999). Adding to the confusion is the fact that what may be high in blood is not necessarily so in the marrow and vice versa. As far as the apoptotic cytokines are concerned, it is probable that TNF-α is acting as the master switch responsible for turning the inflammatory cascade on or off, which immediately makes it the prime therapeutic target. In fact, clinical trials directed at neutralizing TNF activity have resulted in improved cytopenias in a sub-set of MDS patients already and will be discussed in detail below. One possible conclusion of this baffling cytokine milieu is that there is an immune-mediated inflammatory process at work in the marrows of MDS patients.

Cytogenetic abnormalities in MDS

Certain non-random, recurrent cytogenetic abnormalities most commonly affecting chromosomes 5, 7, 8 and 20 have been described in the marrow cells of approximately 50% patients with primary MDS (Rubin et al., 1990; Michalova et al., 1991; Heim, 1992; Ohyashiki et al., 1993; Verhoef & Googaerts, 1996; West et al., 2000). Sub-clones with additional complex abnormalities can continue to appear as the disease progresses, frequently heralding transformation to acute leukemia (White et al., 1992). An important question is whether these represent cause or effect of the disease. There are two problems in trying to associate cytogenetic abnormalities with disease etiology. First, since interstitial deletions in the long arms of chromosomes 5 and 7 are most commonly seen, it was hypothesized that these may harbor a tumor suppressor gene (TSG). Despite concerted efforts of dedicated investigators over the last two decades, no such TSG has been identified. Second, most karyotypic abnormalities are found in a sub-set of cells belonging to an otherwise monoclonal marrow. This appears to indicate that cytogenetically abnormal cells represent derivative populations of evolving sub-clones and are not etiologically related. More recently, there is a report focusing on identifying the cell of origin in patients with 5q- syndrome, a distinct clinical entity well recognized for its relatively better prognosis and low incidence of transformation to overt leukemia. The majority of highly purified CD34+/CD38- hematopoietic stem cells showed the presence of 5q-, while pluripotential stem cells (CD34+, CD19+, pro-B cells) in 3/5 such patients were found to have the 5q- abnormality in 25-90% of the cells examined (Ohyashiki et al., 1993). This suggests that at least in this unique sub-type of MDS, the majority of stem cells contain the 5q- abnormality. Several questions remain unanswered in this study. First, it is not known whether the stem cells without 5q- abnormality were also clonal in nature. Second, B and T cells in these very patients were found to be non-clonal even though they were expected to be clonal since the abnormality was clearly identified in the vast majority of lympho-myeloid parent cells. In addition, other studies have provided contradictory findings as well. All that can be concluded from the above studies is that cytogenetic abnormalities have been traced to some hematopoietic stem cells in the clinically distinct 5q- form of MDS, but for other categories, little is known about the level of stem cells involved in the disease process.

The paradox of robust stem cell proliferation in vivo and their failure to grow in vitro

The ultimate cause of MDS presumably lies in a stem cell defect since the marrow is entirely populated by the daughters of an expanded clone and at least all measurable non-lymphoid hematopoiesis is monoclonal. Despite this exuberant proliferation in vivo, progenitor MDS cells fail to grow well in vitro (Ohmori et al., 1991; Richert-Boe & Bagby, 1992; Aizawa et al., 1999; Flores-Figueroa et al., 1999; Aizawa et al., 2000; Tennant et al. 2000). In fact proliferation defects involving both the hematopoietic stem cell responsible for establishing long-term cultures in vitro as well as in the stromal cells have been described suggesting that the basic abnormality is situated in a parent of both stroma and parenchyma (Alvi et al., 2000). Paradoxically, in vivo studies designed to measure proliferation kinetics in MDS marrows have consistently demonstrated a higher than normal cell birth rate in all three lineages of hematopoietic cells (Raza et al., 1996c; Raza et al., 1997a and b). If anything, the marrow cells in vivo are in a state of heightened proliferation or overdrive. Inability to form colonies in vitro suggests that apoptosis must be occurring even earlier in these cells, probably due to the artificial nature of ex-vivo culture conditions. The in vitro growth defect in other words, parallels the in vivo apoptosis, only in a more profound manner.

A new paradigm

Based upon studies described above, it was hypothesized that an event or series of events confers a growth advantage upon an early pluripotential marrow stem cell. Clonal expansion, accompanied by dysplastic maturation eventually produces monoclonal hemopoiesis. Cytokines whose source is most probably the stroma or accessory cells such as monocytes, serve the dual function of stimulating the dividing cells to proliferate faster while causing apoptosis in their differentiating daughters. The end result is appearance of pancytopenia in the setting of a hyper-proliferative, hyper-cellular, monoclonal bone marrow. The question of what the initial event is begs immediate investigation because of obvious therapeutic implications.

The paradox of malignant transformation in an excessively apoptotic marrow

The increased incidence of transformation to acute leukemia in MDS patients at first glance appears incongruous. How is it possible that a population whose hallmark is excessive apoptosis generates a cell which not only remains immature, but which instead of dying prematurely develops an enormous growth advantage over its siblings, seizing numerical superiority from its parent and overwhelming the marrow with its daughters? A closer examination of the events leading to this situation can clarify some of the confusion at least. The first step in the evolution of a secondary hematopoietic disorder such as MDS may well be the acquisition of a growth advantage by a stem cell leading to its unchecked clonal expansion and eventual monoclonal hematopoiesis. This monoclonal status has been repeatedly demonstrated in some patients who are at high risk for developing MDS by virtue of the fact that they have been heavily pre-treated for a prior malignancy such as lymphoma (Gale et al., 1996). A large number of cells belonging to this expanded clone undergo apoptosis while still in the marrow, most probably due to the effects of pro-apoptotic cytokines in the vicinity. The constant pressure to commit suicide strains the population to the point where a maximally stressed cell eventually rebels by successfully developing a survival phenotype, perhaps through silencing a tumor suppressor gene. A survival phenotype is a malignant phenotype. In fact, a higher incidence of malignancy has historically been associated with chronically irritated or inflamed tissues most probably for the same reason as hypothesized above. Which brings us to the next obvious question of what exactly is the dysplastic marrow telling us about the nature of the underlying pathology in MDS.

MDS marrow as the site of an intense inflammatory reaction

Realistically speaking, the bizarre morphologic changes in the MDS marrow with trilineage malfunction, anarchic clonal proliferation, pathologic suicidal cellular self-destruction, infiltration by plasma cells and lymphocytes, and above all the striking increase in amounts of the signature pro-apoptotic cytokines make the organ look like a war zone. One explanation for this curious state may be that the MDS marrow biopsy compartment is home to an intense inflammatory reaction, resulting in a peculiar cytopathic effect upon the non-lymphoid cells in general, and the erythroid series in particular. Added, albeit circumstantial, support for this possibility is derived from an examination of other dysplastic tissues in the body. Given that Nature is highly parsimonious, it was hypothesized that there may be common and unifying themes threading the biology and pathology of various dysplastic states together. A comparative analysis of dysplasias affecting the BM, liver cells, cervix, esophagus and stomach demonstrated an extraordinary set of molecular, genetic and biologic similarities (Raza, 2000c). In each case, the dysplastic tissue was monoclonal in nature, accompanied by an increased cellular apoptosis-proliferation activity. Pro-inflammatory cytokines were abundant in all dysplasias examined and in each instance, there was an approximately 30% incidence of transformation to an overt malignancy. Finally, all dysplastic states save MDS are associated with an infectious agent. Cervical dysplasia is linked to human papilloma virus (HPV), and human herpesvirus (HHV) 1 and 4, liver cell dysplasia with hepatitis B virus (HBV), and HCV, and stomach cell dysplasia with helicobacter pylori (H. pylori). Thus excessive apoptosis of cells resulting from a persistent infection could predispose the organ towards developing a cancer phenotype as described above. Although no infectious agent has so far been uniquely associated with MDS, there is ample evidence to suspect a pathogen induced inflammatory process in the bone marrow.

ETIOLOGY OF MDS

Myelodysplastic syndromes are a heterogeneous group of disorders where patients differ widely in terms of their clinical presentation, response to therapy, and course or natural history of the illness. Even within a uniform sub-category of MDS, there are likely to be patients with one versus multiple cytopenias, a hyper- versus a hypo-cellular marrow, normal versus complex karyotypes, and minimal versus grotesque dysplastic features. It is therefore unrealistic to expect that a single etiology will explain all cases of MDS. A constellation of etiologic factors such as hereditary pre-disposition, toxic exposure especially to benzene, chemotherapy treatment and ionizing radiation have been proposed as putative causes of MDS and discussed in great detail elsewhere. For two decades, entirely based on hypothetical grounds, it has been fashionable to search for a tumor suppressor gene on chromosomes 5 or 7. The basis for suspecting an infectious etiology for MDS is just as biologically sound as the tumor suppressor gene hypothesis.

Infectious insult may provide the initial event in MDS

It is being hypothesized that the initial event in MDS may be infectious. It can be argued that the infectious agent must be a highly evasive pathogen such as a virus since the organism would have been identified by now if it were bacterial, fungal or parasitic in nature. This may not be exactly true since many of these latter organisms can assume a myriad of disguises. The case of cell wall deficient bacteria is an obvious example. For the moment, we propose that MDS may begin as a viral disease. There are a variety of reasons to raise a high index of suspicion. As summarized above, other dysplastic tissues in the body are invariably associated with a pathogen implying that dysplastic morphology may be a subtle manifestation of some sly and crafty infectious agent. Second, the marrow pathology suggests a chronic inflammatory process. Third, the marrow looks very dysplastic in another retroviral disease, acquired immune deficiency syndrome (AIDS). In fact the marrows of patients with MDS and AIDS are quite indistinguishable from each other in late stages of AIDS (Moses et al., 1998). Another common feature between AIDS and MDS is the cytopathic effect as manifested by excessive apoptosis of CD4+ T cells in the former and all myeloid as well as stromal cells in the latter. These two diseases in fact best demonstrate in vivo, the signature cytopathic effects commonly associated with a retrovirus. In AIDS, a virus has been isolated following a concerted search for it by the best minds in the world. In MDS, the search has not even begun. Given the many similarities between the two disorders, it is possible that a certain missing link can be extrapolated for one if it has already been demonstrated for the other. Or, as Occam's principle states, "what can be done with fewer assumptions is done in vain with more". Fourth, another feature unique to MDS, and suggestive of an inflammatory process rather than a malignant disease is the phenomenon of "signal antonymy". In MDS, we have demonstrated S-phase cells to be simultaneously apoptotic. This peculiar situation of a cell being engaged in two opposing pathways of proliferation and apoptosis (thus the word antonym as opposed to synonym) was absent from malignant cells of patients with lymphoma, acute myeloid leukemia, breast cancer, brain tumors and head and neck cancers. We have further shown that signal antonymy in MDS is also associated with the presence of an altered E2F1 transcript. Involvement of this pathway is also highly suggestive of a pathogen practiced at co-opting normal cellular mechanisms for its own survival and propagation. Fifth, there are a number of patients with MDS who present with unexplained fevers whose cause cannot be identified despite exhaustive efforts. Finally, 20% of children who present with pancytopenia and a dysplastic bone marrow end up with a viral infection suggesting the association between an infectious agent and the presence of pancytopenia and dysplasia.

Reactivation of a dormant pathogen or a new virus?

The disease may result from the re-activation of a dormant virus which had found sanctuary in one of the BM stem cells, or it may be a newly acquired, exogenous agent. In this context, it would be instructive to recapitulate certain counter-intuitive facts regarding micro-organisms in general. First, there are more micro-organisms in our bodies than there are actual cells. If the human body has a 100 trillion cells, it also harbors 1000 trillion micro-organisms. Second, 10% of our dry body weight consists of micro-organisms, and one human's mouth contains more bacteria than all humans who ever lived on this planet. Third, micro-organisms are 25 times the mass of all animal life on Earth, and equal the plant life. An acre of good agricultural soil contains more than 500 pounds of micro-organisms. Finally, over millennia of evolution, many invading micro-organisms have been prevented from practicing a hostile take-over of the human body by being subdued and converted into symbiotic partners forced to provide essential services. An obvious example is that of mitochondria which were once independently living bacteria and now form a vital intracellular organelle. The point in reviewing these somewhat sensational facts is that it is time to accord due respect to our microscopic fellow passengers and cease from thinking of them as mere agents of disease. In fact their role is equally critical in maintaining the normal homeostasis of not only our bodies, but also our planet. In other words, it can safely be concluded that germs are us! The other side of the coin is that since so many micro-organisms maintain a permanent abode within the human body, it is highly likely that a disturbance within their natural symbiotic partnership could lead to an undue growth advantage for one such organism. This could act as the initiation point for a series of subsequent events resulting both from abnormal activity of the micro-organism and the body's attempt to control its expansion that culminates in a slowly progressive, insidious disease like MDS. In other words, reactivation of a dormant pathogen within our bodies is likely to occur if we change the conditions around it by toxic, chemical exposure, or weakened immune system, resulting in a redistribution of growth advantage amongst the resident micro-flora, much like the antibiotic induced diarrhea. Another example of this phenomenon is the appearance of shingles upon reactivation of the measles virus residing in a latent state in the neural ganglia decades after the initial case of measles. If this were the case, then organisms like the herpesviruses would be prime candidates for the role. Epstein-Barr virus (EBV) has found sanctuary in bone marrow cells of almost all of us. Its role in non-lymphoid diseases must be aggressively investigated since in the final analysis, most pathogens would prefer a non-myeloid cell for sanctuary because myeloid cells are too short-lived. Finally, it could be a new virus, and that would include both a retrovirus as well as a DNA virus. Evidence is beginning to accumulate in support of both possibilities.

Stromal versus parenchymal cells as the seat of infection?

So far, most studies in MDS patients have been conducted on parenchymal cells. It may be equally possible that a stromal cell is the source of all trouble. There are several features of MDS which at first glance render a stromal cell etiology appear highly unlikely, if not impossible. First, the hematopoietic cells are monoclonal suggesting that transformation has occurred in an early progenitor as discussed above, while practically nothing is known about the clonality of stromal cells in MDS. We propose that an infectious agent residing in as few as 1-2% stromal cells such as fibroblasts or dendritic cells, along with the resulting immune reaction, could alter the cytokine milieu in such a way that it is no longer suitable for supporting the growth of normal hematopoietic cells. On the other hand, a rapidly proliferating stem cell could thrive in this modified, BM microenvironment, even as its daughters undergo premature apoptosis. Detection of clonal switching at different stages of the disease in an MDS patient supports this possibility. A second objection relates to cures being achieved in MDS via allogeneic transplantation if stromal cells are diseased since stromal cells maintain their recipient origin. A closer look at which MDS patients are being cured with this procedure would shed more light on this critical question. To begin with this procedure is an option for a highly select group of MDS patients, making up less than 5% of all cases. Furthermore, allogeneic transplantation is more than just the preparative regimen followed by an infusion of cells. Other pre-therapy manipulations as well as the concomitant and post-transplant administration of antibiotics, anti-virals, anti-fungals, and immune-suppressive agents may all play an equally important role in altering the host-parasite relationship to tip the balance in favor of the host with resulting long term remissions. This suggestion is not as incredible as it may appear at first glance if one remembers that long term responses are being seen in MDS patients treated with immune modulatory agents such as thalidomide and anti-thymocyte globulin. Finally, the majority of long-term survivors after transplant are patients with low risk refractory anemia, while those with excess of blasts have a higher incidence of relapse after successful engraftment. It is possible that in the highly select sub-group of MDS patients who eventually experience long remissions post-transplant (since it is too early to know if they are actually cured), the stromal cells are not the source of disease. The important point to be emphasized here is that MDS is a heterogeneous disease with a variety of clinical forms that may parallel an equal variety of etiologies. Consequently, some MDS patients may have disease restricted to a hematopoietic progenitor cell and others solely to stromal cells, while in still others it may involve both. It is extremely important to fully appreciate the intimate relationship between stromal and parenchymal cells in the marrow, and appreciate the possibility that the functional integrity of each may be highly dependent on the health of the other. In this regard, greater efforts must be devoted to a closer and more thorough investigation of the previously ignored, poorly characterized hematopoietic stromal compartment in MDS patients.

THERAPEUTIC STRATEGIES IN MYELODYSPLASTIC SYNDROMES

Patients with MDS do not fail therapies. Rather, we the physicians have failed to provide adequate therapies to MDS patients. Our relative ignorance regarding a precise treatment recommendation is best reflected in the fact that therapeutic options range from supportive care to transplantation with all manner of clinical trials testing the efficacy of differentiating agents, recombinant human growth factors, anti-cytokine therapies and cytotoxic drugs thrown in the middle. Stem cell or bone marrow transplantation (BMT) is the only curative therapy. Thus, if the MDS patient at diagnosis is 60 years of age or less, and a matched related donor can be identified, then this remains the option of choice and the patient must be referred to the nearest center excelling in such procedures. This therapeutic approach has been discussed at length elsewhere and will not be described here.

Frustration in designing effective therapies is largely related to the biologic complexity of the disease with the resulting existence of multiple therapeutic targets, and little to guide the optimal choice for an individual patient. Targeted interventional approaches to date have failed to provide long term, substantial benefit in terms of prolonging survival such that the majority of patients at the present time are encouraged to participate in experimental clinical trials. Another confounding factor is that many of the low risk MDS patients survive for years, and are therefore, potential candidates for sequential therapeutic trials during the course of their illness. Finally, even if the patient shows a clinical evolution, this does not necessarily portend a relentless progression to the terminal stage since a state of "punctuated equilibrium" may be attained in the all too disorderly hematopoiesis so that the next "event" or deterioration may not be apparent for a prolonged period. It will be helpful here to review the survival and incidence of transformation according to the French-American-British or FAB classification as well as the prognosis/survival as predicted by the International Prognostic Scoring System or IPSS:

The FAB classification of MDS

Depending upon the morphology and the percentage of blasts in the bone marrow, a group of French, American and British (FAB) hematologists proposed uniform criteria to classify MDS into five main subtypes (Bennett et al., 1982). In refractory anemias (RA), patients suffer from an anemia that is resistant or refractory to treatment with iron and/or vitamins, and there are less than 5% blasts in the marrow. There may be mild to moderate leukopenia and/or thrombocytopenia There is refractory anemia, and in addition, >15% ringed sideroblasts are found in the marrow. Blasts again constitute less than

5% of the marrow. In RA with ringed sideroblasts (RARS), >15% ringed sideroblasts are found in the marrow in addition to other features of RA. When RA patients present with either 1-5% circulating blasts or 5-20% blasts in their marrow, the sub-type is called RA with excess blasts (RAEB). When the percentage of circulating blasts exceeds 5%, or there are 20-30% blasts in the marrow, the patients are considered as transforming towards acute leukemia (RAEB-t). More recently, another classification proposed by WHO considers patients with 20% or more blasts as having acute leukemia. In the final category of chronic myelomonocytic leukemia (CMMoL), the bone marrow looks more or less similar to the other types of MDS, except there is an increase in monocytes in both blood and marrow, and the total WBC count is increased as well. The blasts are usually between 5-20% in the marrow.

***Table 1**. Survival and incidence of leukemic transformation in MDS by FAB Type*

FAB	Median Survival (months)	% Leukemic Transformation
RA	37	11
RARS	49	5
CMMoL	22	20
RAEB	9	23
RAEB-t	6	48

The International Prognostic Scoring System or IPSS

This new system has been proposed to predict disease outcome more accurately (Greenberg et al., 1997). Important variables used in this classification include cytogenetics, percentage of bone marrow blasts, and the number of cytopenias. The following table shows the relative risk of developing acute leukemia as well as the median survival for each IPSS category.

***Table 2.** Median Survival and Risk of Acute Leukemia by IPSS*

MDS by IPSS Risk Category				
IPSS Risk Category	**% Patients**	**Median Survival (months)**	**% Developing AML**	**MDS→AML Interval (months)**
Low	33	68	7	34.0
*Int-1	39	42	10	6.5
*Int-2	22	42	40	4.5
High	7	5	54	2.0

**Intermediate*

There are a number of excellent recent reviews describing the therapeutic strategies commonly employed in MDS, and summarizing the results of these carefully conducted clinical trials. In this review, we wish to take a more practical and problem oriented approach to devise a useful algorithm for the step-wise management of MDS patients as they almost invariably progress towards a worsening state of ineffective hematopoiesis. In order to develop working guidelines for the clinician, the management of each FAB category will be described separately. Great confusion could exist in the mind of a practicing, busy hematologist who may only see a handful of MDS cases a year, but who is nonetheless faced with the tedious, time-consuming ordeal of making the "right" choice of therapy for their patient, from a mountain of experimental approaches being tested. Another source of great frustration is how to identify patients requiring treatment versus those who can be followed with observation alone. The following provides a practical guide for hematologists regarding the management of MDS patients. The treatment options are summarized in the accompanying figure:

Which patients should be treated?

One of the most therapeutically challenging and frustrating problems in MDS is the observation that the best outcome for almost all therapies is seen in early disease, non-transfusion dependent patients with refractory anemia being their sole presenting cytopenia. Non-toxic therapies such as recombinant growth factors as well as invasive procedures like transplantation, all work best in these low risk individuals thereby underscoring the need for screening the population at risk for an early diagnosis. More profound the cytopenias, worse is the response rate. Given the current state of available therapies, all of which are of palliative benefit at best, MDS patients who present without an excess of blasts should only be treated if they show worsening cytopenias, are transfusion dependent, or demonstrate complications related to their cytopenias. RAEB patients with <10% blasts can be followed carefully for disease progression if they are transfusion independent. Otherwise, these individuals should be considered for experimental trials. The following describes our recommendation for therapy according to the FAB sub-type:

Refractory anemia or RA

Uncomplicated refractory anemia at presentation is quite often an accidental diagnosis, highlighting the benign initial course of the disease, especially in a number of elderly patients. Given the fact that the median age at diagnosis is approximately 70 years, such individuals with isolated non-transfusion-dependent anemia should preferably be watched and followed periodically with complete blood counts (CBC). Careful monitoring of the CBC in this period also provides some insight into the natural history as well as the probable course of the disease in individual patients. In case of worsening anemia, supportive care with packed red blood cell (PRBC) transfusions is an eminently reasonable option although consideration must be given to a trial of erythropoietin alone or in combination with granulocyte colony stimulating factor (G-CSF), especially if the serum erythropoietin level is found to be low (Hellstrom-Lindberg, 1995; Hellstrom-Lindberg et al., 1998). If the patient chooses supportive care only, then it is wise to institute iron chelation therapy before the serum ferritin reaches dangerously high, organ-damaging levels. Regular desferrioxamine administration either via a continuous pump, or bolus injections subcutaneously has been associated with organ damage reversal, improvement in anemia as well as a reduction in PRBC transfusion requirements (Jensen et al., 1996).

Refractory anemia patients with a poor prognosis such as those with multiple cytopenias, frequent transfusion requirements and/or adverse cytogenetics should be considered for experimental therapies from the very start. The choice here ranges between anti-cytokine approaches, differentiating agents, immune modulators, and other novel biologic, non-cytotoxic therapies.

Refractory anemia with ringed sideroblasts or RARS

This group of patients is notoriously refractory to therapy including erythropoietin, and has posed a continuing therapeutic challenge for the clinician. Fortunately, they are also the least likely to transform into an acute leukemia. As with refractory anemia patients, non-transfusion dependent individuals should be watched, and followed with periodic CBCs. Those who are transfusion dependent, or who have adverse cytogenetic abnormalities or multiple cytopenias are candidates for experimental trials. The good news is that some of the newer approaches such as those using thalidomide, have provided substantial benefit to these individuals.

Experimental therapies available for RA and RARS patients

These can safely be divided into several categories, and are listed along with the expected response rates:

Table 3. *Response to different experimental therapeutic agent(s) in RA and RARS patients*

Therapy	**Expected Response Rate in Selected Subgroups**	**Reference**
A. Recombinant Human Growth factors		
Erythropoietin (Epo)	20%	Hellstrom-Lindberg, 1995
Epo + GCSF	40%	Hellstrom-Lindberg et al., 1995
IL3 or IL6	10%	Ganser et al., 1993; Nimer et al., 1994; Gordon et al., 1995
B. Differentiating Agents		
Retinoic acid, ATRA Other retinoids	10%	Aul, Runde, and Gatterman, 1993; Ohno, 1994
5-azacytidine	25-45%	Wijermans et al., 1997
C. Immune Suppressive Therapies		
Anti-thymocyte globulin or ATG	30-50%	Molldrem et al., 1997
Cyclosporin	?	Jonasova et al., 1998
Cyclosporin + ATG	?	Biesma, Van den Tweel, and Verdonck, 1997
D. Cytoprotective Therapies		
Pentoxifylline + Cipro + Decadron (PCD)	30-50%	Raza et al., 1998
Amifostine	40-50%	List et al., 1997
Amifostine + PCD	40-50%	Raza et al., 2000a
E. Anticytokine Therapies		
Enbrel	30%	Raza et al., 2000b
Thalidomide	30-40%	Raza et al., 1999
F. Others		
Farnesyl Tranferase Inhibitors Interleukin 1β receptor antagonist Hexamethylene bisacetamide (HMBA)		Andreeff et al., 1992; Karp , 1998

Refractory anemia with excess of blasts

Only rarely do RAEB patients with >10% blasts demonstrate stable disease for any substantial period of time, therefore these patients are candidates for experimental therapies from the start. Those with <10% blasts may be watched only if they are transfusion independent and serial blood counts do not indicate disease progression. Those with 20% or more blasts in their marrows are candidates for acute leukemia like remission induction therapies.

<u>RAEB with <10% blasts</u>:

Many of the approaches described above for RA/RARS patients have been tried in these individuals as well with mixed results. Most protocols combine some form of chemotherapy, albeit in lower doses, with growth factors, anti-cytokine/cytoprotective therapies or differentiating agents. Once disease progression is documented, these patients are candidates for trials containing some form of cytotoxic therapy as part of the regimen.

<u>RAEB with >10% blasts</u>

When the blast count in the marrow is greater than 10%, it is unlikely that the disease will be controlled with non-toxic measures alone. The problem is that use of chemotherapy in MDS has never been shown to improve survival. Some groups regularly treat these individuals with high dose chemotherapy, while others are trying low dose cytosine arabinoside, topotecan, VP-16, and more recently, the anti-CD33 antibody (Mylotarg). None can be recommended unequivocally as the treatment of choice. It is best to enroll these patients onto ongoing clinical trials.

Chronic myelomonocytic leukemia or CMMoL

Perhaps the most difficult category of MDS patients to treat is CMMoL. Results with biologic agents have been less than optimal since frequently the disease acquires a proliferative form, and the rapidly increasing count is difficult to control without the addition of a cytotoxic agent. Chemotherapy is less than ideal because the results are never as good as those seen in RAEB patients until recently. With the introduction of topotecan in the MDS armament, these results have improved considerably, but longer follow-up is needed to determine whether an improvement has been noted in survival or not. It is recommended that CMMoL patients should also be encouraged to participate in clinical trials, especially in the early phases when the disease is not rapidly progressive.

Novel therapies and translational research in MDS

Perhaps the most exciting recent approach to therapy has been directed at reversing the excessive intramedullary apoptosis in hematopoietic cells. Because apoptosis appears to be cytokine mediated, it is logical to try and suppress apoptosis by neutralizing the activity of the dominant pro-apoptotic cytokine. Unfortunately, there are a number of pro-apoptotic cytokines that are upregulated in MDS and therefore would serve as poor therapeutic targets. Recognition that TNF-α may be the proximal initiator of this cascade makes it an excellent target since it is the master switch responsible for turning the pro-apoptotic cytokines on or off. In the last few years then, a series of clinical trials have been conducted to determine the efficacy of this approach to therapy of myelodysplastic syndromes. Agents such as pentoxifylline in combination with ciprofloxacin and dexamethasone (PCD) were used initially for lack of having more specific anti-TNF therapies (Raza et al., 1998). Pentoxifylline interferes with the second messenger pathways for TNF-α, IL1β, and TGF-β, while ciprofloxacin blocks its metabolism by blocking the P450 reductase system in the liver. MDS patients did show an improvement in their cytopenias (30-40%), however the regimen could not be continued for long due to the frequent and often severe side effects of dexamethasone in this older group of patients. The cytoprotective drug amifostine showed activity in MDS as well (List et al., 1997), and was subsequently combined with PCD with encouraging results (Raza et al., 2000a). The problem with amifostine is that it needs to be administered intravenously thrice a week for long periods of time, and most elderly patients prefer a periodic transfusion to this time consuming therapy. A more direct attempt at neutralizing the activity of TNF-α was tested by treating MDS patients with the soluble TNF receptor Enbrel (Immunex). Improvements were noted in ANC and platelets, but no patient showed an increase in hemoglobin (Raza, 2000b). Thalidomide was tried next on the basis of its anti-cytokine, anti-angiogenic and immune modulatory actions, and as a single agent, appears to be the most effective anti-cytokine therapy to date. It is well tolerated in lower doses of 100-200mg/day, and can be administered safely for prolonged periods. Between 30-40% patients show improvement in their hemoglobin levels and/or reduction in transfusion requirements (Raza et al., 1999). Most responders belong to the low risk category of MDS, the good news being that even RARS patients appear to respond as well as RA patients. Thalidomide is now being combined with PCD, Enbrel and arsenic toxide in ongoing trials. It must be remembered that even though the anti-cytokine approach alone may be effective in improving the cytopenias of a sub-set of MDS patients, it is by no means curative and does little for the higher risk patients. In fact, patients with RAEB improve their cytopenias, but often continue to show an increase in blasts in their marrows. To overcome this problem, a dual approach of sequentially using low dose chemotherapy to reduce blast count followed by anti-cytokine drugs to improve cytopenias is also currently being tried. Finally, given the large scale increase in neo-angiogenesis that has been demonstrated in the marrows of MDS patients, newer anti-angiogenic agents must be tested for the treatment of this frustrating hematopoietic disease.

SUMMARY

Myelodysplastic syndromes continue to be "a riddle, wrapped in a mystery inside of an enigma". Clearly, MDS represent a heterogeneous group of disorders, and no uniform etiology or treatment can be prescribed for all patients. This further underscores the need for MDS patients to be seen at specialized centers and placed on experimental protocols if they need treatment. The important thing to remember is that ultimately, the patient must remain the measure of all things, and must be given all the therapeutic choices including that of waiting and watching with supportive care alone. Recent biologic insights have expanded the therapeutic options, but no curative therapies except stem cell transplants are available at this time. By dissecting the biology and focusing efforts towards understanding the etiology of the cytopenias, significant therapeutic advances are being made in this disease. The momentum built up so far must not be lost now.

REFERENCES

Abruzzese E, Buss D, Rainer R, Rao NP, & Pettenati MJ. (1996) Study of clonality in myelodysplastic syndromes: detection of trisomy 8 in bone marrow cell smears by fluorescence in situ hybridization. *Leukemia Research,* **20**:551-557.

Allampallam K, Shetty V, Hussaini S, Mazzoran L, Zorat F, Huang R, & Raza A. (1999) Measurement of mRNA expression for a variety of cytokines and its receptors in bone arrows of patients with myelodysplastic syndromes. *Anticancer Research,* **19**:5323-5328.

Alvi S, Shaher A, Henderson B, Dar S, Zorat F, Broderick E, Lisak L, Du Randt M, Reddy P, Mundle S, Galili N, Borok RZ, & Raza A. (2000) Improved growth of stromal cells in long term bone marrow cultures (LTBMC) of myelodysplastic syndrome (MDS) patients treated with thalidomide. *Blood*, **96**:359a, Abstract #1547.

Aizawa S, Nakano M, Iwase O, Yaguchi M, Hiramoto M, Hoshi H, Nabeshima R, Shima D, Handa H, & Toyama K. (1999) Bone marrow stroma from refractory anemia of myelodysplastic syndrome is defective in its ability to support normal CD 34-positive cell proliferation and differentiation in vitro. *Leukemia Research*, **23**:239-246.

Aizawa S, Hiramoto M, Hoshi H, Toyama K, Shima D, & Handa H. (2000) Establishment of stromal cell line from an MDS RA patient which induced an apoptotic change in hematopoietic and leukemic cells in vitro. *Experimental Hematology*, **28**:148-155.

Anan K, Ito M, Misawa M, Ohe Y, Kai S, Kohsaki M, & Hara H. (1995) Department of Transfusion Medicine and Second Department of Internal Medicine, Hyogo College of Medicine, Hyogo, Japan. Clonal analysis of peripheral blood and haemopoietic colonies in patients with aplastic anaemia and refractory anaemia using the polymorphic short tandem repeat on the human androgen-receptor (HUMARA) gene. *British Journal of Haematology*, **89**:838-844.

Andreeff M, Stone R, Michaeli J, Young CW, Tong WP, Sogoloff H, Ervin T, Kufe D, Rifkind RA, & Marks PA (1992) Hexamethylene bisacetamide in myelodysplastic syndromes and acute myelogenous leukemia: a phase II clinical trial with a differentiating agent. *Blood,* **80**: 2604-2609.

Anzai N, Kawabata H, Hishita T, Yoshida Y, Ueda Y, & Okuma M. (1997) Ca^{2+}/ Mg^{2+} dependent endonuclease in marrow CD34 positive and erythroid cells in myelodysplasia. *Leukemia Research*, **21**:731-734.

Aul C, Runde V, & Gatterman N (1993) All-trans-retinoic acid in patients with myelodysplastic syndromes: results of a pilot study. *Blood*, **82**: 2967-2974.

Bennett JM, Catovsky D, Flandrin DMT, Galton DGAD, Gralnick HR, & Sultan C (1982) Proposal for the classification of myelodysplastic syndromes. *British Journal of Haematology* **51**: 189-199.

Biesma DH, van den Tweel JG, & Verdonck LF. (1997) Immunosuppressive therapy for hypoplastic myelodysplastic syndrome. *Cancer,* **79:** 1548-1551.

Busque L, & Gilliland GD. (1993) Clonal evolution in acute myeloid leukemia. *Blood*, **82**:337-342.

Clark DM, & Lampert IA. (1990) Apoptosis is a common histopathological finding in myelodysplasia: The correlate of ineffective haematopoiesis. *Leukemia and Lymphoma*, **2**:415-418.

Flores-Figueroa E, Gutierrez-Espindola G, Guerrero-Rivera S, Pizzuto-Chavez J, & Mayani H. (1999) Hematopoietic progenitor cells from patients with myelodysplastic syndromes: In vitro colony growth and long term proliferation. *Leukemia Research*, **23**:385-394.

Freedman MH, Cohen A, Grunberger T, Bunin N, Luddy RE, Saunders FE, Shahidi N, Lau A, & Estrov Z. (1992) Central role of tumour necrosis factor, GM-CSF, and interleukin 1 in the pathogenesis of juvenile chronic myelogenous leukaemia. *British Journal of Haematology*, **80**:40-48.

Gale RE, Bunch CE, Moir DJ, Patterson KG, Goldstone AH, & Linch DC. (1996) Demonstration of developing myelodysplasia/acute myeloid leukemia in hematologically normal patients after high dose chemotherapy and autologous bone marrow transplantation using X chromosome inactivation patterns. *British Journal of Haematology,* **93**: 53-58.

Ganser A, Ottoman OG, Seipelt G, Lindemann A, & Hess U et al (1993) Effects of long-term treatment with recombinant interleukin-3 in patients with myelodysplastic syndromes. *Leukemia*, **7**: 696-701.

Gersuk GM, Beckham C, Loken MR, Kiener P, Anderson JE, Farrand A, Troutt AB, Ledbetter JA, & Deeg JH. (1998) A role for tumour necrosis factor-α, FAS and FAS-Ligand in marrow failure associated with myelodysplastic syndrome. *British Journal of Haematology*, **103**:176-188.

Gordon MS, Nemunitis J, Hoffman R, Paquette RL, Rosenfeld C, Manfrede C, Isaacs R, & Nimer SD. (1995) A phase I trial of recombinant interleukin-6 in patients with myelodysplastic syndromes and thrombocytopenia. *Blood*, **85**: 3066-3076.

Greenberg PL. (1992) In vitro marrow culture studies in myelodysplastic syndromes. *Seminars in Oncology,* **19**: 34-46.

Greenberg PL, Cox C, Le Beau MM, Fenaux P, Morel P, Sanz G, Sanz M, Vellaspi T, Hamblin T, Oscier D, Ohyashiki K, Toyama K, Aul C, Mufti G, & Bennett JM (1997) International scoring system for evaluating prognosis in myelodysplastic syndromes. *Blood* , **89**: 2079-2088.

Heim S. (1992) Cytogenetic findings in primary and secondary MDS. *Leukemia Research* **16**:43-46.

Hellstrom-Lindberg E (1995) Efficacy of erythropoietin in the myelodysplastic syndromes: a meta-analysis of 205 patients from 17 studies. *British Journal of Haematology* **89**: 831-837.

Hellstrom-Lindberg E, Ahlgren T, Beguin Y, Carlsson M, Carneskog J, Dahl IM, Dybedal I, Grimfors G, Kanter-Lewensohn L, Linder O, Luthman M, Lofvenberg E, Nilsson-Ehle H, Samuelsson J, Tangen JM, Winqvist I, Oberg G, & Ost A (1998) Treatment of anemia in myelodysplastic syndromes with granulocte colony-stimulating factor plus erythropoietin: results from a randomized Phase II study and long term follow-up of 71 patients. *Blood*, **92**:68-75.

Hibner U, & Coutinho A. (1994) Signal antonymy: A mechanism for apoptosis induction. *Cell Death and Differentiation,* **1**:33-37.

Horikawa K, Nakakuma H, Kawaguchi T, Iwamoto N, Nagakura S, Kagimoto T, & Takatsuki K. (1997) Apoptosis resistance of blood cells from patients with paroxysmal nocturnal hemoglobinuria, aplastic anemia and myelodysplastic syndrome. *Blood*, **90:**2716-2722.

Hotta T. (1997) Clonality in hematopoietic disorders. *International Journal of Hematology* **66**:403-412.

Jandl JH. (1996) Textbook of Hematology. Second Edition, Little Brown & Co. pp. 830.

Janssen JWG, Buschle M, Layton M, Drexler HG, Lyons J, Van den Berghe H, Heimpel H, Kubanek B, Kleihauer E, Mufti GJ, & Bartram CR. (1989) Clonal analysis of myelodysplastic syndromes: Evidence of multipotent stem cell origin. *Blood,* **73**:248-254.

Jensen PD, Heickendroff L, Pederson B, Bendix-Hansen K, Jensen FT, Christensen T, Boesen AM, & Ellegaard J (1996). The effect of iron chelation on hematopoiesis in MDS patients with transfusion iron overload. *British Journal of Haematology*, **94**: 288-299.

Jonasova A, Neuwirtova R, Cermak J, Vozobulova V, Mocikova K, Siskova M, & Hochova I (1998) Cyclosporin A therapy in hypoplastic MDS patients and certain refractory anemias without hypoplastic bone marrow. *British Journal of Haematology* **100**: 304-309.

Kamp H, Fibbe WE, Jansen RPM, Van derKeur M, Graaff E, Willemze R, & Landegent JE. (1992) Clonal involvement of granulocytes and monocytes, but not of T and B lymphocytes and natural killer cells in patients with myelodysplasia: Analysis by x-linked restriction fragment length polymorphisms and polymerase chain reaction of the phosphoglycerate kinase gene. *Blood,* **80**:1774-1780.

Karp JE (1998) Molecular pathogenesis and targets for therapy in myelodysplastic syndrome (MDS) and MDS-related leukemias. *Current Opinions in Oncology*, **10**: 3-9.

Kitagawa M, Yamaguchi S, Takahashi M, Tanizawa T, Hirokawa K, & Kamiyama R. (1998) Localization of Fas and Fas ligand in bone marrow cells demonstrating myelodysplasia. *Leukemia*, **12**:486-492.

Koike M, Ishiyama T, Tomoyasu S, & Tsuruoka N. (1995) Spontaneous cytokine overproduction by peripheral blood mononuclear cells from patients with myelodysplastic syndromes and aplastic anemia. *Leukemia Research*, **19**:639-644.

List AF, Brasfield F, Heaton R, Glinsman-Gibson B, Crook L, Taetale R, & Capizzi R (1997) *Blood*, **90**: 3364-3369.

Michalova K, Musilova J, Zemanova Z, Czechoslovak MDS Cooperative Group. (1991) Consecutive chromosomal studies in patients with myelodysplastic syndrome (MDS). *Annals of Genetics*, **34**:212-218.

Molldrem JJ, Caples M, Mavroudis D, Plante M, Young NS, & Barrett AJ (1997) Anti-thymocyte globulin for patients with myelodysplastic syndromes. *British Journal of Haematology,* **99**: 699-705.

Moses A, Nelson J, & Bagby Jr GC (1998) The influence of human immunodeficiency virus-1 on hematopoiesis *Blood,* **91**: 1479-1495.

Mundle SD, Clark E, Alvi S, Venugopal P, Gezer S, Borok R, Shetty V, Chopra H, Hines C, Jassak P, Gregory SA, Robin E, Rifkin S, Alston D, Hernandez B, Shah R, & Raza A. (1996a) Spontaneous apoptosis in S-phase (Signal Antonymy): A characteristic in vivo feature of myelodysplasia. *Proceedings of American Society of Clinical Oncology,* **15**:89, Abstract #21.

Mundle SD, Venugopal P, Pandav DV, Broady-Robinson L, Gezer S, Robin EL, Rifkin SR, Klein M, Alston DE, Hernandez BM, Rosi D, Alvi S, Shetty VT, Gregory SA, & Raza A. (1996b) Indication of an involvement of interleukin-1 converting enzyme (ICE)-like protease in intramedullary apoptotic cell death in the bone marrows of patients with myelodysplastic syndromes (MDS). *Blood,* **88**:2640-2647.

Mundle S, Venugopal P, Shetty V, Ali A, Chopra H, Handa H, Rose S, Mativi BY, Gregory SA, Preisler HD, & Raza A. (1999) The relative extent and propensity of CD 34^+ vs. $CD34^-$ cells to undergo apoptosis in myelodysplastic marrows. *International Journal of Hematology,* **69**152-159.

Mundle SD, Mativi BY, Cartlidge JD, Dangerfield B, Broady-Robinson L, Li B, Shetty V, Venugopal P, Gregory SA, Preisler HD, & Raza A. (2000) Signal antonymy unique to myelodysplastic marrows correlates with altered expression of E2F1. *British Journal of Haematology,* **109**:376-381.

Nimer SD, Paquette RL, Ireland P, Testa T, Young D, & Golde DW (1994) A phase I/II study of interleukin-3 in patients with aplastic anemia and myelodysplasia. *Experimental Hematology,* **22**: 875-880.

Ohmori M, Ohmori S, Ueda Y, Yoshida Y, & Okuma M. (1991) Ineffective hematopoiesis in myelodysplastic syndromes (MDS) as studied by daily in situ observation of colony-cluster formation. *International Journal of Cell Cloning,* **5**:521-530.

Ohno R (1994) Differentiation therapy of myelodysplastic syndromes with retinoic acid. *Leukemia and Lymphoma,* **14**: 401-409.

Ohyashiki K, Iwabuchi A, Sasao I, Ohyashiki JH, Ito H, & Toyama K. (1993) Clinical and cytogenetic significance of myelodysplastic syndromes with disease evolution. *Cancer Genetics and Cytogenetics,* **67**:71-79.

Peddie CM, Wolf CR, McLellan LI, Collins AR, & Bowen DT. (1997) Oxidative DNA damage in $CD34^+$ myelodysplastic cells is associated with intracellular redox changes and elevated plasma tumour necrosis factor- concentration. *British Journal of Haematology,* **99**:625-631.

Rajapaksa R, Ginzton N, Rott LS, & Greenberg PL. (1996) Altered oncoprotein expression and apoptosis in myelodysplastic syndrome marrow cells. *Blood,* **88**:4275-4287.

Raza A, Mundle S, Iftikhar A, Gregory S, Marcus B, Khan Z, Alvi S, Shetty V, Dameron S, Wright V, Adler S, Loew J, Schott S, Ali N, & Preisler H. (1995a) Simultaneous assessment of cell kinetics and programmed cell death in bone marrow biopsies of myelodysplastics reveals extensive apoptosis as the probable basis for ineffective hematopoiesis. *American Journal of Hematology,* **48**:143-154.

Raza A, Gezer S, Mundle S, Gao X-Z, Alvi S, Borok R, Rifkin S, Iftikhar A, Shetty V, Parcharidou A, Loew J, Marcus B, Khan Z, Chaney C, Showel J, Gregory S, & Preisler H. (1995b) Apoptosis in bone marrow biopsy samples involving stromal and hematopoietic cells in 50 patients with myelodysplastic syndromes. *Blood,* **86**:268-276.

Raza A, Gregory SA, & Preisler HD. (1996a). The myelodysplastic syndromes in 1996: Complex stem cell disorders confounded by dual actions of cytokines. *Leukemia Research,* **20**:881-890.

Raza A, Mundle S, Shetty V, Alvi S, Chopra H, Dar S, Venugopal P, Borok R, Gezer S, Showel J, Robin E, Rifkin S, Alston D, Hernandez B, & Gregory S. (1996b) Novel insights into the biology of myelodysplastic syndromes: Excessive apoptosis and the role of cytokines. *International Journal of Hematology,* **63**:265-278.

Raza A, Mundle S, Shetty V, Alvi S, Chopra H, Span L, Parcharidou A, Dar S, Venugopal P, Borok R, Gezer S, Showel J, Loew J, Robin E, Rifkin S, Alston D, Hernandez B, Shah R, Kaizer H, & Gregory S. (1996c) A paradigm shift in myelodysplastic syndromes. *Leukemia,* **10**:1648-1652.

Raza A, Alvi S, Broady-Robinson L, Showel M, Cartlidge J, Mundle SD, Shetty V, Borok RZ, Dar SE, Chopra HK, Span L, Parcharidou A, Hines C, Gezer S, Venugopal P, Loew

J, Showel J, Alston D, Hernandez B, Rifkin S, Robin E, Shah R, & Gregory S. (1997a) Cell cycle kinetic studies in 68 patients with myelodysplastic syndromes following intravenous iodo- and/or bromodeoxyuridine. *Experimental Hematology*, **25:** 530-535.

Raza A, Alvi S, Borok RZ, Span L, Parcharidou A, Alston D, Rifkin S, Robin E, Shah R, & Gregory SA. (1997b) Excessive proliferation matched by excessive apoptosis in myelodysplastic syndromes: The cause-effect relationship. *Leukemia and Lymphoma*, **27**:111-118.

Raza A, Venugopal P, Gezer S, Gregory S, Dong LM, Leurgens S, Mundle SD, Shetty VT, Alvi S, Ali A, Span L, Dar SE, Hines C, Hsu WT, Loew J, Borok RZ, Hernandez B, Robin E, Rifkin S, Alston D, Shah R, & Preisler HD. (1998) Pilot study of Pentoxifylline and Ciprofloxacin with or without Dexamethasone produces encouraging results in myelodysplastic syndromes. Acute Leukemias VII: Experimental Approaches and Novel Therapies published by Springer-Verlag Berlin Heideberg, New York, (eds) W. Hiddemann, T. Buchner, B. Wormann, J. Ritter, U. Creutzig, Keating M, Plunkett W, pp 42-51.

Raza A, Lisak L, Andrews C, Little L, Muzammil M, Alvi S, Mazzoran L. Zorat F, Akber A, Ekbal M, Razvi S, & Venugopal P. (1999) Thalidomide produces transfusion independence in patients with long-standing refractory anemias and myelodysplastic syndromes (MDS). *Proceedings of American Society of Clinical Oncology*, **15**:89, Abstract #21.

Raza A, Qawi H, Lisak L, Andric T, Dar S, Andrews C, Venugopal P, Gezer S, Gregory S, Loew J, Robin E, Rifkin S, Hsu W-T, & Huang R-W. (2000a) Patients with myelodysplastic syndromes benefit from palliative therapy with Amifostine, Pentoxyfylline, and Ciprofloxacin with or without Dexamethasone. *Blood*, **95**:1580-1587.

Raza A. (2000b) Anti-TNF therapies in Rheumatoid Arthritis, Crohn's Disease, Sepsis and Myelodysplastic Syndromes. *Microscopy Research and Techchnique*, **50**:229-235.

Raza A. (2000c) Consilience across evolving dysplasias affecting myeloid, cervical, esophageal, gastric and liver cells: Common themes and emerging patterns. *Leukemia Research*, **24**:63-72.

Richert-Boe KE, & Bagby CG Jr. (1992) In vitro hematopoiesis in myelodysplasia: Liquid and soft-gel culture studies. *Hematology Oncology Clinical North America*, **6**:543-556.

Rubin CM, Larson RA, Anastasi J, Winter JN, Thangavelu M, Vardiman JW, Rowley JD, Le & Beau MM. (1990) t(3;21)(q26;q22): A recurring chromosomal abnormality in therapy-related myelodysplastic syndrome and acute myeloid leukemia. *Blood*, **76**:2594-2598.

Saarni MI, & Linman JW. (1973) Preleukemia: The hematologic syndrome preceding acute leukemia. *American Journal of Medicine*, **55**:38-48.

Schmetzer HM, Poleck B, Mittermuller J, Duell T, Wilmanns W, & Gerhartz HH. (1997) Clonality analysis as a tool to study the biology and response to therapy in myelodysplastic syndromes. *Leukemia* **11**:660-666.

Shetty V, Mundle S, Alvi S, Showel M, Broady-Robinson L, Dar S, Borok R, Showel J, Gregory S, Rifkin S, Gezer S, Parcharidou A, Venugopal P, Shah R, Hernandez B, Klein M, Alston D, Robin E, Dominquez C, & Raza A. (1996) Measurement of apoptosis, proliferation and three cytokines in 46 patients with myelodysplastic syndromes. *Leukemia Research*, **20**:891-900.

Tennant GB, Walsh V, Truran LN, Edwards P, Mills KI, & Burnett AK. (2000) Abnormalities of adherent layers grown from bone marrow of patients with myelodysplasia. *British Journal of Haematology*, **3**:853-862.

Verhoef GEG, De Schouwer P, Ceuppens JL, Van Damme J, Goossens W, & Boogerts MA. (1992) Measurement of serum cytokine levels in patients with myelodysplastic syndromes. *Leukemia,* **6**:1268-1272.

Verhoef GE, & Googaerts MA. (1996) Cytogenetics and its prognostic value in myelodysplastic syndromes. *Acta Haematologica*, **95**:95-101.

West RR, Stafford DA, White DT, & Padua RA. (2000) Cytogenetic abnormalities in the myelodysplastic syndromes and occupational or environmental exposure. *Blood* **95**:2093-2097.

White AD, Culligan DJ, Hoy TG, & Jacobs A. (1992) Extended cytogenetic follow-up of patients with myelodysplastic syndrome (MDS). *British Journal of Haematology*, **81**:499-502.

Wijermans PW, Krulder JW, Huijens PC, & Neve P. (1997) Continuous infusion of low dose 5-aza-2-deoxycytidine in elderly patients with high risk myelodysplastic syndromes. *Leukemia*, **11**: 19-23.

Zoumbos N, Symeonidis A, Kourakli A, Katevas P, Matsouka P, Perraki M, & Georgoulias V. (1991) Increased levels of soluble interleukin-2 receptors and tumor necrosis factor in serum of patients with myelodysplastic syndromes. *Blood*, **77**:413-414.

2

IN VITRO BIOLOGY OF THE HEMATOPOIETIC SYSTEM IN MYELODYSPLASTIC SYNDROMES

Hector Mayani
Oncological Research Unit, Oncology Hospital, National Medical Center. Mexican Institute of Social Security. Mexico City, Mexico.

INTRODUCTION

The myelodysplastic syndromes (MDS) comprise a heterogeneous group of hematological disorders characterized by ineffective hematopoiesis with a high frequency of progression into acute myeloid leukemia (AML; Heaney and Golde, 1999). During the last few years, compelling evidence has accumulated indicating the clonal nature of MDS (Kere et al., 1987; Janssen et al., 1989). The identity of the cell in which transformation takes place, however, is still not clear. Some studies suggest that the transformation event in MDS occurs at the level of a committed myeloid progenitor (Kroef et al., 1993; Saitoh et al., 1998); this is supported by the fact that MDS rarely transforms into acute lymphoblastic leukemia. In contrast, a recent study by Nilsson et al (2000) shows evidence that transformation may occur on a lympho-myeloid stem cell, suggesting that the apparent myeloid-lineage restriction is a result of the transforming event itself. Regardless of these two possible scenarios, the fact is that severe hematopoietic alterations exist in MDS, both at the level of hematopoietic progenitors and their marrow microenvironment (Yoshida, 1987; Mayani, 1993).

Most of what we know about the biology of hematopoiesis in MDS has come from in vitro studies, performed during the last 20 years, involving several experimental systems and designs (e.g., using semisolid cultures, stroma-free liquid cultures or Dexter-type long-term marrow cultures; and culturing either total marrow cells, low-density mononuclear cells or purified $CD34^+$ cells). In this context, the major goal of the present chapter is to summarize and discuss the studies reported to date, regarding the in vitro biology of the hematopoietic system in MDS.

ORGANIZATION OF THE HEMATOPOIETIC SYSTEM

Under normal conditions, blood cell production results from the controlled interactions between hematopoietic cells and their marrow microenvironment. Together, they form what is known as the hematopoietic system. The hematopoietic cells are organized within three compartments, all located in the bone marrow (BM). The first compartment corresponds to the hematopoietic stem cells (HSC), a rare population that comprises less than 0.1% of marrow cells (Szilvassy & Hoffman, 1995). HSC are cells capable of sustaining the in vivo production of blood cells of all hematopoietic lineages for extended periods of time, and are presumably also capable of generating daughter cells with similar pluripotent properties (Thomas et al., 1999). These properties can be assessed by transferring human cells into immunodeficient (NOD-SCID) mice. Such human HSC are referred to as SCID-repopulating cells (SRC; Dick, 1996) or competitive-repopulating units (CRU, Conneally et al., 1997). In terms of antigen expression, human HSC have been defined as $CD34^+$ $CD38^-$ $lineage^-$ $CD90^+$ $CD117^+$ $HLA\text{-}DR^{-/low}$ $AC133^+$ KDR^+ (Szilvassy & Hoffman, 1995; Ziegler et al., 1999; Gallacher et al., 2000). It is noteworthy, however, that recent studies have demonstrated the existence of a subset of human HSC that lacks the expression of the CD34 antigen ($CD34^-$ $lineage^-$ cells) (Bhatia et al., 1998; Zanjani et al., 1998). In vitro, human HSC are identified by their ability to initiate and sustain hematopoiesis in long-term marrow cultures (LTMC). Thus, they are referred to as long-term culture initiating-cells (LTC-IC; Sutherland et al., 1989).

The second compartment corresponds to the hematopoietic progenitor cells (HPC), which comprise 0.3% - 0.5% of the nucleated cells in BM. These cells are also characterized by the expression of the CD34 antigen, however, in contrast to HSC, they may express a variety of lineage-restricted antigens (Civin & Gore, 1993). Functionally, HPC are identified by their ability to form colonies in semisolid cultures (Metcalf, 1977). Most HPC have a very limited ability to self-renew; interestingly, a minority of them still retain the capacity to give rise to different hematopoietic lineages –i.e., they are pluripotent- and are known as colony-forming units-granulocyte-erythrocyte-monocyte-megakaryocyte (CFU-GEMM or CFU-MIX). The rest of the progenitors are already committed to a particular lineage of differentiation. Among them, we can find those that are part of the erythroid lineage –i.e., burst-forming unit-Erythroid (BFU-E) and CFU-E- those of the myeloid lineage –including CFU-granulocyte/macrophage (CFU-GM), CFU-M and CFU-G- and those of the megakaryocytic lineage (CFU-MK). Following the differentiation/maturation pathway, progenitor cells give rise to morphologically-recognizable precursors (third compartment), which can be identified by light microscopy. These terminally differentiating cells may only be able to mature or die; since death is normally not a major outcome for most of them, they constitute the vast majority of the cells present in BM. Finally, their progeny (i.e., fully mature blood cells) is released into circulation.

Hematopoiesis takes place in specific organs, known as hematopoietic organs. In man, more than 95% of the hematopoietic activity occurs in BM. Within the medullary cavity, the viability, proliferation and differentiation of hematopoietic cells are regulated by a network of stromal cells, accessory cells, and their products (cytokines and extracellular matrix), known as the hematopoietic microenvironment (Mayani et al., 1992). Stromal cells include fibroblasts, macrophages, endothelial cells, adipocytes and osteoblasts; whereas accessory cells include both monocytes and lymphocytes.

Both stromal and accessory cells produce a great variety of proteins known as hematopoietic cytokines (Murphy, 1994). Some cytokines -including the colony-stimulating factors (CSF), erythropoietin (EPO), thrombopoietin (TPO) and steel factor (SF)- act as stimulators of hematopoiesis, and the way they do it is by inducing proliferation and/or blocking apoptosis (Moore, 1991; Metcalf, 1993). In contrast, cytokines such as tumor necrosis factor-α (TNF-α), transforming growth factor-β (TGF-β), interferon-γ (IFN-γ) and macrophage inflammatory protein-1α (MIP-1α), act as hematopoietic inhibitors, basically by inducing apoptosis (Moore, 1991; Mayani et al., 1995). Thus, in normal hematopoiesis there is a balanced interplay between both positive and negative regulators (Metcalf, 1993). All the hematopoietic regulators described thus far interact with their target cells, and exert their functions, via cytokine-receptors, which are specific proteins located on the cell membrane. To date, more than 30 hematopoietic cytokines have been identified; the proteins have been purified and their genes have been cloned, making them readily available for both in vivo and in vitro studies.

HEMATOPOIETIC STEM AND PROGENITOR CELLS IN MDS

Stem/Progenitor Cell Content

It is clear that not all the cells that express the CD34 antigen are stem or progenitor cells, nevertheless, the number of $CD34^+$ cells has been used as an indicator of the content of HSC and HPC. In normal BM, $CD34^+$ cells correspond to 0.5% - 3.0% of the mononuclear cells (Civin & Gore, 1993). Interestingly, in MDS, such a proportion varies considerably from 0% to almost 50% (Asano et al., 1994; Sawada et al., 1995; Nilsson et al., 2000). It is noteworthy that, as compared to patients with refractory anemia (RA), the percentage of $CD34^+$ cells tends to be higher in MDS patients with refractory anemia with excess of blasts (RAEB) and RAEB in transformation (RAEB-t; Table 1).

Table 1. *$CD34^+$ cell content in BM from MDS patients and normal subjects*

Diagnosis	Asano et al (1994)	Sawada et al (1995)	Nilsson et al (2000)
RA	0.19 (0 – 0.79)	2.1 (0.8 – 3.70)	2.5 (0.7 – 5.9)
RAEB	0.50 (0.12 – 2.88)	20.0 (19.3 – 20.8)	5.6 (2.7 – 24.0)
RAEB-t	3.20 (1.29 – 8.75)	36.4 (20.0 – 49.9)	NA
NBM	0.46*	0.8 (0.5 – 2.0)	2.0 ± 0.3*

*Results correspond to the median (range) percentage of $CD34^+$ cells comprised within the marrow mononuclear cells. *Results shown correspond to mean or mean ± SD. NA, not assessed. NBM, normal BM.*

The elevated relative numbers of $CD34^+$ cells in MDS marrow would suggest elevated levels of HSC and HPC; however, functional in vitro and in vivo assays have demonstrated that this is not the case and that reduced levels of stem and progenitor cells are present in this disorder. Recently, Nilsson and colleagues (2000) reported that, in contrast to normal controls, $CD34^+$ $CD38^-$ cells from most of the 5q-deleted MDS patients analyzed by them failed to show LTC-IC activity. This observation correlated with the fact that such cells were unable to reconstitute hematopoiesis in sublethally irradiated NOD-SCID mice, thus, indicating the reduced numbers (or absence) of SCID-repopulating cells in MDS patients. In keeping with these observations, Sato et al (1998) showed reduced secondary colony formation after a 5-week culture period (an indirect measure of LTC-IC) in long-term marrow cultures from MDS patients.

Abnormalities in the content of hematopoietic progenitors in MDS have also been observed at the level of the cells capable of forming hematopoietic colonies in semisolid cultures (CFC). In the majority of the studies reported to date, and regardless of the culture conditions, most of the patients analyzed in each of them showed reduced numbers of CFC, as compared to normal marrow. This has been observed in cultures of mononuclear cells (Greenberg & Mara, 1979; Mayani et al., 1989; Carlo-Stella et al., 1989; Baines et al., 1990; Dan et al., 1993; Greenberg 1996; Flores-Figueroa et al., 1999), as well as in cultures of $CD34^+$ cells (Asano et al., 1994; Sawada et al., 1993; Sawada et al., 1995; Sawada, 1996). Interestingly, although reduced colony growth in MDS includes all of the hematopoietic lineages, each one of them seems to be affected to a different extent. Indeed, alterations in the erythroid lineage are usually more pronounced than those observed in the myeloid lineage; similarly, reduction in the number of megakaryocytic and multipotent progenitor cells is usually higher than the one found in myeloid progenitors (Figure 1). The fact that these observations have been made not only in cultures of mononuclear cells - in which a variety of cells at different maturation stages are present and the production of different inhibitory cytokines has been demonstrated- but also in cultures of purified $CD34^+$ cells, suggests that such abnormalities are intrinsic to the progenitor cells. The molecular mechanisms involved, however, are still not fully understood.

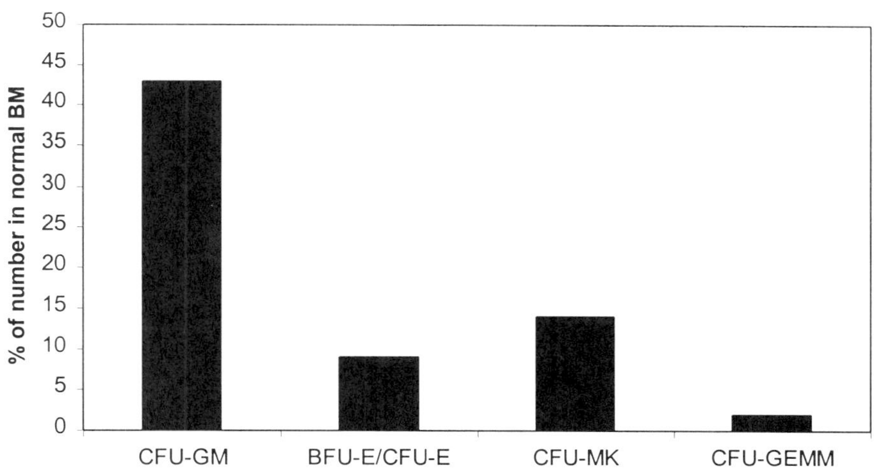

Figure 1. Relative content of hematopoietic progenitor cells (colony-forming cells) in MDS patients. Results shown correspond to the median number of myeloid (CFU-GM), erythroid (BFU-E and CFU-E), megakaryocytic (CFU-MK) and multipotent (CFU-GEMM) progenitor cells in MDS (RA, RAEB and RAEB-t) marrow, and are expressed as percentage of the respective CFC number in normal subjects (100%). Data based on the results reported by Mayani et al (1989); Carlo-Stella et al (1989); Baines et al (1990); Merchav et al (1990); Dan et al (1993); Greenberg (1996) and Flores-Figueroa et al (1999).

To date, a correlation between CFC content and MDS subtype (according to the French-American-British [FAB] classification) is still controversial. Several studies have shown no differences in CFC levels between the different MDS subtypes, thus indicating that such a correlation does not exist (Carlo-Stella et al., 1989; Baines et al., 1990; Coutinho et al., 1990; Greenberg, 1996). In contrast, in the studies by Dan et al (1993), Visani et al (1993) and Flores-Figueroa et al (1999) CFC levels are significantly lower in RAEB and RAEB-t, as compared to RA. These discrepancies seem to reflect the biological complexity of this hematological disorder and the great variability that exists between patients. It is noteworthy that, in contrast to RA, RAEB and RAEB-t, CFC levels in chronic myelomonocytic leukemia (CMML) are usually within or above the normal range (Coutinho et al., 1990; Flores-Figueroa et al., 1999) and their behavior in long-term cultures (see below) differs significantly from that of the progenitors from the other FAB subtypes (Flores-Figueroa et al., 1999; Montesinos et al., 2000). These in vitro observations suggest that, from the biological point of view, CMML should be considered as a separate entity from MDS, a concept that has been previously emphasized by others (Michaux & Martiat, 1993).

Interestingly, colony growth in semisolid cultures has been shown to have prognostic value in MDS. Different groups have presented evidence that MDS patients with normal levels of CFU-GM, BFU-E and CFU-MK had a lower risk of developing leukemia and a longer survival time than those patients with an abnormal colony growth pattern (Shih et al., 1991; Juvonen et al., 1999). Previously, six different studies (reviewed in detailed by Greenberg, 1996), involving about 180 MDS patients with different FAB subtypes, correlated in vitro colony growth and clinical outcome. In those studies, clonal growth in MDS was divided into "leukemic" and "non-leukemic" patterns. The former consisted of microcluster or macrocluster formation with defective maturation or very low colony formation (<2 colonies/10^5 marrow cells). The latter consisted of persisting colony growth even if moderately reduced in frequency. MDS patients with a non-leukemic growth pattern showed a 20% to 40% incidence of leukemic transformation and median survivals of 9 to 50 months. In contrast, patients with leukemic growth patterns showed a 50% to 80% incidence of transformation to AML and median survivals of 5 to 10 months.

Responsiveness To Recombinant Cytokines

Recombinant human GM-CSF, G-CSF and IL-3, alone or in combination, have shown stimulatory effects in vitro on myeloid progenitors from a significant proportion of MDS patients. Usually, combinations of two or three cytokines have stronger affects than each one of them alone. Although a great heterogeneity is evident from those studies, in the majority of the cases a decreased responsiveness of progenitor cells to these recombinant cytokines has been observed. That is to say, the extent to which MDS progenitors respond to the cytokines –in terms of the number of CFC grown in culture and the number of mature cells produced per colony- is usually much lower than that of normal progenitors (Mayani et al., 1989; Carlo-Stella et al., 1989; Baines et al., 1990; Merchav et al., 1991: Schipperus et al., 1990). Most of these observations have been made in cultures of BM mononuclear cells, however, they have been confirmed in studies using purified $CD34^+$ cells, indicating that the functional defects are not due to accessory cells (Sawada et al., 1993; 1996; Tohyama et al., 1994). Furthermore, recent experiments reported by Nilsson et al (2000) demonstrated that such impaired responses to recombinant cytokines are evident even at the level of very primitive hematopoietic cells ($CD34^+$ $CD38^-$ cells) purified from MDS marrow.

The molecular reason for the impaired response of MDS myeloid progenitors to recombinant cytokines is not clear; it may reflect reduced receptor numbers, reduced receptor affinity and/or abnormal signal transduction. In this regard, it is noteworthy that Soligo et al (1996) showed that GM-CSF receptor was overexpressed in those patients that responded to this cytokine, whereas it was absent or downregulated in non-responders. This observation, however, differs from the results by Zwierzina et al (1992) who did not find differences in GM-CSF receptor expression between normal and MDS marrow cells. In any case, it is interesting that some groups have shown that high (supersaturating) doses of GM-CSF, G-CSF or IL-3, although have no further effect on normal progenitors, can increase myeloid progenitor levels, sometimes within the normal range, in a subset of MDS patients (Mayani et al., 1989; Merchav et al., 1991). The actual mechanisms involved in such a response still need to be elucidated.

Decreased responsiveness of erythroid progenitors to EPO has also been documented. Merchav et al (1990) showed that half-maximal growth of CFU-E and BFU-E from MDS patients was detected at 4-fold higher concentration of EPO than the concentration required by normal erythroid progenitors. Although the molecular mechanisms behind this observation are not known, it is noteworthy that MDS erythroid progenitors seem to express normal levels of EPO receptor (Backx et al., 1996); in contrast, alterations at the level of EPO receptor-mediated intracellular signal transduction (involving the STAT5 protein) have recently been reported in a proportion of MDS patients (Hoefsloot, et al., 1997; Fontenay-Roupie et al., 1999).

More recently discovered and characterized early acting cytokines, such as SF and TPO, have already been assessed for their ability to stimulate MDS progenitor cell growth in vitro. SF, alone and in combination with other stimulatory cytokines, proved to be a potent stimulator of myeloid, erythroid and multipotent progenitor cells from MDS patients. Indeed, among all the cytokines tested to date, SF has shown the strongest synergistic activity on MDS CFC growth. In fact, in many cases, SF restored CFC levels within the normal range (Asano et al., 1994; Piacibello et al., 1994; Glinsmann-Gibson et al., 1994; Masters et al., 1995). In spite of the positive response of MDS progenitors to SF, Soligo et al (1994) and Glinsmann-Gibson et al (1994) have shown that only a proportion of MDS patients express the SF receptor (the c-kit oncogene). This latter observation suggests that SF effects on progenitor cells may be both direct and indirect. Interestingly, in the study by Glinsmann-Gibson and colleagues (1994), SF had stimulatory effects in all FAB subtypes analyzed except CMML, despite the fact that 1 out of the 3 CMML patients included in their study showed significant c-kit expression. Once again, alterations at the c-kit-mediated signal transduction level may explain the lack of response. Based on the above results, it seems that SF will prove useful in the clinic.

In a recent study by our own group, a combination of early and late acting stimulatory cytokines was added to liquid cultures of normal and MDS marrow cells enriched for $CD34^+$ cells. After 10 days of culture, there was an increase in total cell number in cultures of patients with RA and RAEB; however, as expected, such an increase was significantly lower than the one observed in normal marrow cultures. Interestingly, total cell numbers in CMML cultures were increased to a significantly higher extent than in cultures from normal marrow cells (Montesinos et al., 2000; Figure 2). Thus, it is clear that this particular disorder has a different physiology in culture, as compared to the rest of the MDS subtypes.

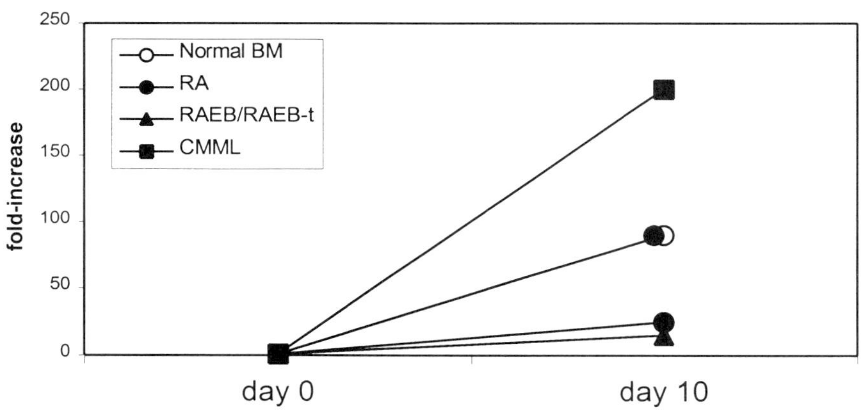

Figure 2. Proliferation of $CD34^+$ cell-enriched populations in liquid cultures from normal and MDS marrow. Cells (10^5/ml) were cultured in 20% serum-containing culture medium in the presence of GM-CSF, G-CSF, IL-3, IL-6, SF (each at 10 ng/ml) and EPO (3 U/ml). After 10 days of culture, total numbers of viable cells were determined. In the absence of cytokines, total cell numbers were 20% to 60% of the input cell number. Data based on the results reported by Montesinos et al (2000).

TPO has also shown stimulatory effects on MDS progenitor cells in vitro. As expected, TPO had significant effects on megakaryocyte progenitors, however, it also increased the stimulatory effects of GM-CSF, G-CSF, IL-3 and SF on myeloid and erythroid CFC (Ferrajoli et al., 1998). Similar to the previously described cytokines, TPO effects were observed only in a proportion of patients (Adams et al., 1997). Interestingly, in the study by Ferrajoli and colleagues (1998), depletion of either T cells or adherent cells abrogated the effect of TPO. This suggests that TPO may not be acting directly on MDS progenitors, but indirectly, via synergistic interactions with other cytokines produced by accessory cells. The fact that TPO may not be able to directly stimulate MDS progenitor cell growth in vitro does not seem to be due to lack of TPO-receptor (c-mpl) expression, but to severe alterations in TPO-receptor-mediated signal transduction (involving STAT3 and STAT5), as recently described by Kalina et al (2000).

Growth Kinetics In Dexter-Type Long-Term Marrow Cultures

Among the different in vitro systems that have been developed to study hematopoiesis, the Dexter-type long-term marrow culture (LTMC) is the one that most closely reproduces the in vivo conditions and dynamics in which blood cell production takes place (Dexter et al., 1977). In LTMC, hematopoiesis can be sustained for several weeks and this is due to the development of an adherent cell layer –similar, in terms of composition, to the marrow stroma- which provides physical support and the hematopoietic cytokines necessary for the growth of hematopoietic cells. Thus, LTMC allows the study and characterization of the interactions between hematopoietic cells and their microenvironment (Mayani et al., 1992).

Proliferation of hematopoietic cells from MDS patients is severely impaired in LTMC (Figure 3). Myelopoiesis is usually sustained at lower levels and for shorter periods of time, than in normal cultures (Borbenyi et al., 1987; Coutinho et al., 1990; Flores-Figueroa et al., 1999). In their study, Coutinho and colleagues observed two distinct growth patterns for myeloid progenitors. In a first group of patients, myelopoiesis was sustained for only 4 weeks and at very low levels; in contrast, a second group of patients showed nearly normal levels of myeloid progenitors for up to 7 weeks. The authors indicate that such growth patterns may reflect the stage of evolution of the disease. In this regard, it is noteworthy that whereas 50% of the patients with RA were included in each one of the two groups, the vast majority of the patients with RAEB (7 out of 8) were included in the group with the poorest growth. The only CMML patient included in this study was part of the first group.

More recently, Flores-Figueroa et al (1999) also showed deficient proliferation of MDS myeloid progenitors in LTMC. In general, patients with RA showed slightly higher levels of progenitors as compared to RAEB(-t) patients. These authors, however, observed increased levels –even higher than in normal cultures- of progenitors from the 2 CMML patients included in their study. These authors also analyzed the growth of erythroid and multipotent progenitor cells and observed severe growth deficiencies; indeed, the former were sustained for 1-4 weeks, whereas the latter were supported for only 2 weeks. Interestingly, the proportion of progenitor cells present in the adherent layer was significantly reduced in the majority of cases, thus suggesting that HPC from MDS patients loose their ability to adhere to the stromal cells in vitro. As reported by Soligo et al (1994), and in keeping with the deficient response of MDS cells to recombinant cytokines, addition of recombinant SF to LTMC from myelodysplastic patients resulted in only a 7% mean increase both in total cell number and CFC levels.

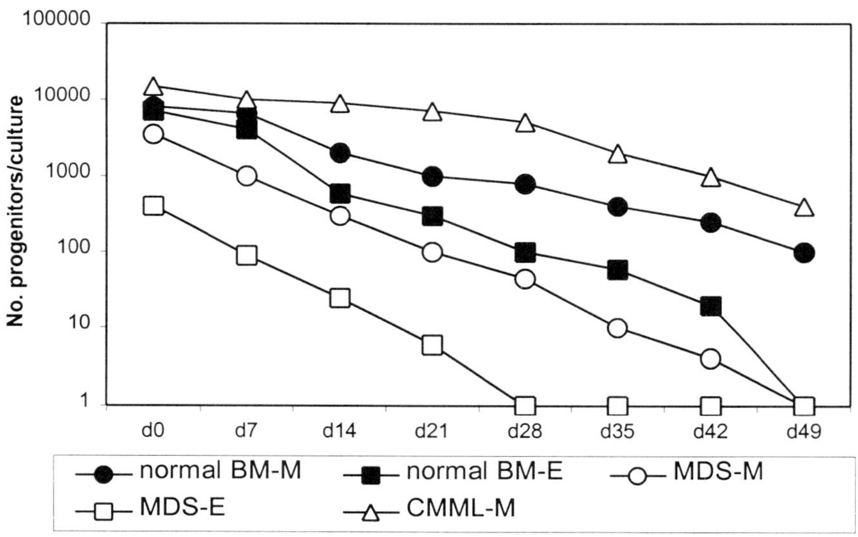

Figure 3. Kinetics of hematopoietic progenitors in LTMC from normal subjects and MDS patients. Results shown correspond to the mean numbers of progenitor cells per culture, throughout 49 days (d0-d49). M, myeloid progenitors; E, erythroid progenitors. Data on myeloid progenitor levels (normal BM-M and MDS-M) are based on the results reported by Borbenyi et al (1987); Coutinho et al (1990) and Flores-Figueroa et al (1999). The values shown for erythroid progenitors (normal BM-E and MDS-E) and myeloid progenitors from CMML patients (CMML-M) are based on the report by Flores-Figueroa et al (1999).

The LTMC system has also been used for cytogenetic and molecular studies on the leukemic transformation from MDS. Kanamaru & Tamura (1993) have demonstrated that novel abnormal karyotypes - not detected at culture onset- can emerge after a few weeks in LTMC from a significant proportion of MDS patients. Interestingly, in 4 of the 32 patients studied, novel karyotypes detected in LTMC emerged in vivo, one to 11 months later. Thus, this in vitro system may provide useful insights into the multistep process of leukemic transformation from MDS.

THE HEMATOPOIETIC MICROENVIRONMENT IN MDS

Since normal hematopoiesis results from the controlled interplay between hematopoietic stem/progenitor cells and their microenvironment, it is clear that alterations in the latter may contribute to the origin and/or progression of hematological diseases. To date, it has been demonstrated that microenvironment abnormalities, both in terms of composition and function, may exist in disorders such as aplastic anemia and myeloid leukemia (Juneja & Gardner, 1985; Mayani, 1996), and as we shall see in this section, important abnormalities are also present in the MDS-derived hematopoietic microenvironment developed in vitro. According to the evidence obtained so far, it seems unlikely that such abnormalities are the cause of any of the disorders analyzed; instead, they seem to contribute to the progression of the disease by (i) inhibiting normal hematopoietic growth and (ii) favoring the expansion of the abnormal cells (Mayani, 1996).

Cellular Composition Of Adherent Stromal Layers

Some studies reported to date indicate that adherent stromal layers from MDS patients are similar to their normal marrow counterparts in terms of cellular composition (Hirayama et al., 1993; Flores-Figueroa et al., 1999). In the report by Hirayama et al (1993), the authors showed similar proportions of fibroblasts (80% vs 77% of the total adherent cells), endothelial cells (12.5% vs 14.5%), macrophages (6% vs 7.5%) and adipocytes (1.5% vs 1%) in LTMC from normal and MDS marrow. In keeping with this study, Flores-Figueroa et al (1999) reported similar adherent cell numbers and morphologic appearance in normal and myelodysplastic LTMC. The lack of significant differences in the composition of adherent cell layers from normal and myelodysplastic LTMC correlates with the fact that the numbers of fibroblastic progenitors (CFU-F) present in BM are similar (4 – 10 CFU-F/10^5 marrow cells) in both conditions, as demonstrated by Coutinho et al (1990) and Flores et al (2000).

It is noteworthy, however, that some differences have also been reported. Coutinho et al (1990) showed that in a proportion of myelodysplastic LTMC no confluence was observed; this was particularly evident in patients with RAEB and CMML. Also, adipocytes were absent in most LTMC from RAEB patients. The differences observed between these reports could reflect the intrinsic heterogeneity of this disease, but also differences in experimental cell processing and culture conditions.

Hematopoietic Supportive Capacity Of Adherent Stromal Layers

A variety of studies have shown functional differences between normal and MDS stromal cells. By means of establishing "chimeric" LTMC (i.e., HPC from one individual are co-cultured onto preformed adherent cells from a different subject), it has been possible to assess the hematopoietic supportive capacity of normal and MDS adherent cell layers. In the study performed by Coutinho et al (1990), BM mononuclear cells from normal subjects were cultured on stromal cell layers from normal and MDS individuals and the numbers of nucleated cells and CFC were determined weekly. As reported by the authors, MDS adherent cell layers were as efficient as normal BM adherent cells in supporting the growth of HPC from normal subjects, during a 7-week culture period, thus suggesting that stroma from MDS is functionally normal.

In contrast to Coutinho's observation, a more recent study by Aizawa et al (1999) presented evidence indicating that MDS stroma is functionally deficient, at least in a group of patients. In their study, $CD34^+$ cells from normal marrow were inoculated onto stroma from normal subjects and patients with RA, and the cultures were maintained for several weeks. The authors observed three distinct patterns of hematopoietic growth. In some patients, HPC were maintained at nearly normal levels; in a second group of patients, HPC numbers increased during the first week of culture and then declined drastically, reaching lower levels than control cultures by week 3. In the third group, HPC numbers declined continuously from the beginning of the culture. In this latter group of cultures, apoptosis was frequently observed. The discrepancy observed between these two reports may be due to the fact that the experimental conditions differed significantly. On the one hand, the cell populations inoculated onto the stroma were different (mononuclear cells in the study by Coutinho et al and $CD34^+$ cells in the study by Aizawa and colleagues). The patients included in the study by Coutinho comprised different FAB subtypes, whereas all the patients included in the study by Aizawa had RA. Finally, these functional differences of the stromal cells may simply reflect the biological heterogeneity and complexity of myelodysplasia.

It is noteworthy that Aizawa et al (2000) have just reported on the development of a stromal cell line (LS801), established from one of the patients with RA included in the previous report. When $CD34^+$ cells from normal BM were co-cultured onto LS801 cells, the latter induced apoptosis in the hematopoietic cells. Interestingly, if direct cell-to-cell contact between stromal and $CD34^+$ cells was prevented, the inhibitory effect of LS801 disappeared. Based on these observations, the authors suggested that stromal cells from some MDS patients are unable to support hematopoiesis due to the fact that they induce apoptosis (via direct contact) in HPC and their progeny.

Cytokine Production By Microenvironment Cells

Production of hematopoietic cytokines –including both stimulatory and inhibitory factors- has been taken as another indicator of the functional integrity of the cells that form part of the hematopoietic microenvironment. In this regard, significant differences have been reported between MDS and normal marrow stromal cells. Several studies have demonstrated that stromal cells from MDS patients produce significantly higher levels of IL-1, IL-6, TNFα and G-CSF than normal BM stromal cells (Hirayama et al., 1993; Wetzler et al., 1995; Shetty et al., 1996; Kitagawa et al., 1997). In some cases, such an increased production has been found to be constitutive, that is to say, cytokines are produced even if the cells are not stimulated. However, it has been shown that LPS-stimulated cytokine production is also higher in cultures of MDS cells than in their normal counterparts. Interestingly, overproduction of these cytokines by MDS cells has also been observed in peripheral blood mononuclear cells (Koike et al., 1995).

Among the above mentioned cytokines, TNFα, a well-characterized hematopoietic inhibitor mainly produced by macrophages, has called the attention of several groups. Considering its effects within the hematopoietic system (i.e., inhibiting progenitor cell growth and inducing apoptosis at different maturation stages), it has been suggested that this cytokine is directly involved in the pathogenesis of myelodysplasia. Indeed, some institutions have already used anti-TNFα therapy for MDS patients (reviewed by Raza et al., 1996). As expected, the main cellular source of TNFα in MDS patients seems to be macrophages, however, as indicated by Flores and colleagues, it is possible that other cell populations (including fibroblasts themselves) may be producing this cytokine as well (Flores et al., 2000). At the moment, the physiological relevance of the increased production of IL-1, IL-6, and G-CSF by MDS stromal cells is not fully clear. The fact that their levels are consistently increased in myelodysplasia suggests that they play a role at some stage in the progression of the disease, however, such a role is not exactly known. In their study, Hirayama et al (1993) observed extremely high levels of IL-6 and IL-8 in two patients with MDS, both with RAEB; interestingly, these patients showed a very rapid evolution to AML. Based on this observation, the authors suggested that active production of certain cytokines by stromal cells may be involved in the progression to overt leukemia.

Other hematopoietic inhibitors shown to be overproduced by MDS cells are TGFβ (Wetzler et al., 1995; Shetty et al., 1996) and IFNγ (Kitagawa et al., 1997). Both of them are well-recognized negative regulators of hematopoiesis (Mayani et al., 1995), thus they may also be involved in the biology of MDS, probably by inhibiting normal progenitor cell growth. It is noteworthy, however, that in contrast to these reports, Ohmori et al (1993) presented evidence indicating that MDS-derived macrophages produce a soluble inhibitory activity that does not seem to contain IFNγ but ferritin, another molecule postulated to inhibit hematopoiesis. Interestingly, these authors observed that such an inhibitory activity only affected myeloid progenitors from normal subjects and not those from MDS patients.

Finally, it is important to mention that deficiencies in the production of some stimulatory cytokines by MDS cells have also been observed. Visani et al (1993) reported on the reduced production of GM-CSF by MDS macrophages, as compared to normal BM-derived macrophages. Thus, taking all of the above data together, it seems reasonable to suggest that dysregulated cytokine production by marrow stromal/accessory cells is one of the mechanisms involved in the development and/or progression of myelodysplasia.

CONCLUDING REMARKS

Most of what we know about the biology of hematopoiesis in MDS has come from in vitro studies, performed during the last 20 years, involving several experimental systems and designs. Based on the information obtained during all these years, it is clear that severe functional abnormalities exist within the hematopoietic system, both at the level of hematopoietic cells and their microenvironment. The numbers of stem and progenitor cells are drastically reduced in the majority of MDS patients; their responsiveness to stimulatory cytokines is impaired, thus addition of recombinant cytokines to cultures may not have a beneficial effect. At least in a subgroup of patients, marrow stromal cells show aberrant patterns of cytokine production (i.e., increased production of hematopoietic inhibitors and reduced production of stimulators), and this seems to contribute to the progression of the disease, probably by inhibiting normal hematopoiesis and favoring neoplastic cell expansion.

Interestingly, in vitro culture of MDS marrow cells may also have a place in the clinic. Indeed, based on the reports from certain groups, semisolid and liquid cultures of myelodysplastic marrow cells may have prognostic value, predicting both disease progression and in vivo response to recombinant cytokines.

To date, however, many questions regarding the biology of MDS remain unanswered. By developing new and more efficient procedures for HSC/HPC purification; by getting a more complete analysis of gene expression of stem/progenitor cells; and by characterizing in more detail the functional integrity of the hematopoietic microenvironment, we should be able, in the short term, to understand in greater detail the biology of myelodysplasia. The next step will be to translate such a knowledge into better diagnostic, prognostic and therapeutic strategies.

REFERENCES

Adams JA, Liu Yin JA, Brereton ML, Briggs M, Burgess R & Hyde K (1997) The in vitro effect of pegylated recombinant human megakaryocyte growth and development factor (PEG rHuMGDF) on megakaryopoiesis in normal subjects and patients with myelodysplasia and acute myeloid leukemia. *British Journal of Haematology* **99**, 139-146

Aizawa S, Nakano M, Iwase O, Yaguchi M, Hiramoto M, Hoshi H, Nabeshima R, Shima D, Handa H & Toyama K (1999) Bone marrow stroma from refractory anemia of myelodysplastic syndrome is defective in its ability to support normal CD34-positive cell proliferation and differentiation in vitro. *Leukemia Research* **23**, 239-246

Aizawa S, Hiramoto M, Hoshi H, Toyama K, Shima D & Handa H (2000) Establishment of stromal cell line from an MDS RA patient which induced an apoptotic change in hematopoietic and leukemic cell in vitro. *Experimental Hematology* **28**, 148-155

Asano H, Hotta T, Ichihara M, Murate T, Kobayashi M & Saito H (1994) Growth analysis of marrow CD34-positive hematopoietic progneitor cells in patients with myelodysplastic syndromes. *Leukemia* **8**, 833-838

Backx B, Broeders L, Hoefsloot LH, Wognum B & Lowenberg B (1996) Erythropoiesis in myelodysplastic syndrome: expression of receptors for erythropoietin and kit ligand. *Leukemia* **10**, 466-472

Baines P, Bowen D & Jacobs A (1990) Clonal growth of haemopoietic progenitor cells from myelodysplastic marrow in response to recombinant haemopoietins. *Leukemia Research* **14**, 247-253

Bhatia M, Bonnet D, Murdoch B, Gan OI & Dick JE (1998) A newly discovered class of human hematopoietic cells with SCID repopulating activity. *Nature Medicine* **4**, 1038-1045

Borbenyi Z, Cinkotai C, Harrison C & Testa NG (1987) The growth of myelodysplastic bone marrow in long-term cultures. *British Journal of Cancer* **55**, 291-293

Carlo-Stella C, Cazzola M, Bergamaschi C, Bernasconi P, Dezza L, Invernizzi R & Pedrazzoli P (1989) Growth of human hematopoietic colonies from patients with myelodysplastic syndromes in response to recombinant human granulocyte-macrophage colony stimulating factor. *Leukemia* **3**, 363-366

Civin CI & Gore SD (1993) Antigenic analysis of hematopoiesis: a review. *Journal of Hematotherapy* **2**, 137-144

Conneally E, Cashman J, Petzer A & Eaves CJ (1997) Expansion in vitro of transplantable human cord blood stem cells demonstrated using a quantitative assay of their lympho-myeloid repopulating activity in nonobese diabetic scid/scid mice. *Proceeding of the National Academy of Sciences, USA* **94**, 9836-9841

Coutinho LH, Geary CG, Chang J, Harrison C & Testa NG (1990) Functional studies of bone marrow haemopoietic and stromal cells in themyelodysplastic syndrome (MDS). *British Journal of Haematology* **75**, 16-25

Dan K, An E, Futaki M, Inokuchi K, Gomi S, Yamada T, Ogata K, Tanabe Y, Ohki I, Shinohara T & Nomura T (1993) Megakaryocyte, erythroid and granulocyte macrophage colony formation in myelodysplastic syndromes. *Acta Hematologica* **89**, 113-118

Dexter TM, Allen TD & Lajtha L (1977) Conditions controlling the proliferation of hemopoietic stem cell in vitro. *Journal of Cellular Physiology* **91**, 335-344

Dick JE (1996) Normal and leukemic human stem cells assayed in SCID mice. *Seminars in Immunology* **8**, 197-206

Ferrajoli A, Talpaz M, Kurzrock R, Harris D, Van Q, Estey EH & Estrov E (1998) Thrombopoietin stimulates myelodysplastic syndrome granulocyte-macrophage and erythroid progenitor proliferation. *Leukemia & Lymphoma* **30**, 279-292

Flores E, Montesinos JJ, Gutierrez G & Mayani H (2000) Functional characterization of bone marrow fibroblasts and macrophages from patients with myelodysplastic síndromes. *Experimental Hematology* **28** (supplement 1), 95 (abstract)

Flores-Figueroa E, Gutierrez-Espindola G, Guerrero-Rivera S, Pizzuto-Chavez J & Mayani H (1999) Hematopoietic progenitor cells from patients with myelodysplastic syndromes: In vitro colony growth and long-term proliferation. *Leukemia Research* **23**, 385-394

Fontenay-Roupie M, Bouscary D, Guesnu M, Picard F, Melle J, Lacon, Gisselbrecht S, Mayeux P & Dreyfus F (1999) Ineffective erythropoiesis in the myelodysplastic syndromes: correlation with Fas expression but not with lack of erythropoietin receptor signal transduction. *British Journal of Haematology* **106**, 464-473

Gallacher L, Murdoch B, Wu DM, Karanu FN, Keeney M & Bhatia M (2000) Isolation and characterization of human $CD34^-$ Lin^- and $CD34^+$ Lin^- hematopoietic stem cells using surface markers AC133 and CD7. *Blood* **95**, 2813-2820

Glinsmann-Gibson B, Spier C, Baier M, Taetle R, Broudy VC & List AF (1994) Mast cell growth factor (c-kit ligand) restores growth of multipotent progenitors in myelodysplastic syndrome. *Leukemia* **8**, 827-832

Greenberg PL (1996) Biologic and clinical implications of marrow culture studies in the myelodysplastic syndromes. *Seminars in Hematology* **33**, 163-175

Greenberg PL & Mara B (1979) The preleukemic syndrome. Correlation of in vitro parameters of granulopoiesis with clinical features. *The American Journal of Medicine* **66**, 951-958

Heaney ML & Golde DW (1999) Myelodysplasia. *New England Journal of Medicine* **340**, 1649-1660

Hirayama Y, Kohgo Y, Matsunaga T, Ohi S, Sakamaki S & Niitsu Y (1993) Cytokine mRNA expression of bone marrow stromal cells from patients with aplastic anemia and myelodysplastic syndrome. *British Journal of Haematology* **85**, 676-683

Hoefsloot LH, van Amelsvoort MP, Broeders LC, van der Plas DC, van Lom K, Hoogerbrugge H, Touw IP & Lowenberg B (1997) Erythropoietin-induced activation of STAT5 is impaired in the myelodysplastic syndrome. *Blood* **89**, 1690-1700

Jacobs A (1985) Myelodysplastic syndromes: pathogenesis, functional abnormalities and clinical implications. *Journal of Clinical Pathology* **38**, 1201-1217

Janssen JW, Buschle M & Layton M (1989) Clonal analysis of myelodysplastic syndromes: evidence of multipotent stem cell origin. *Blood* **73**, 248-254

Juneja H & Gardner FH (1985) Functionally abnormal marrow stromal cells in aplastic anemia. *Experimental Hematology* **13**, 194-199

Juvonen E, Aimolahti A, Volin L & Ruutu T (1999) The prognostic value of in vitro cultures of erythroid and megakaryocyte progenitors in myelodysplastic syndromes. *Leukemia Research* **23**, 889-894

Kalina U, Hofmann W, Koschmieder S, Wagner S, Kauschat D, Hoelzer D & Ottmann OG (2000) Alterations of c-mpl-mediated signal transduction in CD34(+) cells from patients with myelodysplastic syndromes. *Experimental Hematology* **28**, 1158-1163

Kanamura A & Tamura S (1993) Application of long-term bone marrow cultures for studying the leukemic transformation of myelodysplastic syndromes. *Leukemia & Lymphoma* **11**, 345-352

Kere J, Ruutu T & de la Chapelle A (1987) Monosomy 7 in granulocytes and monocytes in myelodysplastic syndrome. *New England Journal of Medicine* **316**, 499-506

Kitagawa M, Saito I, Kuwata T, Yoshida S, Yamaguchi S, Takahashi M, Tanizawa T, Kamiyama R & Hirokawa K (1997) Overexpression of tumor necrosis factor (TNF)-α and interferon (IFN)-γ by bone marrow cells from patients with myelodysplastic syndromes. *Leukemia* **11**, 2049-2054

Koike M, Ishiyama T, Tomoyasu S & Tsuruoka N (1995) Spontaneous cytokine overproduction by peripheral blood mononuclear cells from patients with myelodysplastic syndromes and aplastic anemia. *Leukemia Research* **19**, 639-644

Kroef MJPL, Fibbe WE & Mout R (1993) Myeloid but not lymphoid cells carry the 5q deletion: polymerase chain reaction analysis of loss of heterozygosity using mini repeat sequences on highly purified cell fractions. *Blood* **81**, 1849-1854

Masters GS, Baines P, Tang C, Bowen DT & Burnett AK (1995) Responsiveness to stem cell factor (SCF) of peripheral blood colony forming cells from patients with myelodysplastic syndromes (MDS). *Leukemia Research* **19**, 561-566

Mayani H (1993) Human preleukemia: cellular, molecular and clinical aspects. *Archives of Medical Research* **24**, 317-324

Mayani H (1996) Composition and function of the hemopoietic microenvironment in human myeloid leukemia. *Leukemia* **10**, 1041-1047

Mayani H, Baines P, Bowen DT & Jacobs A (1989) In vitro growth of myeloid and erythroid progenitor cells from myelodysplastic patients in response to recombinant human granulocyte-macrophage colony-stimulating factor. *Leukemia* **3**, 29-32

Mayani H, Guilbert LJ & Janowska-Wieczorek A (1992) Biology of the hemopoietic microenvironment. *European Journal of Haematology* **49**, 225-233

Mayani H, Little MT, Dragowska W, Thornbury G & Lansdorp PM (1995) Differential effects of the hematopoietic inhibitors MIP-1α, TGF-β and TNF-α on cytokine induced proliferation of subpopulations of CD34+ cells purified from cord blood and fetal liver. *Experimental Hematology* **23**, 422-427

Merchav S, Nielsen OJ, Rosenbaum H, Sharon R, Brenner B, Tatarsky I, Scigalla P & Wieczorek L (1990) In vitro studies of erythropoietin-dependent regulation of erythropoiesis in myelodysplastic syndrome. *Leukemia* **4**, 771-774

Merchav S, Wagemarker G, Souza LM & Tatarsky I (1991) Impaired response of myelodysplastic marrow progenitors to stimulation with recombinant haematopoietic growth factors. *Leukemia* **5**, 340-346

Metcalf D (1977) Hematopoietic colonies. In vitro cloning of normal and leukemic cells. Springer-Verlag, Berlin-Heidelberg, p.227.

Metcalf D (1993) Hematopoietic regulators: redundancy or subtlety? *Blood* **82**, 3515-3523

Michaux JL & Martiat P (1993) Chronic myelomonocytic leukemia (CMML)- a myelodysplastic or myeloproliferative syndrome?. *Leukemia & Lymphoma* **9**, 35-41

Montesinos JJ, Flores P, Flores E, Martínez G & Mayani H (2000) In vitro proliferation and expansion of human hematopoietic progenitor cells from normal subjects and patients with hematologic neoplasias. *Experimental Hematology* **28** (supplement 1), 95 (abstract)

Moore MAS (1991) Clinical implications of positive and negative hematopoietic stem cell regulators. *Blood* **78**, 1-19

Murphy MJ (1994) Polyfunctionality of hemopoietic regulators. The Metcalf Forum. AlphaMed Press, Dayton, USA p.326

Nilsson L, Astrand-Grundstrom I, Arvidsson I, Jacobsson B, Hellstrom-Lindberg E, Hast R & Jacobson SEW (2000) Isolation and characterization of hematopoietic progenitor/stem cells in 5q-deleted myelodysplastic syndromes: evidence for involvement at the hematopoietic stem cell level. Blood 96, 2012-2021

Ohmori S, Ohmori M, Yamagishi M & Okuma M (1993) MDS-macrophage derived inhibitory activity on myelopoiesis of MDS abnormal clones. British Journal of Haematology 83, 388-391

Piacibello W, Sanavio F, Bresso P, Severino A, Carlesso N, Pregno P, Stacchini A, Morelli S, Fubini L, Gallo E, Aglietta M & Ferrero D (1994) Stem cell factor improvement of proliferation and maintenance of hematopoietic progenitors in myelodysplastic syndromes. *Leukemia* **8**, 250-257

Raza A, Gregory SA & Preisler HD (1996) the myelodysplastic syndromes in 1996: Complex stem cell disorders confounded by dual actions of cytokines. *Leukemia Research* **20**, 881-890

Saitoh K, Miura I, Takahashi N & Miura AB (1998) Fluorescence in situ hybridization of progenitor cells obtained by fluorescence activated cell sorting for the detection of cells affected by chromosome abnormality trisomy 8 in patients with myelodysplastic syndromes. *Blood* **92**, 2886-2892

Sato T, Kim S, Selleri C, Young NS & Maciejewski JP (1998) Measurement of secondary colony formation after 5 weeks in long-term cultures in patients with myelodysplastic syndrome. *Leukemia* **12**, 1187-1194

Sawada K (1996) Proliferation and differentiation of myelodysplastic CD34+ cells. *Leukemia & Lymphoma* **12**, 43-51

Sawada K, Sato N, Tarumi T, Sakai N, Koizumi K, Sakurama S, Ieko M, Yasukouchi T, Koyanagawa Y, Yamaguchi M, Ohmoto A, Kohno M & Koike T (1993) Proliferation and differentiation of myelodysplastic CD34+ cells in serum-free medium: response to individual colony-stimulating factors. *British Journal of Haematology* **83**, 349-358

Sawada K, Sato N, Notoya A, Tarumi T, Hirayama S, Takano H, Koizumi K, Yasukouchi T, Yamaguchi M & Koike T (1995) Proliferation and differentiation of myelodysplastic CD34+ cells: Phenotypic subpopulations of marrow CD34+ cells. *Blood* **85**, 194-202

Schipperus M, Sonneveld P, Lindemans J, Hagemeijer A, Vink N, Pegels J & Abels J (1990) The effects of interleukin-3, GM-CSF and G CSF on the growth kinetics of colony forming cells in myelodysplastic syndromes. *Leukemia* **4**, 267-272

Shetty V, Mundle S, Alvi S, Showel M, Broady-Robinson L, Dar S, Borok R, Showel J, Gregory S, Rifkin S, Gezer S, Parcharidou A, Venugopal P, Shah R, Hernandez B, Klein M, Alson D, Robin E, Dominguez C & Raza A (1996) Measurement of apoptosis, proliferation and three cytokines in 46 patients with myelodysplastic syndromes. *Leukemia Research* **20**, 891-899

Shih LY, Chiu WF & Lee CT (1991) Diagnostic and prognostic values of in vitro culture growth patterns of marrow granulocyte macrophage progenitors in patients with myelodysplastic syndrome. *Leukemia* **5**, 1092-1098

Soligo D, Servida F, Cortelezzi A, Pedretti D, Uziel L, Morgutti M, Pogliani E & Lambertenghi Deliliers G (1994) Effects of recombinant human stem cell factor (rh SCF) on colony formation and long-term bone marrow cultures (LTBMC) in patients with myelodysplastic síndromes. *European Journal of Haematology* **52**, 53-60

Soligo DA, Campiglio S, Servida F, Bossolasco P, Romitti L, Cortelezzi & Lambertenghi Deliliers G (1996) Response of myelodysplastic syndrome marrow progenitor cells stimulation with cytokine combination in a stroma-free long-term culture system. *British Journal of Haematology* **92**, 548-558

Sutherland HJ, Eaves CJ, Eaves AC, Dragowska W, Lansdorp PM (1989) Characterization and partial purification of human marrow cells capable of initiating long-term hematopoiesis in vitro. *Blood* **74**, 1563-1570

Szilvassy SJ & Hoffman R (1995) Enriched hematopoietic stem cells: Basic biology and clinical utility. *Biology of Blood and Marrow Transplantation* **1**, 3-17

Tohyama K, Ueda T, Yoshida Y & Nakamura T (1994) Altered responses of purified blast cells from the myelodysplastic syndromes to colony-stimulating factors in vitro: comparison with normal blast cells. *Experimental Hematology* **22**, 539-545

Thomas TE, Miller CL & Eaves CJ (1999) Purification of hematopoietic stem cells for further biological study. *Methods. A companion to Methods in Enzymology* **17**, 202-218

Visani G, Zauli G, Tosi P, Fogli M, Cenaucchi A, Finelli C, Gamberi B, Ottaviani E, Manfoi S & Tura S (1993) Impairment of GM-CSF production in myelodysplastic syndromes. *British Journal of Haematology* **84**, 227-231

Wetzler M, Kurzrock R, Estrov Z, Estey E & Talpaz M (1995) Cytokine expression in adherent layers from patients with myelodysplastic syndrome and acute myelogenous leukemia. *Leukemia Research* **19**, 23-34

Yoshida Y (1987) Biology of myelodysplastic syndromes. *International Journal of Cell Cloning* **5**, 356-375

Zanjani ED, Almeida-Porada G, Livingston AG, Flake AW & Ogawa M (1998) Human bone marrow CD34-negative cells engraft in vivo and undergo multilineage expression that includes giving rise to CD34-positive cells. *Experimental Hematology* **26**, 353-360

Ziegler BL, Valtieri M, Almeida Porada G, De Maria R, Müller R, Masella B, Gabianelli M, Casella I, Pelosi E, Bock T, Zanjani ED & Peschle C (1999) KDR receptor: A key marker defining hematopoietic stem cells. *Science* **285**, 1553-1558

Zwierzina H, Schollenberger S, Herold M, Schmalzl F & Besemer J (1992) Endogenous serum levels and surface receptor expression of GM-CSF and IL-3 in patients with myelodysplastic syndromes. *Leukemia Research* **16**, 1181-1186

3

BIOLOGY OF STEM AND MYELOID PROGENITOR CELLS IN MYELODYSPLASTIC SYNDROMES

Lambert F.R. Span and Theo M. de Witte,
Department of Hematology, University Medical Center Nijmegen
Nijmegen, The Netherlands

The myelodysplastic syndromes (MDS) are hyperproliferative, acquired clonal stem cell disorders, associated with massive intramedullary apoptosis or programmed cell death (PCD). A leukemic phenotype, mainly characterized by an increase of blasts showing differentiation arrest, is gradually observed, as MDS progresses from low-risk (LR-MDS) to high-risk MDS (HR-MDS). Three interacting compartments can be distinguished in MDS, the polyclonal, residual normal hematopoiesis, the monoclonal preleukemic compartment, and the blastic leukemic compartment. Within LR-MDS, monoclonal hematopoiesis dominates leukemic blast cell proliferation (<5%), whereas this pattern is reversing during MDS evolution to acute myeloid leukemia (AML). This shift in the balance of proliferation versus apoptosis has to be applied constantly to these three interacting compartments in MDS. For illustration, the following example and nomenclature is used. Stem Cell Factor (SCF) is a major factor to induce differentiation and to mediate the transition from the earliest CD34 negative (CD34–) stem cells to the more differentiated CD34 positive (CD34+) stem cells, whereas IL-6 promotes proliferation and maintains self-renewal of CD34+ stem cells. The balance and interaction between these cytokines may play different roles in normal, monoclonal, and leukemic hematopoiesis *("static profile" of these compartments).* Furthermore, these cytokine levels, their receptor density, and/or their receptor-ligand interaction may *change* within each hematopoietic compartment as MDS progresses, also changing the balance and interaction of these cytokines between these three pools *("dynamic profile").* Genetic or phenotypic changes of the malignant pool and changing interactions with the environment (stroma or different accessory cells) also cause a complex dynamic change in different interactions (cell-cell, cell-stroma, stroma-stroma) between these three pools as MDS progresses *("complex-dynamic profile").*

This chapter describes these complex-dynamic profiles of stem cells and progenitors in MDS. Emphasis is put on the origin of monoclonality and its implications in MDS (Part I) and phenotypic-functional studies to understand the biology (balance of proliferation and apoptosis) of MDS in evolution (Part II). Part III of this chapter discusses the Fas/FasL system as one of the most important members of the nerve-growth factor receptor family for carrying apoptosis signal transduction.

CLONALITY IN MDS

Dysplastic features and an increase of blasts found in hypercellular BM characterize MDS. The IPSS scoring system (Greenberg et al., 1997), based upon the percentage of marrow myeloblasts, cytogenetic characteristics, and the number of cytopenias, defined prognosis and survival of MDS patients with more accuracy than the original FAB-classification. MDS progression to AML is determined by further accumulation of genetic defects in the myelodysplastic clone. Early studies suggested that these aberrant clones may originate in a more committed myeloid stem cell (CFU-GEMM) in most patients, evaluated by immunophenotyping and (fluorescent) in situ hybridization (F)ISH (Gerritsen et al., 1992; Kibbelaar et al., 1992; Kroef et al., 1993). More recent studies proved that cytogenetically aberrant cells could also be detected in the primitive stem cell pool (Mehrotra et al., 1995; Nilsson et al., 2000). Mehrotra et al (1995) found cytogenetically aberrant cells in a primitive (CD34+lin–) stem cell compartment. The percentage abnormal cells was *not* associated with compartment expansion, indicating that these aberrant primitive hematopoietic cells do not show a leukemic phenotype (growth and survival advantage). This primitive compartment (with high MDR1 expression) accounts for the high relapse rate of MDS patients treated with intensive chemotherapy and autologous BM transplantation.

In general, it is hypothesized that a first hit causes inactivation or deletion of tumor suppressor genes (e.g. IRF-1 and EGR-1 at 5q31-33 region),

DNA repair genes (at 7q22 region) or, although less frequently, activating mutations in a proto-oncogene (e.g. N-ras and its association with chromosome 7 deletions). This first hit will subsequently lead to a "controlled" growth advantage of this "damaged" stem cell and its progeny over the normal pool of stem cells (Greenberg, 1983). MDS in preleukemic phase detects *monoclonality* (in females) by X-chromosome inactivation studies (see below), which may occur before the development of karyotypical abnormalities. The growth advantage of these preleukemic CD34+ cells and its progeny may be caused by an increase of the number of S-phase cells (Span et al., 1998a) with or without a substantial survival benefit. This genetically altered progenitor cell pool is more prone to additional mutations or deletions *("genomic instability")*. S-phase cells are more susceptible to detrimental DNA events because of their status of unpacked and uncoiled DNA and intense DNA synthesis with less DNA repair time. The final behavior of the leukemic clone in MDS is determined by its overall make-up of activated genes. Patients with balanced chromosomal translocations seem more likely to present with overt leukemia than patients with unbalanced chromosomal abnormalities (Pederson-Bjergaard & Rowley, 1994; Pederson-Bjergaard et al., 1995).

Interestingly, patients with and without abnormal karyotype have no different levels of *overall apoptosis* (Bogdanovic et al., 1997). It is therefore tempting to speculate that monoclonality by itself induces immune responses leading to overt apoptosis. This apoptotic process is also conferred to the normal, polyclonal hematopoiesis and stromal tissues as innocent bystanders (see Part II). As polyclonal blood cells are dying intramedullary, relatively more apoptosis-resistant blood cells with normal or dysplastic appearance in the peripheral blood are found as the progeny of monoclonal hematopoiesis (Horikawa et al., 1997). Furthermore, the percentage cytogenetically aberrant BM blasts is always considerably higher than the BM mature granulocytes indicating a partial maturation arrest (and decreased PCD) of monoclonal hematopoiesis in MDS (van Lom et al., 1996). Above all, anti-apoptotic therapy in MDS patients sometimes results in disappearance of cytogenetically aberrant clones and resumption of polyclonal hematopoiesis (Reza et al., 1998). The role of Fas/FasL in MDS is probably a double-edged sword: a tool of immune surveillance by NK-cells and/or cytotoxic T cells with enhanced mFasL attacking the preleukemic clone(s), which in their turn show decreasing Fas and increasing FasL expression during leukemic progression. This process gradually leads to an escape of the leukemic cells with high FasL expression from immunoregulatory cells and probably contributes to progressive PCD of normal and monoclonal preleukemic hematopoiesis with enhanced Fas expression (see part III).

The HUMARA assay which uses a polymorphic gene on the X-chromosome showing a high rate of heterozygosity (>90%) is the most used assay to study *X Chromosome Inactivation Patterns* (XCIP) to detect monoclonality. The presence of monoclonality is an early feature in MDS. However, differentiation from constitutional excessive Lyonization and acquired skewing associated with increasing age, is a major limitation in interpretation of these assays (total skewing 15-40%). The use of T lymphocytes as control cells and sequential analyses may solve this practical problem. On the other hand, no specific genetic marker is needed for assessment of monoclonality with XCIP. The different XCIP assays used on different sorted subsets of BM and blood in MDS patients have shown monoclonality originating in a primitive (CD34+Lin–/Thy1+) or early committed (CD34+CD33+) stem cell.

BIOLOGICAL FEATURES OF CD34+ CELLS AND THEIR MYELOID PROGENY IN MDS EVOLUTION

Characteristics Of CD34+ Cells In MDS

The percentage CD34, CD33, and CD13 positive bone marrow mononuclear cells (BMMNC) increased as patients progressed to HR-MDS, and correlated with shorter survival (Guyotat et al., 1990; Kerndrup et al., 1988; Kristensen & Hokland, 1990; Gersuk et al., 1998). Also co-expression of CD13 (mean ±90%) was significantly increased in MDS CD34+ cells. This was associated with a predominant outgrowth of CFU-GM, usually showing undifferentiated clusters, as hardly any erythroid aggregates were found (Sawada et al., 1995). Furthermore, abnormally high ratios of pro- versus anti-apoptotic proteins (c-Myc/Bcl-2 and Bax+Bad/Bcl-2+Bcl-X) were found within the CD34+ cells of especially LR-MDS patients (Parker et al., 2000; Rajapaksa et al., 1996). These ratios reversed in advanced MDS and AML.

The size of the CD34+ pool is rapidly increasing during MDS progression in the majority of patients (Span et al., 1998a), and a concomitant rise in the number of *aberrant* blasts occurred, as was detected by flow cytometry (FCM) side scatter and CD45 expression (Gersuk et al., 1998). The morphologically "normal" CD34+ blast cells may contain monoclonal, cytogenetically normal CD34 cells, but this remains to be proven. The presence of circulating CD34+ cells in MDS correlated with leukemic progression, even better than cytogenetics and CFU-GM growth in vitro (Sullivan et al., 1992). It may indicate that cell-stroma interactions have changed in HR-MDS, and this may contribute to leukemic evolution.

Proliferation Of CD34+ Cells And Their Progeny In MDS

In vivo thymidine analogue (BrdU/IUdR) incorporation studies in MDS patients (Shetty et al., 1996; Raza et al., 1997) followed by BM immunohistochemistry (IH) have shown an increment of *overall proliferation of BMMNC*. These studies demonstrated a higher than normal overall myeloid growth fraction (median percentage S-phase cells 25-30%, range 13-49%) with a decreasing trend towards HR-MDS. Furthermore, the total cell cycling times (Tc) increased when RA progressed to RAEB-t (Tc of 37.5 and 56.6 hrs, respectively). Within the myeloid compartment, a rapid increment of the percentage of *CD34+ cells* (from 1.67 to 8.69% from LR- to HR-MDS, respectively) and the percentage *CD34+ cells in S-phase* (from 0.19 to 0.43%, respectively) was observed during the evolution of MDS (Span et al., 1998a). A concomitant rise was also found in the percentage *proliferating CD34+ cells* within the *proliferating* myeloid compartment during MDS progression (from 0.35 to 1.44%, respectively). These patterns clearly illustrate a growth advantage within the CD34+ pool, which only partially explains the exponential growth of the size of the CD34+ pool during MDS evolution. Using FCM with Ki-67, Parker et al (2000) found increasing percentages of *proliferating* (G_1) CD34+ cells (range 10-70%) within the (growing) CD34+ compartment during MDS progression, as the percentage *S-phase* cells in the CD34+ pool was hardly changing in our study (mean 5-10%, Span et al., 1998a). As the nuclear antigen Ki-67 is not an excellent proliferation marker for myeloid cells and it only distinguishes non-cycling (G_0) from cycling (G_1) cells, the differences between these two studies can be explained by enhanced PCD of CD34+ cells in G_1. Thus, the CD34+ compartment expands as MDS progresses with a tendency to cycle slower than their more mature CD34– progeny. Furthermore, also the differentiation arrest in leukemic blasts (Gersuk et al., 1998), and their progressive survival benefit account for this expansion of CD34+ cells and blasts. It is important to stress that proliferation and differentiation are progressively uncoupled mechanisms during the evolution of the leukemic clone(s) as MDS progresses.

Proliferation And Apoptosis Of CD34+ Cells And Their Progeny In MDS: *dynamic profiles in vitro*

In vitro studies with *BMMNC* of MDS patients have shown decreased colony and increased cluster formation with slower growth kinetics, delayed and disturbed differentiation or arrest at the stage of myelo-monocytic blasts (Sawada, 1994), as well as increased apoptosis (Span et al., 1998b). This leukemic growth pattern in vitro was associated with an increase of blasts and CD34+ BM cells, and correlated with a higher incidence of leukemic transformation with shorter survival (Guyotat et al., 1990; Raymakers et al.,

1991; Sawada et al., 1996). We studied the profiles of proliferation and PCD (by ISEL) of BMMNC of MDS patients in vitro (Span et al., 1998b). The proliferation defined by the total number of clusters and colonies was initially enhanced as compared to normals. But this was rapidly followed by a concomitant increased apoptosis: 75% of clusters and more than 40% of colonies showed more than 50% PCD. In contrast, normal controls showed a median PCD of 50% in clusters and 17% in the colonies. AML patients showed delayed and low colony growth in vitro, because of enhanced apoptosis at cluster level (60-80%) compared to a relative low PCD in colonies (20%). Interestingly, some colonies of AML patients showed no apoptosis at all (Span et al., 1998b).

Single cell assays of CD34+ BM cells in MDS showed a similar biological profile: increased proliferation and apoptosis at cluster level and decreased colony formation showing decreased cell numbers. These colonies showed less overall PCD than normal colonies (Span et al., 1999). As neither stromal interactions nor accessory cell influences are involved in this system, probably (pre)leukemic clones with longer cell cycling time (43.7 hrs in MDS versus 33.8 hrs in normal colonies) and less PCD can evolve in this system. It implies that the patterns observed are intrinsic properties of MDS progenitor cells. (F)ISH studies have to be performed to distinguish growth patterns of chromosomal aberrant from normal clones.

Long-term bone marrow cultures (LTBMC), analyzing *MDS stromal* influences on normal CD34+ cells, have shown defective surface coverage and support in promoting proliferation and differentiation (Novitzky et al., 2000), leading to increased levels of Fas and apoptosis (Aizawa et al., 1999). In contrast, Deeg et al (2000) found stimulatory effects of MDS stroma on normal CD34+ or MDS CD34+ cells. They suggested that accessory mononuclear (non-stromal) cells or abnormal hematopoietic precursors in the non-adherent marrow fraction provided the inhibitory effects as they produced TNF-α at maximal levels.

LTBMC (with *normal stroma*) were capable of detecting latent subclones with abnormal karyotypes in the majority of MDS patients with normal cytogenetics. In some patients (25%) these karyotypes also became apparent in vivo (Tamura et al., 1992). Furthermore, LTBMC detected profound deficiencies in the number of secondary colony-forming cells and in long-term proliferation of multipotent MDS progenitors, together with disturbed differentiation and stromal interference (Sato et al., 1998; Flores-Figueroa et al., 1999; Novitzky et al., 2000).

Stroma-free LTBMC with a combination of four growth factors (GF) showed a normal expansion of MDS progenitor cells with normal or dysplastic differentiation in 50% of cases. Complete unresponsiveness and progressive leukemic growth with 100% immature blasts was found in 30% and 20% of MDS cases, respectively (Soligo et al., 1996). Furthermore, Novitzky et al. (2000) showed that the subgroup of MDS patients with the highest overall BMMNC apoptosis had the best clonogenic growth in vitro and showed the best response to anti-TNF-α therapy in vivo. This shows that the inhibitory and PCD-inducing cytokines and their corresponding cells outweigh their stimulating counterparts in MDS marrows. A high proliferative potential continues to be present in MDS hematopoiesis.

Several mechanisms may explain these altered growth patterns in vitro. MDS CD34+ cells with enhanced co-expression of CD13 form predominantly nonerythroid clusters with impaired differentiation (Sawada et al., 1995). MDS progenitors show a diminished response to G-CSF (Sawada, 1994), and GM-CSF (Mayani et al., 1989), which could be reversed by supersaturating doses in some patients (Merchav et al., 1991). Stem cell factor (SCF) promotes cluster growth, whereas in combination with other GF undifferentiated colonies are promoted. SCF may in part be responsible for the growth advantage of MDS clonogenic cells over normal blasts, although no differences in c-kit expression were observed (Sawada et al., 1996; Tohyama et al., 1994; Sawada et al., 1999). Enhanced apoptosis detected in the progeny of BMMNC and CD34+ cells of MDS patients may explain this decreased colony formation. In serum-free cultures and LTBMC, MDS CD34+ cells showed poor or no growth of *differentiated* colonies, irrespective of their growth type, suggesting the defective support of accessory and stromal cells (Sawada et al., 1999, Aizawa et al., 1999). Influences of stromal and accessory cells are not the only explanation of increased PCD as it was also found in single cell assays of MDS CD34+ cells. Differentiation between cytokine-mediated and/or Fas-FasL mediated PCD is warranted!

Apoptosis Of CD34+ Cells And Their Progeny In MDS: *dynamic profiles and controversies*

Apoptosis can be triggered by a variety of circumstances like GF deprivation, receptor interaction like TNFR1 and Fas, and cell damage causing molecular and or genomic damage beyond repair. Several quantitative techniques have been developed to measure apoptosis like immunohistochemistry (IH) or flowcytometry (FCM) by in situ end-labeling (ISEL) or TdT-mediated dUTP nick-end labeling (TUNEL). ISEL and TUNEL detect specific DNA fragmentation products developed after the activation of different endonucleases. These techniques proved enhanced intramedullary PCD (Raza et al., 1995; Mundle et al., 1999a), as it was postulated before (Yoshida, 1993).

Overall apoptosis detected by the ISEL technique on plastic embedded BM biopsies was excessive in MDS. More than 50% of patients showed ≥ 75% ISEL+ cells (Raza et al., 1995; Raza et al., 1996). In general, less apoptosis was found with TUNEL (mean range 12-46%), especially when bone marrow smears were used (Lepelley et al., 1996; Bouscary et al., 1997; Kitagawa et al., 1998; Bouscary et al., 2000, Novitzky et al., 2000). The detection of PCD by morphology (±3%) underestimates the amount of apoptosis (Bogdanovic et al., 1997). This phenomenon is explained by the short duration of the apoptotic process. In addition, early apoptotic cells present phosphatidylserine on their outer membrane, signaling macrophages for engulfment, often before clear apoptotic morphology can be detected. Apoptosis was observed in clusters of marrow cells in BM biopsies and the amount of PCD was positively and significantly correlated with the level and localization of TNF-α expression (Shetty et al., 1996). Both trilineage parenchymal and stromal cells are dying (Raza et al., 1995, Aizawa et al., 1999). The number of macrophages was clearly increased, showing massive ISEL-positive apoptotic bodies of captured, dead cells (Shetty et al., 1996). PCD was inversely correlated with leukocyte count (Bogdanovic et al., 1997).

Overall apoptosis of BMMNC measured by *TUNEL* on BM *aspirates* (range 20-46%) and BM *biopsies* (range 47-69%) is high in LR-MDS and decreases during progression of MDS (Lepelley et al., 1996; Bouscary et al., 1997; Hellström-Lindberg et al., 1997; Bouscary et al., 2000). High rates of overall PCD were correlated with low Bournemouth scores (Bouscary et al., 1997) and were significantly correlated with low blast numbers (Bouscary et al., 2000). In contrast, a large number of BM *biopsies* treated with *ISEL* showed massive apoptosis (>75%) in most HR-MDS patients. ISEL-positivity decreased towards intermediate levels (range 33-67%) in low-risk MDS, although both high and low ISEL positivity (ISEL+) was found in LR-MDS (Raza et al., 1995; Shetty et al 1996). The most likely explanation for these discrepancies in PCD is the difference in used material. More apoptotic cells in MDS marrow aspirates were found in the high-density fraction of mononuclear cells than in the mostly used low-density fraction (Shetty et al., 2000). A considerable amount of apoptotic cells is damaged and lost during the work-up of marrow aspirates. Differences in the detection of different DNA fragmentation products by ISEL and TUNEL is another fair explanation (Mundle et al., 1999a). Another explanation may be the heterogeneity of MDS. The apoptotic degree is different in the various compartments (CD34+ vs. CD34–, and leukemic vs. monoclonal vs. polyclonal) in time. These compartments also change in size during MDS progression.

In MDS, various levels of apoptosis within the *CD34+ pool* were found with different techniques. Massive PCD of CD34+ progenitors was found in LR-MDS, as it decreased towards HR-MDS (Parker et al., 2000; Rajapaksa et al., 1996). Parker et al (2000) showed excessive apoptosis (median range 50-60%) by FCM using Annexin-V (AnV), whereas Rajapaksa et al. (1996) showed a sub-G1 peak of 9%, both detected in the CD34+ subset in early MDS. In contrast, TUNEL performed on cytospin preparations of sorted CD34+ cells of MDS patients showed a lower mean PCD of 24%, not significantly different from normals. In general, lower values were found in LR- versus HR-MDS (Novitzky et al., 2000). Increased c-myc/Bcl-2 ratios of CD34+ cells were correlated with enhanced PCD in LR-MDS patients (Rajapaksa et al., 1996). In addition, pro-apoptotic (Bax+Bad) versus anti-apoptotic (Bcl-2+Bcl-x) ratios were increased in CD34+ cells of patients with LR-MDS. Disease progression was associated with significantly reduced ratios, due to increased Bcl-2 and a reduction in Bad expression (Parker et al., 2000). Surprisingly, as these ratios play an eminent role as molecular death switches, they were *not* associated with apoptosis measured by AnV, whereas they were inversely correlated with IPSS score and cytogenetic risk group. AnV detects phosphatidylserine on the outer membrane of cells. This is probably a marker *before* the point of "no-return" of PCD, as a fraction of thawed AnV+CD34+ cells showed proliferation in single cell assays (own observation).

Conflicting results were found when CD34+ and CD34– cell populations were compared with TUNEL by FCM and ISEL by IH (Mundle et al., 1999b). In general, CD34– cells showed more PCD with TUNEL than CD34+ cells, but this difference was not significant, whereas 56% CD34– cells versus an occasional CD34+ cell showed ISEL+ in BM biopsies. Different types of nuclear endonucleases found in CD34+ and CD34- cells causing different DNA fragmentation products may explain this. Above all, ISEL positivity was decreased in blast clusters of advanced MDS and in AML blasts in BM biopsies (Raza et al., 1995).

The *overall balance* of these dynamic profiles between increased proliferation and apoptosis results in ineffective hematopoiesis with cytopenias in the peripheral blood. A significant positive correlation was observed between the degree of PCD and proliferation (Raza et al., 1995). Also anti-PCD treatment studies (Reza et al., 1998) clearly showed that PCD and proliferation were correlated phenomena. Parker et al (2000) found the following apoptosis/proliferation ratios in the MDS CD34+ cells: 2.08 (RA/RARS), 1.14 (RAEB), and 1.7 (MDS-AML). Maximum PCD was found in RA/RARS, whereas proliferation peaked in RAEB, and both processes declined towards MDS-AML. Signal antonymy is an unique feature for MDS (Mundle et al., 1994). It means that the cell is dying in S-phase as a result of concomitant engagement into incompatible pathways like proliferation and cell cycle arrest. Signal antonymy in MDS (mean of 54% of S-phase cells) was found in all hematopoietic lineages as well as stromal cells. The explanation for this phenomenon is still unknown.

Complex Dynamic Profiles In MDS: *interactions*

Growth factors (GF) and cytokines play an important role in the apoptotic processes in MDS. In general, GF can be considered as survival factors. The end result is determined by the balance between levels of positive and negative hematopoietic GF and cytokines and their receptor status. Enhanced expression of *TNF-α and IFN-γ* was detected in BM biopsies of MDS patients (Shetty et al., 1996, Kitagawa et al., 1997). TNF-α expression was significantly correlated with PCD. TNF-α-induced cytotoxicity is mediated by reactive oxygen intermediates generated in the mitochondrial respiratory chain. Anti-apoptotic therapy by TNF-α-lowering regimens in MDS patients resulted in decreased TNF-α levels followed by decreased PCD in BM, and clinical responses in 40-50% of patients (Reza et al., 1998; Novitzky et al., 2000; Raza et al., 2000). These results led to Raza's postulation of *a dual role of elevated TNF-α* (and IL-1β) levels in the hematopoiesis of MDS patients: stimulation of proliferation of CD34+ stem and early progenitor cells, but inducing apoptosis in their CD34– progeny (Raza et al., 1996). One contributing link interacting in this paradigm has been found: TNF-α (and IFN-γ) upregulates Fas/CD95 expression, which is one of the main pathways of introducing cell death signals to cells. Sometimes a decrease or disappearance of cytogenetically aberrant clone(s) was observed during TNF-α-lowering therapy (Reza et al., 1998). These effects suggest that anti-TNF-α treatment may favor normal rather than aberrant hematopoiesis.

THE Fas/FasL SYSTEM

Introduction Of Normal Physiology

All members of the nerve growth factor receptor family play dual roles as they can trigger both apoptosis as well as proliferation (Wallach et al., 1996). One of the members is *Fas (CD95, APO-1),* a 45kDa type I transmembrane glycoprotein. The Fas receptor is expressed on a wide range of mature blood cells (monocytes, neutrophils, NK cells, B and T cells), and highly expressed on activated lymphocytes. In contrast, Fas is weakly expressed on immature BM cells. CD34+/CD38+ cells have two-fold higher expression than CD34+/CD38– cells (Maciejewski et al., 1995; Nagafuji et al., 1995; Josefsen et al., 1999). The receptor density increases from early CD34+ stem cells to more mature progenitors, and it is particularly upregulated on proliferating myeloid progenitors (Stahnke et al., 1998). Cytokines known to mediate proliferation, maturation, and survival of hematopoiesis facilitate negative growth regulation by the Fas pathway in activated cells (Stahnke et al., 1998). This effect could serve as a negative feedback mechanism by T cells on activated hematopoiesis (Degliantoni et al., 1985; Pantel & Nakeff, 1993). These findings suggest that the Fas/FasL system plays a role in the homeostasis of hematopoiesis (Niho & Asano, 1998). Furthermore, Fas expression is upregulated in a dose-dependent fashion in IFN-γ and TNF-α treated marrow CD34+ stem cells and it facilitates Fas-induced PCD (Maciejewski et al., 1995; Nagafuji et al., 1995). The combination of TNF-α and IFN-γ had a synergistic effect on the induction of Fas expression on progenitors (Nagafuji et al., 1995). Activated peripheral blood mononuclear cells were able to produce soluble Fas isoforms (Knipping et al., 1995). Soluble Fas (sFas) inhibits apoptosis in vitro (Cheng et al., 1994).

Fas Ligand (FasL) is a 40kDa type II transmembrane protein. FasL is predominantly expressed in activated T cells (CTL's), B cells, and NK cells, but it is also expressed on monocytes, neutrophils and tumor cells. Membrane FasL (*mFasL*) induces PCD by trimerization or cross-linking of the Fas receptor in some Fas-expressing cell lines or memory T cells (Tanaka et al., 1995). It works as a cytotoxic effector molecule of CTL and NK cells, and probably of AML tumor cells. Membrane-bound FasL can be cleaved into a soluble form (*sFasL*) by a metalloproteinase (Kayagaki et al., 1995). Membrane-bound FasL is more potent in promoting PCD than sFasL (Suda et al., 1997). The shedding of FasL from the membrane is a mechanism for downregulating its killing activity: sFasL competitively inhibits the killing of T cells by mFasL (Suda et al., 1997; Tanaka et al., 1998). Above all, Josefsen et al. (1999) found that sFasL promoted cell survival of human BM CD34+CD38– progenitor cells by suppressing PCD in suspension cultures as well as in single cell assay, whereas PCD was slightly increased in the more mature CD34+CD38+ cells. These studies demonstrate that the delicate balance between mFasL and sFasL levels represents a (paracrine and/or autocrine) regulator of early hematopoiesis: survival and proliferation promotion by sFasL versus apoptosis induction by mFasL.

Interaction of Fas with its natural ligand (FasL) or with agonistic anti-Fas monoclonal antibodies (like CH11) causes homotrimerization of CD95 and triggers PCD by activation of the FADD/MORT-1 cascade (Nagata, 1997). Concurrent expression of Fas and FasL on the same cell leads to PCD after interaction by membrane folding, although monocyte-derived macrophages could escape from spontaneous or anti-Fas IgM induced apoptosis (Kiener et al., 1997).

Enhanced Fas expression on *BM progenitors* seems to play a role in ineffective hematopoiesis (Maciejewski et al., 1995). They showed that IFN-γ and TNF-α mediated suppression of colony formation from immature (CD34+CD38–) and mature (CD34+CD38+) progenitors was enhanced by

FasL without the presence of accessory cells. IFN-γ and TNF-α cause cell cycle inhibition of hematopoietic cells, upregulate Fas expression on CD34+ cells, and induce ICE expression in these cells which subsequently led to PCD in vitro when CH-11 was added (Maciejewski et al., 1995; Nagafuji et al., 1995; Sloand et al., 1998). Above all, tumor cells with FasL expression escape from the T cell-mediated immune surveillance, while they maintain the ability to induce Fas-mediated apoptosis in normal cells, especially in activated lymphocytes (Nagata & Golstein, 1995; Villunger et al., 1997).

The Fas/FasL System In MDS

Immunohistochemical (IH) stained MDS BM sections showed positive staining for Fas (and FasL), whereas BM samples of normals showed no staining (Kitagawa et al., 1998). These findings were confirmed by RT-PCR for Fas (and FasL) mRNA (Kitagawa et al., 1998; Gersuk et al., 1998). Fas+ cells were found in all cell lineages, including CD34+ cells. Also Lepelley et al (1996) observed increased Fas expression in BM cells (by IH) in about 40% of MDS, whereas a variable proportion of blasts showed weak Fas expression. Gersuk et al. (1998) found increased Fas expression of BMMNC by FCM in MDS. They observed that considerably more CD34+ blasts showed Fas expression in MDS as compared to normal BM (87% vs 25%), but Fas expression intensity on CD34+ cells was negatively correlated to the BM blast number. Leukemic blasts apparently loose Fas expression with progression of MDS (Bouscary et al., 1997). Interestingly, significantly more CD3+ activated T cells with Fas expression were found in MDS BM in comparison to normal BM (Gersuk et al., 1998).

Regarding the function of Fas, not all Fas+ BM cells showed TUNEL positivity (Kitagawa et al., 1998). Furthermore, MDS BMMNC showed increased caspase-3 mRNA (Gersuk et al., 1998; Mundle et al., 1999c) with a lower to absent FAP-1 expression, which is an inhibiting modulator of the Fas signal transduction pathway (Sato et al., 1995). Bouscary et al. (2000) found clearly enhanced apoptosis by TUNEL associated with significantly increased levels of caspase-3 activity and low blast numbers in LR-MDS patients.

Although overall Fas expression on hematopoietic progenitors was increased in MDS, it was not correlated with FAB subtype, the Bournemouth score, apoptosis rates or peripheral cytopenias (Bouscary et al., 1997; Lepelley et al., 1996). In contrast, in vitro culture studies in MDS have shown decreased clonogenic capacity of CFU-GM and the involvement of enhanced Fas expression on proliferation and PCD (Nagler et al., 1995; Lepelley et al., 1996; Bouscary et al., 1997; Gersuk et al., 1998). The erythroid lineage seems to be more sensitive for Fas-mediated apoptosis than the myeloid lineage (Lepelley et al., 1996; Bouscary et al., 1997; Gupta et al., 1999). Also LTBM cultures with MDS stroma have shown defective support in promoting proliferation and differentiation in combination with increased levels of Fas and apoptosis of these normal progenitors (Aizawa et al 1999). Higher levels of TNF-α and sTNF-R1 were found in marrow plasma of MDS patients as compared to normals (Gersuk et al., 1998). The addition of anti-TNF-α mAb or soluble rhuTNFR:Fc to Dexter cultures increased colony numbers (Gersuk et al., 1998).

FasL expression in MDS was increased in BM cells of all lineages, irrespective their maturation state, but it was even higher in AML blasts (Kitagawa et al., 1998; Gupta et al., 1999). This increase in FasL expression was significantly correlated with FAB subtype, the number of abnormal metaphases, and survival (Gupta et al., 1999). Furthermore, overall FasL expression in de novo AML was comparable to AML after MDS (Gupta et al., 1999), whereas primary MDS had significantly lower FasL+ aberrant blasts compared to secondary MDS (Gersuk et al., 1998). Gersuk et al (1998) observed variable and increased amounts of FasL on MDS CD34+ blasts in contrast to normal CD34+ cells. FasL expression was inversely associated with TNF-α levels and Fas expressing during MDS progression. Furthermore, considerably more BM FasL+ CD3+ cells in MDS (17%) were found as compared with normal BM (2%) (Gersuk et al., 1998). The majority of apoptotic cells by TUNEL were also FasL+ with the exception of macrophages (Kitagawa et al., 1998). Macrophages showed considerably more staining for FasL than for Fas. In addition, significantly higher levels of *soluble FasL* were found in marrow plasma of MDS patients (Gersuk et al., 1998). Soluble FasL seems to be functional in MDS as it inhibited the growth of clonogenic CD34+/HLA-DR+ progenitors in a dose-dependant way (Gupta et al., 1999). Similarly, suppression of apoptosis of BM mononuclear cells was observed by treatment with anti-FasL (Mundle et al., 1999c).

Overexpression (by RT-PCR and IH) of TNF-α was detected more often than overexpression of IFN-γ in BMMNC of MDS patients (79% vs. 42%, respectively), in contrast to observations in normal BM (Kitagawa et al., 1997). The majority of TNF-α and IFN-γ producing cells were CD68+ macrophage lineage cells. TNF-α and IFN-γ upregulate Fas expression in a wide array of hematopoietic cells. A significant correlation was found between TNF-α protein levels in marrow plasma and Fas expression on MDS marrow blasts (Gersuk et al.,1998) and between TNF-α expression (by IH) and the extent of apoptosis in BM biopsies (Raza et al., 1996).

The following model of immunoregulatory mechanisms in MDS can be postulated from all these observations. Monoclonality develops as one of the first hallmarks in early MDS. The immune system probably detects these aberrant cells and an immune response is triggered. Activated CTL's and NK-cells show increasing expression of mFasL, whereas activated monocytes and macrophages produce increasing amounts of TNFα and IFN-γ. Subsequently, upregulation of Fas occurs, especially in the more mature cells. Massive apoptosis develops in both normal and monoclonal compartments by enhanced TNF-α levels as well as by increased Fas/FasL interactions. Upregulated Fas-bearing mature and immature normal and stromal BM cells die as innocent bystanders and subsequently proliferation increases to compensate for their loss. As particularly proliferating myeloid progenitors have enhanced Fas expression, they also die in increasing numbers (causing signal antonymy). Upregulation of mFasL (subsequently leading to soluble FasL) is a way to defend them against attacking FasL-bearing CTL's, NK cells or macrophages. The same happens to the rapidly dividing monoclonal cells, but as a consequence of additional mutations / deletions during high mitotic pressure they acquire a differentiation defect and a survival benefit. These cells are capable of turning down their Fas expression. Alternatively, they develop non-functional truncated Fas splicing variants leading to a survival benefit and consequently a growth advantage. On the other hand, as these blasts maintain enhanced mFasL in order to escape from the triggered immune-surveillance, their enhanced mFasL expression may also contribute to the increased killing of polyclonal hematopoiesis and imunoregulatory cells with increased expression of Fas. During MDS progression, evolution of leukemic clones with decreasing Fas and increasing mFasL switch off their PCD machinery by acquiring additional genetic aberrances. These leukemic clones progressively develop growth advantage at the expense of increasing death of monoclonal preleukemic and normal hematopoiesis.

REFERENCES

Aizawa, S., Nakano, M., Iwase, O., Yaguchi, M., Hiramoto, M., Hoshi, H., Nabeshima, R., Shima, D., Handa, H., Toyama, K. (1999) Bone marrow stroma from refractory anemia of myelodysplastic syndrome is defective in its ability to support normal CD34 positive cell proliferation and differentiation. *Leukemia Research*, **23**, 239-246.

Bogdanovic, A.D., Tripnac, D.P., Jankovic, G.M., Bumbasirevic, V.Z., Obradovic, M., Colovic, M.D. (1997) Incidence and role of apoptosis in myelodysplastic syndrome: morphological and ultrastructural assessment. *Leukemia*, **11**, 656-659.

Bouscary, D., De Vos, J., Guesnu, M., Jondeau, K., Viguier, F., Melle, J., Picard, F., Dreyfus, F., Fontenay-Roupie, M. (1997) Fas/APO-1 (CD95) expression and apoptosis in patients with myelodysplastic syndromes. *Leukemia*, **11**, 839-845.

Bouscary, D., Chen, Y.L., Guesnu, M., Picard, F., Viguier, F., Lacombe, C., Dreyfus, F., Fontenay-Roupie, M. (2000) Activity of the caspase-3/CPP32 enzyme is increased in "early stage" myelodysplastic syndromes with excessive apoptosis, but caspase inhibition does not enhance colony formation in vitro. *Experimental Hematology*, **28**, 784-791.

Cheng, J., Zhou T., Liu, C., Shapiro, J.P., Brauer, M.J. Kiefer, M.C., Barr, P.J., Mountz J.D. (1994) Protection from Fas-mediated apoptosis by a soluble form of the Fas molecule. *Science*, **263**, 1759-1762.

Deeg, H.J., Beckham, C., Loken, M.R., Bryant, E., Lesnikova, M., Shulman H.M., Gooley, T. (2000) Negative regulators of hematopoiesis and stroma function in patients with myelodysplastic syndrome. *Leukemia Lymphoma*, **37**, 405-414.

Degliantoni, G., Perussia, B., Mangoni, L., Trinchieri G. (1985) Inhibition of bone marrow colony formation by human natural killer cells and by natural killer cell-derived colony-inhibiting activity. *Journal of Experimental Medicine*, **161**, 1152-1168.

Flores-Figueroa, E., Gutierrez-Espindola, G., Guerrero-Rivera, S., Pizzuto-Chavez, J., Mayani H. (1999) Hematopoietic progenitor cells from patients with myelodysplastic syndromes: in vitro colony growth and long-term proliferation. *Leukemia Research*, **23**, 385-394.

Gerritsen, W.R., Donohue, J., Bauman, J., etal (1992) Clonal analysis of myelodysplastic syndrome: monosomy 7 is expressed in the myeloid lineage, but not in the lymphoid lineage as detected by fluorescent in situ hybridization. *Blood*, **80**, 217-224.

Gersuk, G.M., Beckham, C., Loken M.R., Kiener, P., Anderson J.E., Farrand, A., Troutt, A.B., Ledbetter, J.A., Deeg H.J. (1998) A role for tumour necrosis factor-a, Fas and Fas-Ligand in marrow failure associated with myelodysplastic syndrome. *British Journal of Hematology*, **103**, 176-188.

Greenberg, P.L. (1983) The smoldering myeloid leukemic states: clinical and biological features. *Blood*, **61**, 1035-1044.

Greenberg, P., Cox, C., LeBeau, M.M., Fenaux, P., Morel, P., Sanz, G., Sanz, M., Vallespi, T., Hamblin, T., Oscier, D., Ohyashiki, K., Toyama, K., Aul, C., Mufti, G., Bennett, J. (1997) International scoring system for evaluating prognosis in myelodysplastic syndromes. *Blood*, **89**, 2079-2088.

Gupta, P., Niehans, G.A., LeRoy, S.C., Gupta, K., Morrison, V.A., Knapp, D., Kratzke, R.A. (1999) Fas ligand expression in the bone marrow in myelodysplastic syndromes correlates with FAB subtype and anemia, and predicts survival. *Leukemia*, **13**, 44-53.

Guyotat, D., Campos, L., Thomas, X., Vila, I., Shi, Z.-H., Charrin, C., Gentilhomme, O., Fiere, D. (1990) Myelodysplastic syndromes: A study of surface markers and in vitro growth patterns. *American Journal of Hematology*, **34**, 26-31.

Hellstrom-lindberg, E., Kanter-Lewensohn, L., Ost, A. (1997) Morphological changes and apoptosis in bone marrow from patients with myelodysplastic syndromes treated with G-CSF and erythropoitin. *Leukemia Research*, **21**, 415-425.

Horikawa, K., Nakakuma, H., Kawaguchi, T., Iwamoto, N., Nagakura, S., Kagimoto, T., Takatsuki, K. (1997) Apoptosis resistance of blood cells from patients with paroxysmal nocturnal hemoglobinuria, aplastic anemia and myelodysplastic syndrome. *Blood*, **90**, 2716-2722.

Josefsen, D., Myklebust, J.H., Lynch, D.H., Stokke, T., Blomhoff, H.K., Smeland, E.B. (1999) Fas ligand promotes cell survival of immature human bone marrow CD34+CD38– hematopoietic progenitor cells by suppressing apoptosis. *Experimental Hematology*, **27**, 1451-1459.

Kayagaki, N., Kawasaki, A., Ebata, T., Ohmoto, H., Ikeda, S., Inoue, S., Yoshino, K., Okumura, K., Yagita, H. (1995) Metalloproteinase-mediated release of human Fas ligand. *Journal of Experimental Medicine*, **182**, 1777-1783.

Kerndrup, G., Bendix-Hansen, K., Pedersen, B., Ellegaard, J., Hokland, P. (1988) Analysis of leukocyte differentiation antigens in blood and bone marrow in patients with refractory anaemia (RA) and RA with sideroblasts. Prognostic indications of sequential and follow-up data. *European Journal of Haematology*, **41**, 368-374.

Kibbelaar, R.E., van Kamp, H., Dreef, E.J. et al (1992) Combined immunophenotyping and DNA in situ hybridization to study lineage involvement in patients with myelodysplastic syndromes. *Blood*, **79**, 1823-1828.

Kiener, P.A., Davis, P.M., Starling, G.C., Mehlin, C., Klebanoff S.J., Ledbetter, J.A., Liles, W.C. (1997) Differential induction of apoptosis by Fas-Fas ligand interactions in human monocytes and macrophages. *Journal of Experimental Medicine*, **185**, 1511-1516.

Kitagawa, M., Saito, I., Kuwata, T., Yoshida, S., Yamaguchi S., Takahashi, M., Tanizawa, T., Kamiyama, R., Hirokawa, K. (1997) Overexpression of tumor necrosis factor (TNF)-alpha and interferon (IFN)-gamma by bone marrow cells from patients with myelodysplastic syndromes. *Leukemia*, **11**, 2049-2054.

Kitagawa, M., Yamaguchi, S., Takahashi, M., Tanizawa, T., Hirokawa, K., Kamiyama, R. (1998) Localization of Fas and Fas ligand in bone marrow cells demonstrating myelodysplasia. *Leukemia*, **12**, 486-492.

Knipping, E., Debatin, K-M., Stricker, K., Heilig, B., Eder, A., Krammer, P.H. (1995) Identification of a soluble APO-1 in supernatants of human B- and T-cell lines and increased serum levels in B- and T-cell leukemias. *Blood*, **85**, 1562-1569.

Kristensen, J.S. & Hokland, P. (1990) Monoclonal antibody ratios in malignant myeloid diseases: diagnostic and prognostic use in myelodysplastic syndromes. *British Journal of Haematology*, **74**, 270-276.

Kroef, M.J., Fibbe, W.E., Mout, R., Jansen, R.P., Haak, H.L., Wessels, J.W. Van Kamp, H., Willemze, R., Landegent, J.E. (1993) Myeloid but not lymphoid cells carry the 5q deletion: polymerase chain reaction analysis of loss of heterozygosity using mini-repeat sequences on highly purified cell fractions. *Blood*, **81**, 1849-1854.

Lepelley, P., Campergue, L., Grardel, N., Preudhomme, C., Cosson, A., Fenaux, P. (1996) Is apoptosis a massive process in myelodysplastic syndromes? *British Journal of Haematology*, **95**, 368-371.

van Lom, K., Hagemeijer, A., Vandekerckhove, F., Smit, E.M.E., Lowenberg, B. (1996) Cytogenetic clonality analysis: typical patterns in myelodysplastic syndrome and acute meyloid leukemia. *Britisch Journal of Haematology*, **93**, 594-600.

Maciejewski, J., Selleri, C., Anderson, S., Young, N.S. (1995) Fas antigen expression on CD34+ human marrow cells is induced by interferon gamma and tumor necrosis factor alpha and potentiates cytokine-mediated hematopoietic suppression in vitro. *Blood*, **85**, 3183-3190.

Mayani, H., Baines, P., Bowen, D.T., Jacobs, A. (1989) In vitro growth of myeloid and erythroid progenitor cells from myelodysplastic patients in response to recombinanthuman granulocyte-macrophage colony-stimulating factor. *Leukemia*, **3**, 29-32.

Mehrotra, B., George T.I., Kavanau, K., Avet-Loiseau, H., Moore II, D., Willman, C.L., Slovak, M.L., Atwater, S., Head, D.R., Pallavicini, M.G. (1995) Cytogenetically aberrant cells in the stem cell compartment (CD34+lin–) in acute myeloid leukemia. *Blood*, **86**, 1139-1147.

Merchav, S., Wagemarker, G., Souza, L.M., Tatarsky, I. (1991) Impaired response of myelodysplastic marrow progenitors to stimulation with recombinant hematopoietic growth factors. *Leukemia*, **5**, 340-346.

Mundle, S., Iftikhar, A., Shetty, V., Dameron, S., Wright-Quinones, V., Marcus, B., Loew, J., Gregory, S., Raza, A. (1994) Novel in situ double labeling for simultaneous detection of proliferation and apoptosis. *Journal of histochemistry and Cytochemistry*, **42**, 1533-1537.

Mundle, S.D., Ali, A., Cartlidge, J.D., Reza, S., Alvi, S., Showel, M.M., Mativi, B.Y., Shetty, V.T., Venugopal, P., Gregory, S.A., Raza, A. (1999a) Evidence for involvement of tumor necrosis factor-alpha in apoptotic death of bone marrow cells in myelodysplastic syndromes. *American Journal of Hematology*, **60**, 36-47.

Mundle, S., Venugopal, P., Shetty, V., Ali, A., Chopra, H., Handa, H., Rose, S., Mativi, B.Y., Gregory, S.A., Preisler, H.D., Raza, A. (1999b) The relative extent and propensity of CD34+ vs. CD34– cells to undergo apoptosis in myelodysplastic marrows. *International Journal of Hematology*, **69**, 152-159.

Mundle, S.D., Mativi, B.Y., Bagai, K., Feldman, G., Cheema, P., Gautam, U., Reza, S., Cartlidge, J.D., Venugopal, P., Shetty, V., Gregory, S.A., Robin, E., Rifkin, S., Shah, R., Raza, A. (1999c) Spontaneous down-regulation of Fas-associated phosphatase-1 may contribute to excessive apoptosis in myelodysplastic marrows. *International Journal of Hematology*, **70**, 83-90.

Nagafuji, K., Shibuya, T., Harada, M., Mizuno, S.I., Takenaka, K., Miyamoto, T., Okamura, T., Gondo, H., Niho, Y. (1995) Functional expression of Fas antigen (CD95) on hematopoietic progenitor cells. *Blood*, **86**, 883-889.

Nagata, S. (1997) Apoptosis by death factor. *Cell*, **88**, 355-356.

Nagata, S. & Golstein, P. (1995) The Fas death factor. *Science*, **267**, 1449-1456.

Nagler, A., MacKichan, M.L., Negrin, R.S., Donlon, T., Greenberg, G.L. (1995) Effects of granulocyte colony-stimulating factor therapy on in vitro hemopoiesis in myelodysplastic syndromes. *Leukemia*, **9**, 30-39.

Niho, Y. & Asano, Y. (1998) Fas/Fas ligand and hematopoietic progenitor cells. *Current Opinion in Hematology*, **5**, 163-165.

Nilsson, L., Xstrand-Grundstr m, I., Arvidsson, I., Jacobsson, B., Hellstr m-Lindberg, E., Hast, R., Jacobsen, S.E.W. (2000) Isolation and characterization of hematopoietic progenitor/stem cells in 5q–deleted myelodysplastic syndromes: evidence for involvement at the hematopoietic stem cell level. *Blood*, **96**, 2012-2021.

Novitzky, N., Mohamed, R., Finlayson, J., du Toit, C. (2000) Increased apoptosis of bone marrow cells and preserved proliferative capacity of selected progenitors predict for clinical response to anti-inflammatory therapy in myelodysplastic syndromes. *Experimental Hematology*, **28**, 941-949.

Pantel, K. & Nakeff, A (1993) The role of lymphoid cells in hematopoietic regulation. *Experimental Hematology*, **21**, 738-742.

Parker, J.E., Mufti, G.J., Rasool, F., Mijovic, A., Devereux, S., Pagliuca, A. (2000) The role of apoptosis, proliferation, and the Bcl-2-related proteins in the myelodysplastic syndromes and acute myeloid leukemia secondary to MDS. *Blood*, **96**, 3932-3938.

Pederson-Bjergaard, J. & Rowley J.D. (1994) The balanced and the unbalanced chromosome aberrations of acute myeloid leukemia may develop in different ways and may contribute differently to malignant transformation. *Blood*, **83**, 2780-2786.

Pederson-Bjergaard, J., Pedersen, M., Roulston, D., Philip, P. (1995) Different genetic pathways in leukemogenesis for patients presenting with therapy-related myelodysplasia and therapy-related acute myeloid leukemia. *Blood*, **86**, 3542-3552.

Rajapaksa, R., Ginzton, N., Rott, L.S., Greenberg, P.L. (1996) Altered oncoprotein expression and apoptosis in myelodysplastic syndrome marrow cells. *Blood*, **88**, 4275-4287.

Raymakers, R., de Witte, T., Joziasse, J., van der Lely, N., Boezeman, J. and Haanen, C. (1991) In vitro growth pattern and differentiation predict for progression of myelodysplastic syndromes to acute nonlymphocytic leukaemia. *British Journal of Haematology*, **78**, 35-41.

Raza, A., Gezer, S., Mundle, S., Gao, X.-Z., Alvi, S., Borok, R., Rifkin, S., Iftikhar, A., Shetty, V., Parcharidou, A., Loew, J., Marcus, B., Khan, Z., Chaney, C., Showel, J., Gregory, S., Preisler, H. (1995) Apoptosis in bone marrow biopsy samples involving stromal and hematopoietic cells in 50 patients with myelodysplastic syndromes. *Blood*, **86**, 268-276.

Raza, A., Mundle, S., Shetty, V., Alvi, S., Chopra, H., Span, L., Parcharidou, A., Dar, S., Venugopal, P., Borok, R., Gezer, S., Showel, J., Loew, J., Robin, E., Rifkin, S., Alston, D., Hernandez, B., Shar, R., Kaizer, H., Gregory, S. (1996) Novel insights into the biology of myelodysplastic syndromes: excessive apoptosis and the role of cytokines. *International Journal of Hematology*, **63**, 265-278.

Raza, A., Alvi, S., Borok, R.Z., Span, L., Parcharidou, A., Alston, D., Rifkin, S., Robin, E., Shah, R., Gregory, S.A. (1997) Excessive proliferation matched by excessive apoptosis in myelodysplastic syndromes: the cause-effect relationship. *Leukemia and Lymphoma*, **27**, 111-118.

Raza, A., Qawi, H., Lisak, L., Andric, T., Dar, S., Andrews, C., Venugopal, P., Gezer, S., Gregory, S., Loew, J., Robin, E., Rifkin, S., Hsu, W.T., Huang, R.W. (2000) Patients with myelodysplastic syndromes benefit from palliative therapy with amifostine, pentoxifylline, and ciprofloxacin with or without dexamethasone. *Blood*, **95**, 1580-1587.

Reza, S., Shetty, V., Dar, S., Qawi, H., Raza, A. (1998) Tumor necrosis factor-alpha levels decrease with anticytokine therapy in patients with myelodysplastic syndromes. *Journal of Interferon and Cytokine Research*, **18**, 871-877.

Sato, T., Irie, S., Kitada, S. & Reed, J.C. (1995) FAP-1: a protein tyrosine phosphatase that associates with Fas. *Science*, **268**, 411-415.

Sato, T., Kim, S., Selleri, C., Young, N.S., Maciejewski, J.P. (1998) Measurement of secondary colony formation after 5 weeks in long-term cultures in patients with myelodysplastic syndrome. *Leukemia*, **12**, 1187-1194.

Sawada, K.-I. (1994) Impaired proliferation and differentiation of myelodysplastic CD34+ cells. *Leukemia and Lymphoma*, **14**, 37-47.

Sawada, K., Sato, N., Notoya, A., Tarumi, T., Hirayama, S., Takano, H., Koizumi, K., Yasukouchi, T., Yamaguchi, M., Koike, T. (1995) Proliferation and differentiation of myelodysplastic CD34+ cells: Phenotypic subpopulations of marrow CD34+ cells. *Blood*, **85**, 194-202.

Sawada, K., Ieko, M., Notoya, A., Tarumi, T., Koizumi, K., Kitayama, S., Nishio, H., Fukada, Y., Yasukouchi, T., Yamaguchi, M., Katoh, S., Koike, T. (1996) Role of cytokines in leukemic type growth of myelodysplastic CD34+ cells. *Blood*, **88**, 319-327.

Sawada K.-I., Koizumi, K., Tarumi, T., Takano, H., Ieko, M., Nishio, M., Fukada, Y., Yasukouchi, T., Yamaguchi, M.,Koike, T. (1999) Role of physiological concentrations of stem cell factor in leukemic type growth of myelodysplastic CD34+ cells. *Leukemia Research*, **23**, 1-11.

Schulze-Osthoff, K. (1994) The Fas/APO-1 receptor and its deadly ligand. *Trends in Cell Biology*, **4**, 421-426.

Selleri, C., Sato, T., Raiola, A.M., Rotoli, B., Young, N.S., Maciejewski, J.P. (1997) Induction of nitric oxide synthase is involved in the machanism of Fas-mediated apoptosis in haematopoietic cells. *British Journal of Haematology*, **99**, 481-489.

Shetty, V., Mundle, S., Alvi, S., Showel, M., Broady-Robinson, L., Dar, S., Borok, R., Showel, J., Gregory, S., Gezer, S., Venugopal, P., Shah, R., Hernandez, B., Klein, M., Robin, E., Dominquez, C., Raza, A. (1996) Measurement of apoptosis, proliferation and three cytokines in 46 patients with myelodysplastic syndromes. *Leukemia Research*, **20**, 891-900.

Shetty, V., Hussaini, S., Broady-Robinson, L., Allampallam, K., Mundle, S., Borok, R., Broderick, E., Mazzoran, L., Zorat, F., Raza, A. (2000) Intramedullary apoptosis of hematopoietic cells in myelodysplastic syndrome patients can be massive: apoptotic cells recovered from high-density fraction of bone marrow aspirates. *Blood*, **96**, 1388-1392.

Sloand, E.M., Young, N.S., Sato, T., Kim, S., Maciejewski, J.P. (1998) Inhibition of interleukin-1beta-converting enzyme in human hematopoietic progenitor cells results in blockade of cytokine-mediated apoptosis and expansion of their proliferative potential. *Experimental Hematology*, **26**, 1093-1099.

Soligo, D.A., Campiglio, S., Servida, F., Bossolasco, P., Romitti, L., Cortelezzi, A., Lambertenghi Deliliers, D. (1996) Response of myelodysplastic syndrome marrow progenitor cells to stimulation with cytokine combinations in a stroma-free long-term culture system. *British Journal of Haematology*, **92**, 548-558.

Span, L.F.R., Dar, S.E., Shetty, V., Mundle, S.D., Broady-Robinson, L., Alvi, S., Raymakers, R.A.P., de Witte, T., Raza, A. (1998a) Apparent expansion of CD34+ cells during the evolution of myelodysplastic syndromes to acute myeloid leukemia. *Leukemia*, **12**,1685-1695.

Span, L.F.R., Raymakers, R.A.P., Rutten, E.S.M., de Witte, Th. (1998b) Proliferation and apoptosis characteristics in vitro in myelodysplasia, AML, and normal bone marrow. (Abstract). *British Journal of Haematology*, **102**, P-1358.

Span, L.F., Vierwinden, G., Pennings, A.H., Boezeman, J.B., Raymakers, R.A., de Witte, T.J. (1999) Programmed cell death of CD34+ cells in MDS is clearly enhanced in cluster forming cells but remarkably decreased in colony forming cells. (Abstract). *Blood*, **94**, Suppl. 1, #467.

Stahnke, K., Hecker, S., Kohne, E., Debatin K-M (1998) CD95 (APO-1/FAS)-mediated apoptosis in cytokine-activated hematopoietic cells. *Experimental Hematology*, **26**, 844-850.

Suda, T., Hashimoto, H., Tanaka, M., Ochi, T., Nagata, S. (1997) Membrane Fas Ligand kills human peripheral blood T lymphocytes and soluble Fas Ligand blocks the killing. *Journal of Experimental Medicine*, **86**, 2045-2050.

Sullivan, S.A., Marsden, K.A., Lowenthal, R.M., Jupe, D.M.,Jones, M.E. (1992) Circulating CD34+ cells: an adverse prognostic factor in myelodysplastic syndromes. *American Journal of Hematology*, **39**, 96-101.

Tamura, S., Kanamaru, A., Kakishita, E., Nagai, K. (1992) Detection of latent subclones with abnormal karyotypes by long-term bone marrow cultures in cases of myelodysplastic syndrome. *British Journal of Haematology*, **81**, 353-361.

Tanaka, M., Suda, T., Takahashi, T., Nagata, S. (1995) Expression of the functional soluble form of human Fas Ligand in activated lymphocytes. *European. Mol. Biol. Organ.*, *14*, 1129-1135.

Tanaka, M., Itai, T., Adachi, M., Nagata, S. (1998) Downregulation of Fas ligand by shedding. *Nature Medicine*, **4**, 31-36.

Tohyama, K., Ueda, T., Yoshida Y., Nakamura, T. (1994) Altered responses of purified blast cells from the myelodysplastic syndromes to colony-stimulating factors in vitro: Comparison with normal blast cells. *Experimental Hematology*, **22**, 539-545.

Verma, D.S., Spitzer, G., Dicke, K.A., McCredie, K.B. (1979) In vitro agar culture patterns in preleukemia and their clinical significance. *Leukemia Research*, **3**, 41-49.

Villunger, A., Egle, A., Marschitz, I., Kos, M., Bock, G., Ludwig, H., Geley, S., Kofler, R., Greil, R. (1997) Constitutive expression of fas (APO-1/CD95) ligand on multiple myeloma cells: a potential mechanism of tumor-induced suppression of immune surveillance. *Blood*, **90**, 12-20.

Wallach, D., Boldin, M., Goncharov, T., Goltsev, Y., Mett, I., Malinin, N., Adar, R., Kovalenko, A., Varfolomeev, E. (1996) Exploring cell death mechanisms by analyzing signaling cascades of the TNF/NGF receptor family. *Behring Inst Mitt*, **97**, 144-155.

Yoshida, Y. (1993) Hypothesis: apoptosis may be the mechanism responsible for the premature intramedullary cell death in the myelodysplastic syndrome. *Leukemia*, **7**, 144-146.

4

NOVEL IN VITRO CULTURE AND ULTRASTRUCTURAL TECHNIQUES TO STUDY THE BIOLOGY OF MYELODYSPLASTIC SYNDROMES (MDS)

Sairah Alvi, Laurie A. Lisak and Vilasini T. Shetty
MDS Center and Section of Myeloid Diseases, Department of Medicine
Rush University, Chicago, IL

INTRODUCTION

MDS is a heterogeneous clonal stem cell disorder with trilineage dysplasia resulting in ineffective, monoclonal hematopoiesis (Resegotti et al., 1993). Extensive studies over the decade have led to better understanding of cell proliferation, differentiation, cytokine production and apoptosis in MDS (Greenburg et al., 1987; Shetty et al., 1996; Clark et al., 1990; Yoshida et al., 1993; Raza et al., 1995). However there has been limited information in the literature regarding long term bone marrow cultures and ultrastructural studies performed on MDS. In the past, it has been difficult to grow MDS bone marrow (BM) cells as the progenitor cells have a great propensity to undergo programmed cell death (Ohmori et al., 1991; Aizawa et al., 1999; Raza et al., 1996). On the other hand the role of electron microscopy has not been clearly established in MDS either, other than few individual cases on BM aspirate because of the failure to overcome the technical impediment of maintaining the ultrastructural details in decalcified tissues (Guccion et al., 1992; Gerrad et al., 1992; Cohen et al., 1997; Payne et al., 1987). As a result very little is known about the association between the hematopoietic cells and their microenvironment especially in a disease like MDS where both the parenchymal and stromal cells may be involved in the disease process (Coutinho et al., 1990; Sawada et al., 1998)). The present chapter focuses on novel techniques where primarily the MDS core bone marrow biopsy was used to maintain long term bone marrow cultures followed by ultrastructural studies, hence preserving the BM architecture and the geographical distribution of the hematopoietic and stromal cells as they exist *in vivo*. A number of novel and interesting observations were made which are summarized here.

BONE MARROW CULTURES IN MDS

The long term bone marrow cultures (LTBMC) first described by Dexter et al., (Dexter et al., 1979; Lanotte et al., 1981; Blazsek et al., 1995) have often been used as an in vitro model to understand hematopoiesis (Greenburg et al., 1992; Chang et al., 1991). We have developed a novel technique of using the core bone marrow biopsies from MDS patients and normal donors in LTBMC as the primary source for stromal cells instead of bone marrow mononuclear cells (BMMNC) (Diana et al., 2000). Freshly obtained bone marrow biopsy sample from MDS patients were teased and cultured in complete medium without cytokines or growth factors at 37° in a humidified 5% CO_2 chamber for 8-22 weeks. The bone marrow piece latches onto the dish in the first week of culture and majority of the sample plates were 30-50% confluent in four weeks with bipolar, tripolar or multipolar monolayers followed by the appearance of preadipocyte or adipocytes (Figures 1 & 2). The cultures were 80-100% confluent in eight to ten weeks with compact parallel multiple layers of fibroblasts, macrophages and large adipocytes (Figure 3). Most of the stem cells and maturing myeloid cells were released from the adherent layer into the growth medium. The main feature of the long term bone marrow culture is the initial establishment of an adherent cellular environment with four major cell types; epithelial fibroblast like cells, endothelial cells, phagocytic cells and adipocytes (Duhrsen et al., 1996; Coutinho et al., 1990; Gidali et al., 1996).

The MDS patient cultures were maintained in vitro for six months. Their ultrastructural morphology and growth characteristics were studied and compared to hematologically normal subjects (Figures 4 & 5). The following parameters were used to measure the growth pattern of all the samples over three to six months in LTBMC. Initially the time required for the bone marrow biopsy to latch onto the culture plate was recorded. Next, the appearance of radiating stromal cells followed by preadipocytes and adipocytes was observed and lastly, the confluency of the culture plates was evaluated. The growth was termed "good growth" when biopsy piece latched by second week, the adipocytes appeared by week four and the plates appeared 80-90% confluent by eight weeks.

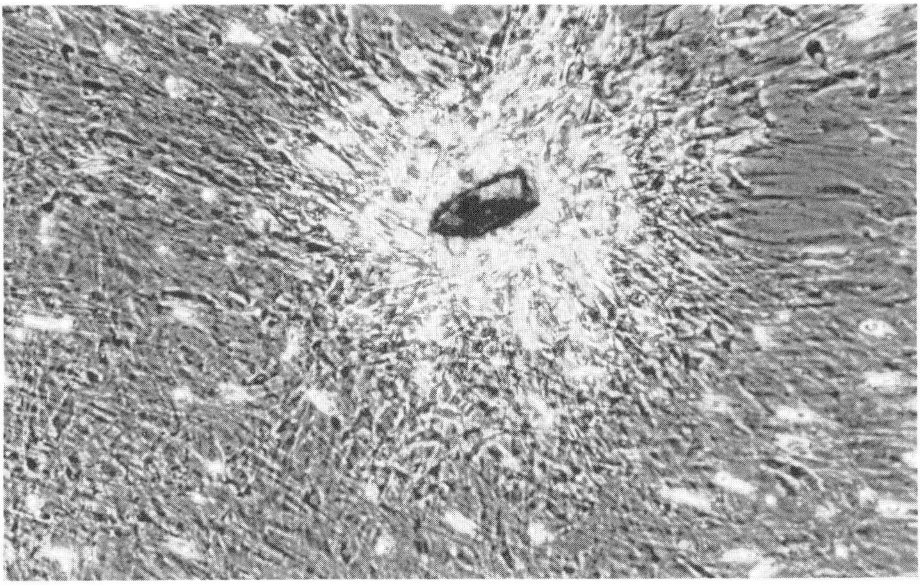

Figure 1. MDS Bone marrow biopsy piece after 3 weeks in LTBMC with streaming stromal and hematopoietic cells and preadipocytes/adipocytes (original magnification x 10).

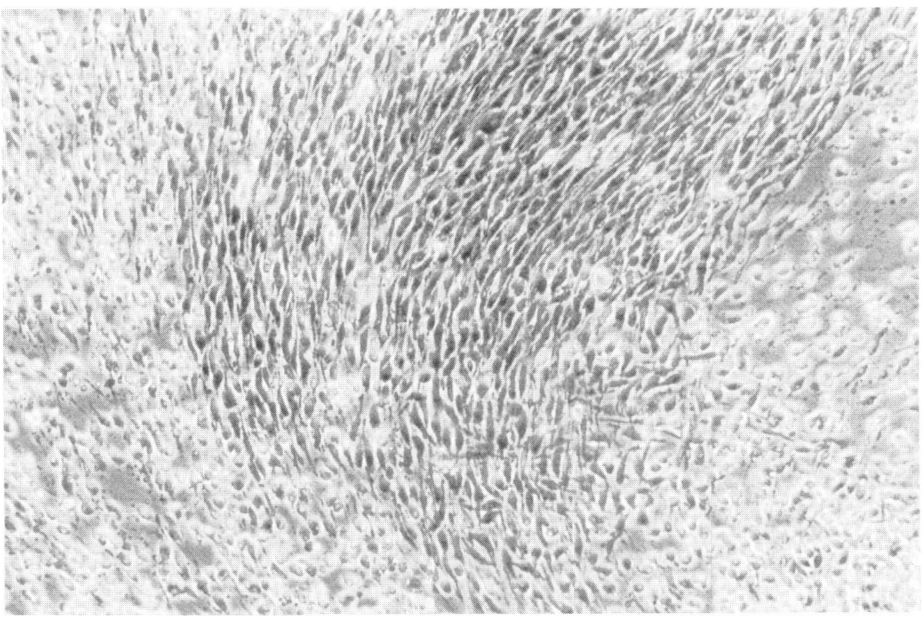

Figure 2. MDS patient after 5 weeks in LTBMC with 60% confluent bipolar and tripolar monolayers (original magnification x 10).

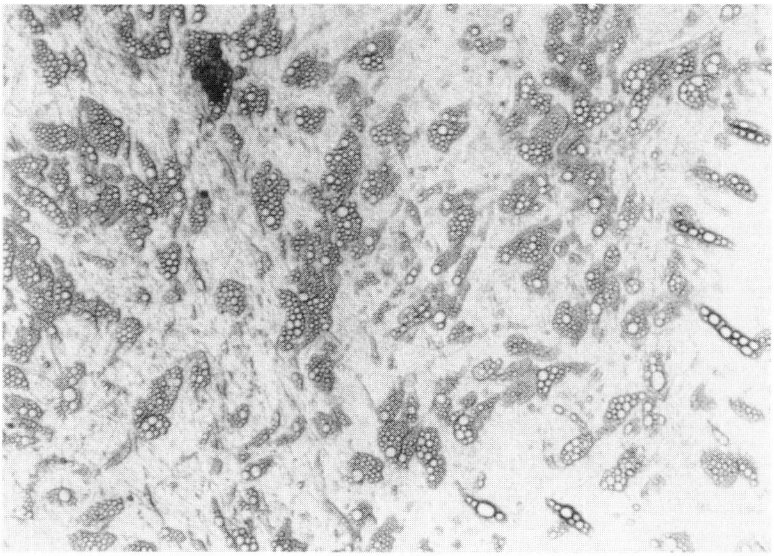

Figure 3. Bone marrow biopsy culture of MDS patient with 90% confluency accompanied by sheet of adipocytes (original magnification x 10).

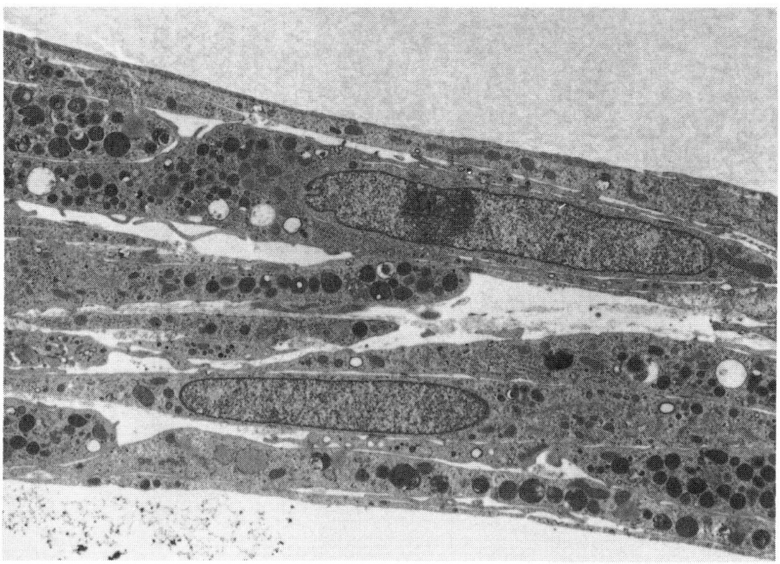

Figure 4. Ultrastructural morphology of long term bone marrow cultures using BM biopsy tissue from MDS patients; multilayer BM cultures with spindle shaped fibroblasts with one or more nucleoli (original magnification x 3,300).

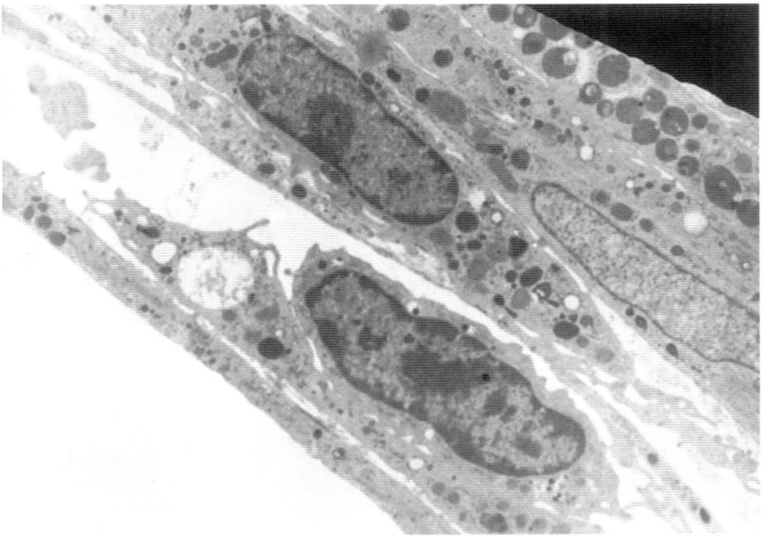

Figure 5. Endothelial cells presented with classical morphology in MDS bone marrow cultures (original magnification x 3,300).

Similarly the growth was considered "fair growth" if culture was only 40-50% confluent by eighth week and termed "poor growth" when the culture was 10-30% confluent by week eight. French American British (FAB) classification and karyotypic analyses were performed on the diagnostic bone marrow aspirates of each patient (Verhoef et al., 1995; Bennett et al., 1982; Pedersen-Bjergaard et al., 1993). The type of culture growth according to FAB sub-categories and karyotypic abnormalities can be summarized as follows. In low risk MDS patients (RA and RARS) 53% had "good growth", 12% "fair growth" and 33% showed "poor growth" after eight weeks in culture. In the high risk group of MDS patients (RAEB, RAEB-t and CMMoL) 47% presented with "good growth", 23% had "fair growth" and 28% showed "poor growth" in LTBMC after eight weeks. The FAB categories and karyotypic abnormalities did not appear to influence the potency of stromal cell growth in culture. The use of bone marrow biopsy tissue is recommended instead of BMMNC to generate robust stromal cells in MDS patients.

CYTOGENETIC ABNORMALITIES IN MDS STROMAL CELLS

To date clonality studies have been confined to bone marrow aspirate cells and the clonal nature of bone marrow stromal cells have not been intensively investigated. Evidence for the clonal nature of MDS is provided by nonrandom cytogenetic abnormalities that are detected in 50% of patients with primary MDS and in about 90% of patients with secondary MDS (Vallespi et al., 1998). Long term bone marrow culture using bone marrow biopsy of MDS patients with known karyotypic abnormalities were routinely cultured to obtain stromal cells in vitro. The adherent cultured layers predominantly consisted of fibroblast/macrophages and were usually confluent in about 7-8 weeks (Alvi et al., 2000). The confluent plates were sacrificed and cytospin preparation was made from both adherent and non-adherent layers followed by FISH to detect cytogenetic abnormalities. MDS samples were probed with CEP7, CEP 8, CEP X/Y, LSI5q EGR1/D5S23, D20S108 to detect monosomy 7, trisomy 8, deletions of chromosome Y, 5q and 20q (Lai et al., 1997; Weimar et al., 1994). On average 300-400 stained cells/slide were counted and it was observed that anywhere from 3% to 69% of the adherent layer cells carried the same cytogenetic abnormality as the non adherent cells (Figure 6). Further more a double label for FISH and the immunohistochemical studies revealed that stromal cells belonged to both fibroblast as well as monocyte/macrophage lineage. These studies for the first time show that both the cultured parenchymal and stromal cells carry similar karyotypic abnormality as the bone marrow mononuclear cells therefore they must all belong to the same MDS clone. We concluded that at least in some MDS patients, a subset of fibroblasts and monocytes/macrophages appear to be clonal in nature and perhaps the *in vivo* stromal cells may also be clonal during disease progression

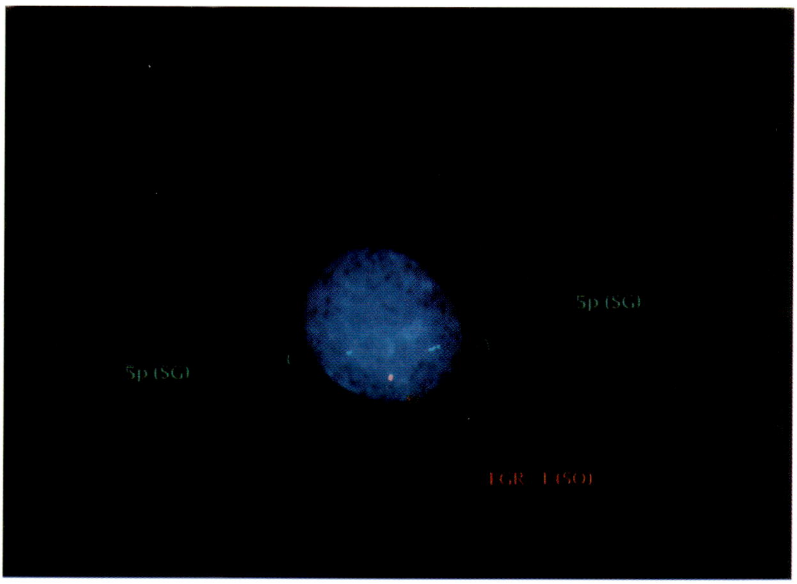

Figure 6. MDS patient adherent layer cultured cells demonstrating the presence of 5q deletion by FISH technique.

ULTRASTRUCTURAL STUDIES IN MDS

In the past most of the ultrastructural studies have been carried out on mouse and rat marrow (Weiss et al., 1976; Seed et al., 1986), because of the feasibility to process the tissue directly due to the fact that they have active hematopoiesis without the trabecular bone and very little fat. A detailed explanation of the human BM biopsy at the ultrastructural level was difficult because of the hindrance bone provides to fixation and sectioning for electron microscopy. In order to overcome the standard process of decalcification for the elimination of bone from biopsies, a modification of previously described technique (Polli et al., 1995) was used to study MDS BM biopsies that consisted of tediously dissecting out bone pieces from a large core biopsy without subjecting the biopsy to decalcification thus maintaining the architecture of the BM biopsy. The biopsy tissue thus obtained could then be embedded directly for ultrastructural studies. Studies were also carried out on LTBMNC and BM aspirates. Briefly the culture plates were fixed in situ with 1.5% gluteraldehyde at room temperature followed by gentle scraping and both the BM aspirate and the stromal layer from the culture plates were processed for routine electron microscopic (EM) studies.

The ultrastructural details in the MDS BM biopsy were very well preserved. The stromal and parenchymal cells could be clearly identified (Figure 7).

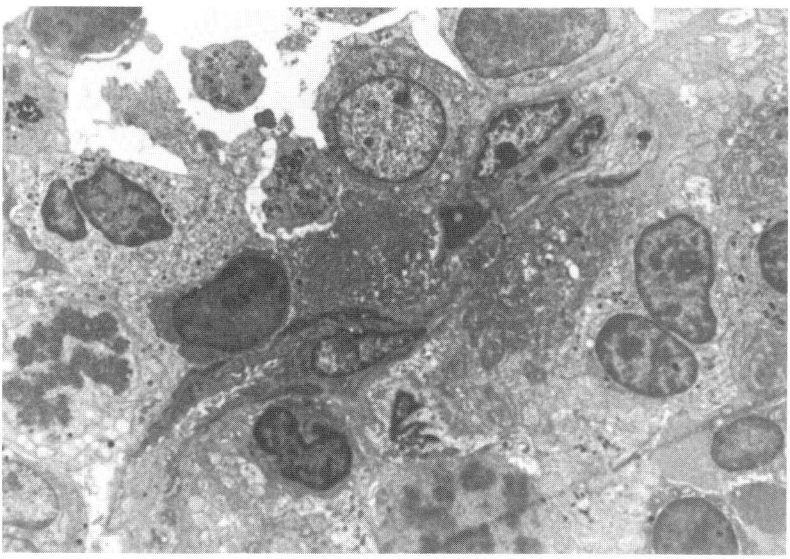

Figure 7. Ultrastructural details in an MDS biopsy. Note the cells showing dysplastic features in the parenchymal cells. The stromal cells are also identified (Magnification X 2,600).

Various degrees of dysplasia were noted in the BM biopsy, which could be appreciated at the ultrasructural level. The dysplastic features included morphological abnormalities seen in the erythroid series. They may have finely granular flocculent chromatin. At times irregularly shaped nuclei and cytoplasmic alterations were noted (Figure 7), Abnormal megakaryocytes were seen. The appearance of the cytoplasm with blocks of glycogen or vacuolization and characteristic smaller size makes it possible to identify these cells as megakaryocytes (Figure 8). Although positive peroxide reaction is required to identify them, they could also be recognized by ultrastructural features more easily on BM biopsies as compared to the BM aspirate.

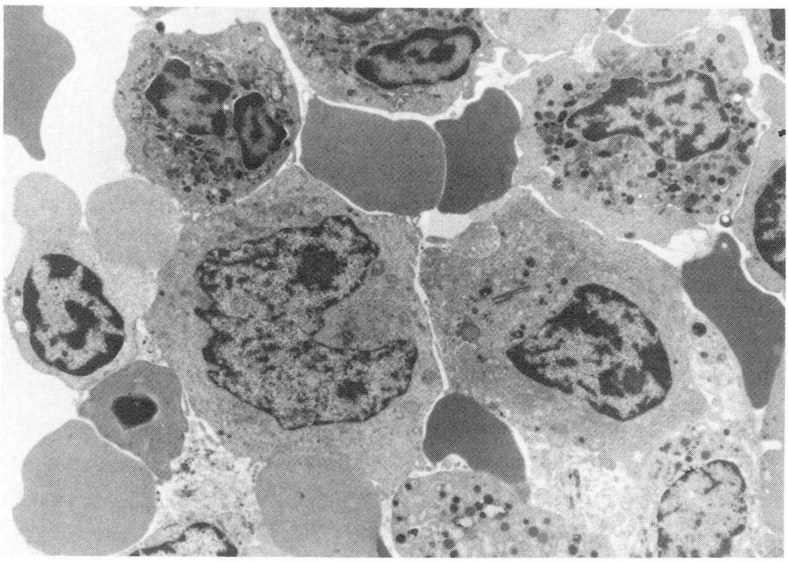

Figure 8. MDS BM Bx showing dysgranulopoiesis and abnormal megakaryocytes (Magnification X 2,600).

Dysgranulopoiesis which included an increase in the number of immature cells, a decrease of cytoplasmic granules (Kouides et al., 1992, Davey et al., 1988) was seen. Highly active and enormously increased amount of phagocytic activity was observed in the MDS BM biopsies (Figure 9).

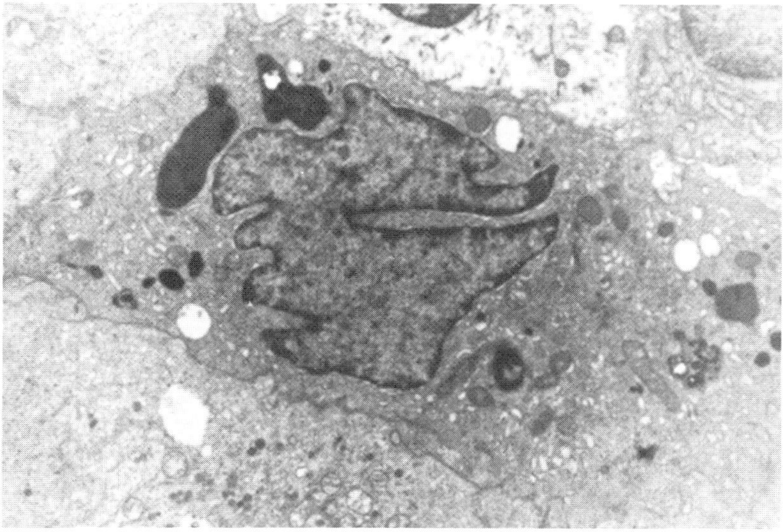

Figure 9. Macrophages engulfing the phagocytosed material (Magnification 5,000).

Another interesting feature was the presence of ring sideroblasts in this modified preparation of BM biopsy (Figure 10). The preparation made it possible to observe iron-laden mitochondria because of the absence of decalcification.

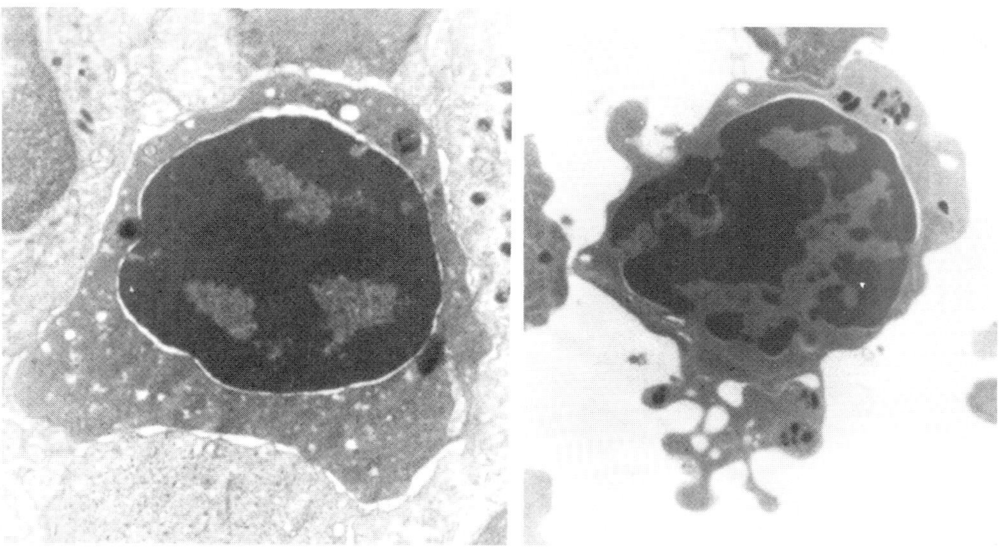

Figure 10. Iron laden mitochondria in a ringed sideroblast from an MDS BM biopsy (Magnification 10,000 & 8,300).

The detailed ultrastructural features were very well preserved in the decorticated tissue in MDS biopsy. Both the stromal and parenchymal cells could be identified in various forms. This is the first study to look directly at the MDS BM biopsy at the ultrastructural level.

ULTRASTRUCTURAL EVIDENCE OF APOPTOSIS IN MDS

Studies in the past have shown that there is an increased rate of apoptosis in MDS BM biopsies compared to the BM aspirate by using a variety of techniques (Raza et al., 1997; Bogdanovic. et al., 1996; Parcharidou et al., 1996). The MDS BM biopsy showed an abundance of apoptotic cells predominantly in the myeloid and erythroid lineage (Figure 11). It was seen that the early progenitor cells as well as the terminally differentiated cells were undergoing apoptosis.

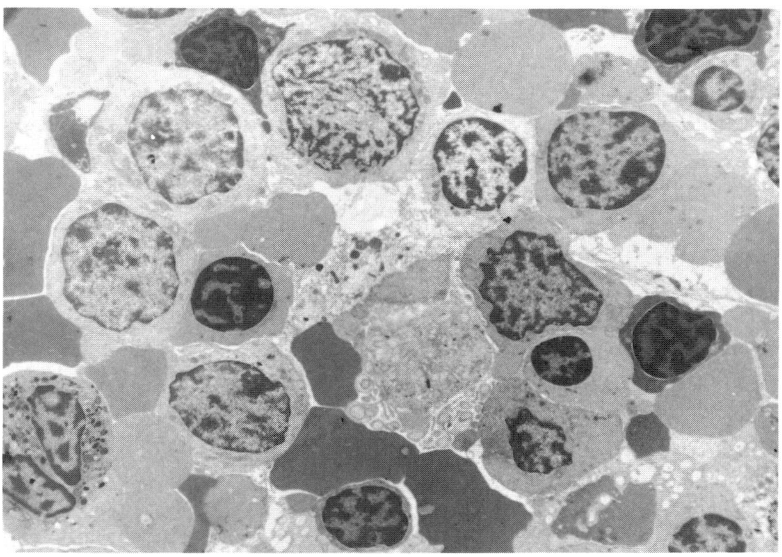

Figure 11. MDS BM Bx showing excessive apoptosis in the myeloid and erythroid lineages. The classical apoptotic features of condensed chromatin in the nucleus of the cells was noted (Magnification 2,600).

Not only the parenchymal cells but also the stromal cells such as the endothelial cells (Figure 12) were undergoing programmed cell death.

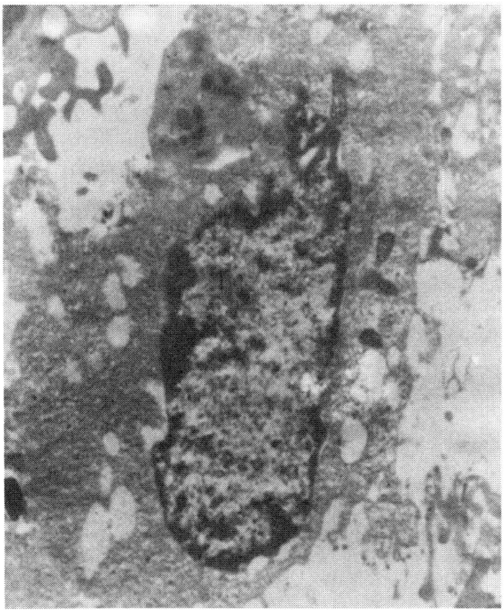

Figure 12. An endothelial cell undergoing apoptosis in an MDS BM biopsy (Magnification x 5,000).

In the BM aspirates of MDS patients, most of the studies have been carried out on the low-density fraction (LDF) mononuclear cells following density separation to look for the apoptotic index (AI). These studies including the earlier studies from our group have found that there was a discrepancy in the AI between the BM aspirate cells and the BM biopsies (Raza et al., 1995, Bogdanovic et al., 1996, Lepelley et al., 1995). Ultrastructurally when both the HD and LD fraction of the BM aspirate was studied it was found that cells from all the lineage were undergoing apoptosis with the myeloid and the erythroid cells showing maximum apoptosis (Figures 13 & 14).

However a significantly higher rate of apoptosis was seen in the HD fraction as compared to the LD fraction. It seems that the mature or maturing cells have a higher tendency to undergo apoptosis as compared to less mature cells. Ultrastructurally it was seen that the BM biopsies still showed higher degree of apoptosis as compared to BM aspirates even after taking into consideration the LDF. This could be because of the higher concentration of the proapoptotic signals in the BM biopsies of MDS patients.

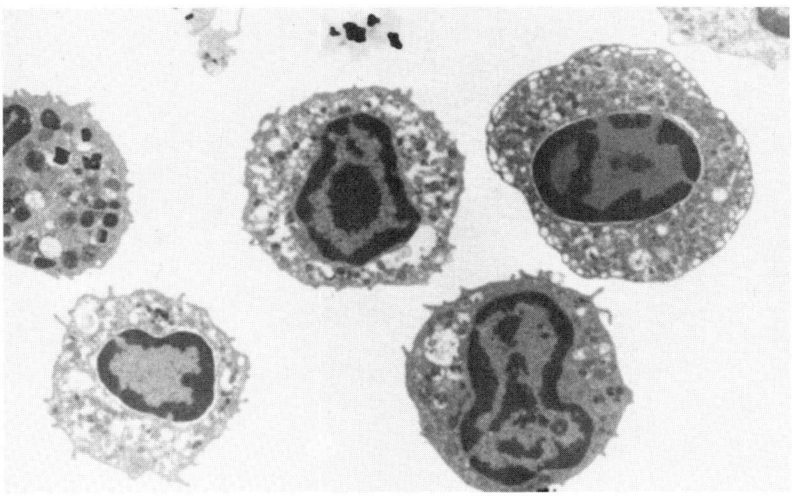

Figure 13. Low magnification of BM aspirate cells exhibiting apoptosis (Magnification 3,300)

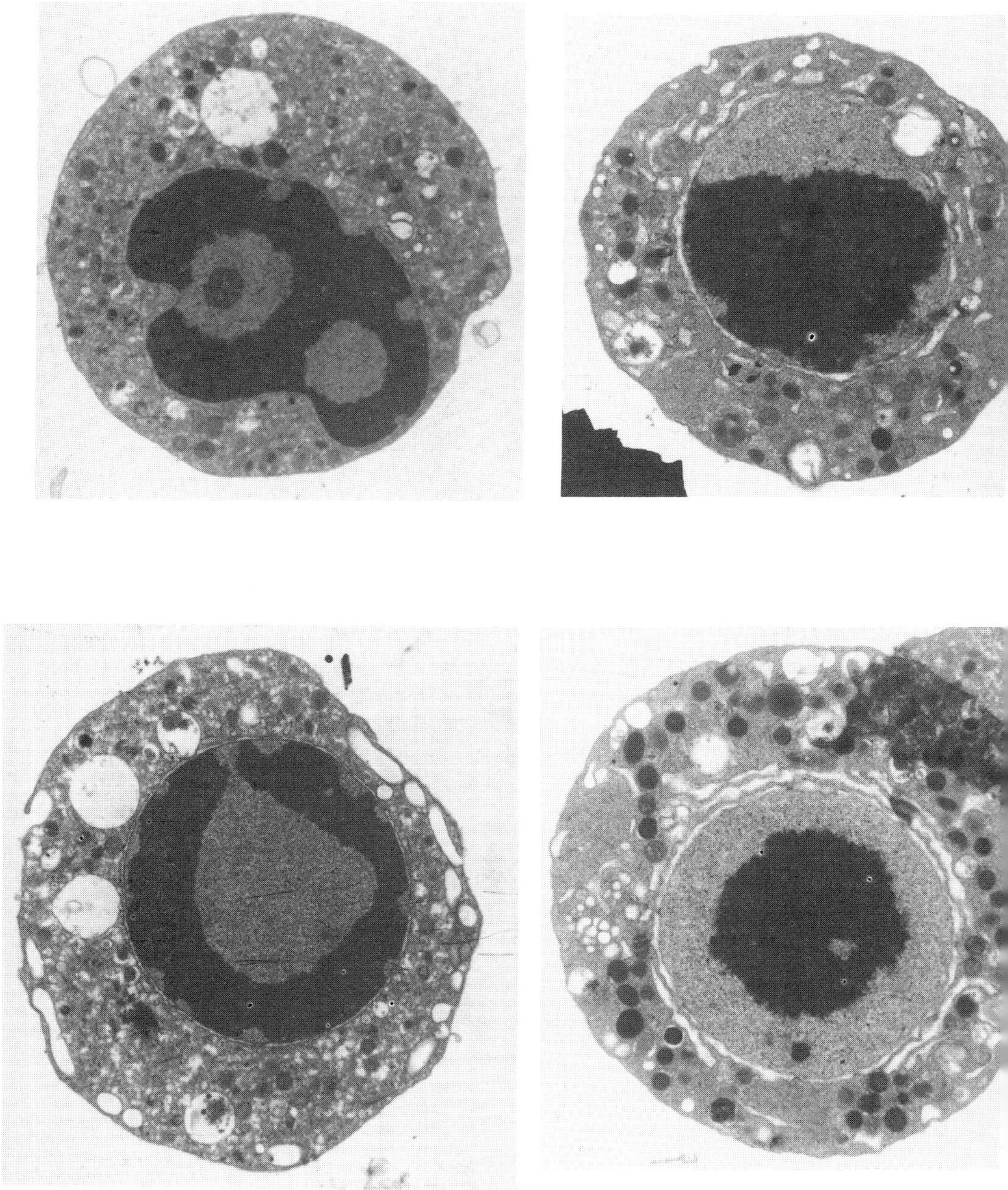

Figure 14. Different apoptotic cells in HD and LD fractions of MDS BM aspirate showing morphological characteristics like chromatin condensation of the nucleus, vacuoles and swollen mitochondria in the cytoplasm (Magnification x8,300)

CONCLUSION

Bone marrow biopsies from patients belonging to all FAB sub-categories of myelodysplastic syndromes (MDS) and normal controls were used to maintain long term cultures as well as extensive ultrastructural studies were performed on cultured and decorticated BM tissue. The prominent stromal cells observed in LTBMC were fibroblasts, macrophages, endothelial cells and adipocytes; while the FAB categories and cytogenetics were not co-related with the potency of growth in culture. The immunohistochemical and electron microscopic studies provided morphology, lineage confirmation, while the FISH studies demonstrated clonal nature of stromal cells in some MDS patients. The ultrstructural studies showed that both the stromal and hematopoietic cells exhibited extensive apoptosis in the MDS bone marrow biopsies. Furthermore to have an accurate estimate of the Apoptotic index (AI) in the BM aspirate of MDS patients, it is important to investigate both high and low density fractions of BM aspirate. Interestingly however, in LTBMC the MDS stroma was able to support normal hematopoiesis and appeared to be both morphologically and functionally normal though it may be clonal in nature. This perhaps may be due to either elimination of apoptotic cells from the cultures or low activity of proapoptotic cytokine in the culture microenvironment. In future, the MDS LTBMC studies may present an ideal in vitro model to study hematopoiesis in various myeloproliferative disorders.

REFERENCES

Aizawa, S., Nakano, M., Iwase, O., Yaguchi, M., Hiramoto, M., Hoshi, H., Nabeshima, R., Shima, D., Handa, H., & Toyama, K, (1999) Bone marrow stroma from refractory anemia of myelodysplastic syndrome is defective in its ability to support normal CD34-positive cell proliferation and differentiation in vitro. *Leukemia Research*, **23**, 239-246.

Alvi, S., Shaher, A., Henderson, B., Dar, S., Zorat, F., Broderick, E., Lisak, L., Du Randt, M., Reddy, P., Mundle, S., Galili, N., Borok, R.Z., & Raza, A, (2000) Improved growth of stromal cells in long term bone marrow cultures (LTBMC) of myelodysplastic syndrome (MDS) patients treated with thalidomide. *Blood*, **96**, 359a. Abstract #1547.

Bennett, J.M., Catovsky, D., Flandrin, D.M.T., Galton, G.D.A.G., Gralnick, H.R., & Sultan, C., (1982) Proposal for the classification of the myelodysplastic syndromes. *British Journal of Haematology*, **51**,189-199.

Blazsek, I., Liu, X.H., Anjo, A., Quittet, P., Comisso, M., Kim-Triana, B,, & Misset, J.L, (1995) The hematon, a morphogenetic functional complex in mammalian bone marrow, involves erythroblastic islands and granulocytic cobblestones. *Experimental Hematology*, **23**, 309-319.

Bogdanovic, A.D., Jankovic, G.M., Colovic, M.D., Trpinac, D.P., & Bumbasirevic, V.Z, (1996) Apoptosis in bone marrow of myelodysplastic syndrome patients. *Blood*, **87**, 3064.

Bouscary, D., De Vos, J., Guesnu , M., Jondeau, K., Viguier, F., Melle, J., Picard, F., Dreyfus, F., & Fontenay-Roupie, M, (1997) Fas/Apo-1 (CD95) expression and apoptosis in patients with myelodysplastic syndromes. *Leukemia*, **11**, 839-845.

Chang, J., & Dexter, T.M. (1991) Long–term cultures: in vitro purging of leukemic cells. *Baillieres Clinical Haematology*, **3**:775-788.

Clark, D.M., & Lampert, I.A., (1990) Apoptosis is a common histopathological finding in myelodysplasia: the correlate of ineffective hematopoiesis. *Leukemia Research*, **2**, 415-418.

Cohen, A., Alexandrova, S., Bessler, H., Mittelman, M., Cycowitz, Z., & Djaldetti, M, (1997) Ultrastructural observation on bone marrow cells of 26 patients with myelodysplastic syndromes. *Leukemia &Lymphoma*, **27**, 165-172.

Coutinho, L.H., Geary, C.G., Chang, J., Harrison, C., & Testa, N.G, (1990) Functional studies of bone marrow haemopoietic and stromal cells in the myelodysplastic syndromes (MDS). *British Journal of Haematology*, **75**, 16-25.

Davey, F. R., Erber, W. N., & Gatter, K.C., (1988) Abnormal neutrophils in acute leukemia and myelodysplastic syndrome. *Human Pathology*, **19**, 454-459.

Dexter, T.M, (1979) Haemopoiesis in long term bone marrow cultures. *Acta Haematologia*, **62**, 299-305.

Diana, C., Dominici, M., Lanza, F., Punturieri, M., Pauli, S., Tieghi, A., Dabusti, M., Scapoli, G., & Castoldi, G, (2000) Impairment of stromal cells compartment in hypoplastic myelodysplastic syndromes. *Blood*, **96**, 357a. Abstract # 1541.

Duhrsen, U., & Hossfeld, D.K, (1996) Stromal abnormalities in neoplastic bone marrow diseases. *Annals of Hematology*,**73**, 53-70.

Gerrad, J.M., & McNicol, A, (1992) Platelet storage pool deficiency, leukemia, and myelodysplastic syndromes. *Leukemia & Lymphoma*, **8**, 277-281.

Gidali, J., Feher, I,, & Hollan, S.R, (1996) Blast colony forming cell-binding capacity of bone marrow stroma from myelodysplastic patients. *Stem Cells*, **14**, 577-583.

Greenburg, P.L, (1992) In vitro marrow culture studies in the myelodysplastic syndromes. *Seminars in Oncology*, **1**, 34-46.

Greenburg, P.L. (1987) Biologic nature of the myelodysplastic syndromes. *Acta Haematologica*, **78**, 94-99.

Guccion, J.G., Schechter, G.P., & Zeller, J, (1992) Cytomembranous inclusions in myelodysplastic syndromes. *Ultrastructural Pathology*, **16**, 521-527.

Kouides, P.A., & Bennett, J.M, (1992) Morphology and classification of myelodysplastic syndromes [review]. *Hematology Oncology Clinics of North America*, **6**, 485-499.

Lanotte, M., Allen, T.D., & Dexter, M.T., (1981) Histochemical and ultrastructural characteristics of a cell line from human bone marrow stroma. *Journal of Cell Science*, **50**, 281-297.

Lai, J.L., & Fenaux, P, (1997) Cytogenetics of myelodysplastic syndromes. *Pathological Biology*, **45**, 550-555.

Lepelley, P., Campergue, L., Grardel, N., Preudhomme,C., Cosson, A., Fenaux, P, (1996) Is apoptosis a massive process in myelodysplastic syndromes? *British Journal of Haematology*, **95**, 368-371.

Ohmori, M., Ohmori, S., Ueda, Y., Yoshida, Y., & Okuma, M, (1991) Ineffective hematopoiesis in myelodysplastic syndromes (MDS) as studied by daily in situ observation of colony-cluster formation. *International Journal of Cell Cloning*, **9**, 521-530.

Payne, C.M., Greenberg, B., Cromey, D., & Woo, L, (1987) Morphological evidence of an altered bone marrow microenvironment in patients with acute nonlymphoblastic leukemia and myelodysplastic disorders. *Experimental. Hematolo*gy, **15**, 143-153.

Parcharidou, A., Raza, A., Economopoulos, T., Papageorgiou, E., Anagnostou, D., Papadaki, T., & Raptis, S, (1999) Extensive apoptosis of bone marrow cells as evaluated by in situ end-labeling (ISEL) technique may be the basis for ineffective haematopoiesis in patients with myelodysplastic syndromes. *European Journal of Haematology*, **62**, 19-26.

Pedersen-Bjergaard, J., Philip, P., Larsen, S.O., Anderson, M., Daugaard, G., Ersboll, J., Hansen, S.W., Hou-Jensen, K., Nielsen, D., Sigsgaard, T.C., Specht, L., & Osterlind, K, (1993) Therapy related myelodysplastic syndromes and acute myeloid leukemia. Cytogenetic characteristics of 115 consecutive cases and risk in seven cohorts of patients treated intensively for malignant diseases in the Copenhagen series. *Leukemia*, **7**, 1975-1986.

Polli, N., O'Brien M., Tavares, de., Castro, J., Matutes, E., San Miguel, J.F., & Catovsky, D, (1995) Characterization of blast cells in chronic granulocytic leukemia in transformation, acute myelofibrosis and undifferentiated leukemia. 1. Ultrastructural Morphology and Cytochemistry. *British. Journal Haematol*ogy, **59**, 277-296.

Raza, A., Mundle, S., Iftikhar, A., Gregory, S., Marcus, B., Khan, Z., Alvi, S., Shetty, V., Dameron, S., Wright, V., Adler, S., Loew, J., Scott, S., Ali, S.N., & Preisler, H.D., (1995) Simultaneous assessment of cell kinetics and programmed cell death in bone marrow biopsies of myelodysplastics reveals extensive apoptosis as the probable basis for ineffective hematopoiesis. *American Journal of Hematology*, **48**, 143-154.

Raza, A., Gezer, S., Mundle, S., Gao, X.Z., Alvi, S., Borok, R., Rifkin, S., Iftikhar, A., Shetty, V., Parcharidou, A., Loew, J., Marcus, B., Khan, Z., Chaney, C., Showel, J., Gregory, S.,& Preisler, H.D, (1996) Apoptosis in bone marrow biopsy samples involving stromal and hematopoietic cells in 50 patients with myelodysplastic syndromes. *Blood*, **86,** 268-276.

Raza, A., Alvi, S., Borok, R.Z., Span, L., Parcharidou, A., Alston, D., Rifkin, S., Robin, E., Shah, R., & Gregory, S.A, (1997).Excessive proliferation matched by excessive apoptosis in myelodysplastic syndromes: The cause-effect relationship. *Leukemia & Lymphoma*, **27**(1-2), 111-118.

Resegotti, L., (1993) The nature and natural history of myelodysplasia. *Haematologia*, **25**, 191-204.

Sawada, K, (1998) Growth characteristics of myelodysplastic CD34+ cells. *Leukemia & Lymphoma*,, **29**, 49-60.

Seed, T.M., Husseini, S.G., & Knospe, W.H, (1986) Hematopoiesis on cellulose ester membranes: VII. Ultrastructure of stroma of marrow enriched membranes with trilineal hematopoiesis. *Experimental Hematology*, **14**, 108-118.

Shetty, V., Mundle, S, Alvi, S., Showel, M., Broady-Robinson, L., Dar, S., Borok, R., Showel, J., Greagory, S., Rifkin, S., Gezer, S., Parcharidou, A., Venugopal, P., Shah, R., Hernandez, B., Klein, M., Alston, D., Robin, E., Dominguez, C., & Raza, A, (1996) Measurement of apoptosis, proliferation and three cytokine in 46 patients with myelodysplastic syndromes. *Leukemia Research*, **20**, 891-900.

Vallespi, T., Imbert, M., Mecucci, C., Preudhomme, C., & Fenaux, P, (1998) Diagnosis, classification, and cytogenetics of myelodysplastic syndromes. *Haematologica,* **83**, 258-275.

Verhoef, G.E.G, Pittaluga, S., De Wolf- Peters, C., & Boogaerts, M.A., (1995) FAB classification of myelodysplastic syndromes: merits and controversies. *Annals of Hematology*, **71**, 3-11.

Weimar, I. S., Bourhis, J..H., De Gast, G.C., & Gerritsen, W.R, (1994) Clonality in myelodysplastic syndromes. *Leukemia & Lymphoma*, **13**, 215-221.

Weiss, L., (1976) The hematopoietic microenvironment of the bone marrow: An ultrastructural study of the stroma in rat. *Anatomica. Records*, **186**, 161-184.

Yoshida, Y., (1993) Apoptosis may be the mechanism responsible for the premature intramedullary cell death in myelodysplastic syndromes. *Leukemia*, **7**, 144-146.

5

THE MONOCYTIC COMPONENT IN MYELODYSPLASTIC SYNDROMES

Gianluigi Castoldi and Gian Matteo Rigolin
Hematology Section, University of Ferrara, Italy

INTRODUCTION

The involvement of the monocytic component in myelodysplastic syndromes (MDS) was confined for a long time mainly to the identification of a single disease, the Chronic Myelo-Monocytic Leukemia (CMML). However, more recently, the monocytes have been re-evaluated in other MDS as possible target cells directly participating into the clonal process. In MDS other than CMML, monocytes reflect the abnormality of the progenitor cells even though their contribution to the pathological aspects of the disease is sometimes not clearly expressed. Immunophenotypic and molecular studies have demonstrated that, in MDS, the malignant transformation occurs mainly at the level of the myeloid stem cells. In particular fluorescent in situ hybridization (FISH) analysis of progenitor cells sorted by FACS has shown that, in MDS patients with trisomy 8, only the stem cells at the CFU-GEMM level (CD34+/CD33+ cells) presented the +8 chromosome abnormality while the pluripotent stem cells (CD34+/Thy1+), the lymphoid B (CD34+/CD19+) and T (CD34+/CD7+) cells did not show the trisomy 8 (Saitoh et al., 1998). However, more recently, it has been demonstrated that, in 5q- MDS, the deletion occurrred in hemopoietic cells endowed with lympho-myeloid potential even though these CD34+CD38- cells were inefficient at reconstituting hemopoiesis in a NOD/SCID mouse model (Nilsson et al.,

2000). Whatever the case, monocytes which directly derive from the CFU-GEMM progenitor cells, are part of the malignant clone.

BIOLOGICAL ASPECTS OF MONOCYTES IN MDS

Morphology

The French-American-British (FAB) classification of MDS is based on the recognition of morphological abnormalities, which, for the diagnosis of myelodysplasia, should be present in at least 10% of the cells of a single lineage (Kouides & Bennett, 1996; Castoldi & Cuneo 1996). While well-defined criteria have been established as far as the erythroid, the granulocytic and the megakaryocytic lineages are concerned, only quantitative aspects have been considered in the evaluation of the monocytic component. Despite the lack of precise and diagnostic morphological abnormalities, peripheral blood monocytes may exhibit several dysplastic features such as abnormal nuclear lobations, cytoplasmic granules, and increased basophilia. Peripheral and bone marrow preparations may frequently show an increased percentage of immature monocytes (promonocytes) which sometimes are erroneously classified as blasts. Cytochemical stainings such as peroxidase, Sudan B Black, NaF sensitive non specific esterases and double esterases may help to distinguish monocytic cells from abnormal myeloid elements.

Histological aspects

The evaluation of bone marrow biopsies has revealed that in most of the severe forms of MDS there is a topographic distortion of the bone marrow architecture. In a normal healthy subject the bone marrow presents a well-organized spatial distribution of the hematopoietic progenitors: in particular erythropoietic islands and megakaryocytes are localized in the central regions of marrow cavities in the proximity of the sinusoids, while early granulocyte precursors are close to the endosteal surfaces and more mature granulocytes are in the central inter-trabecular areas. By contrast, in MDS there is a displacement of myeloid progenitor cells from the peri-trabecular towards the inter-trabecular areas. This abnormal localization of bone marrow precursors in the bone marrow has been historically named ALIP (Abnormal Localization of Immature Precursors, Tricot et al., 1984). A combined morphologic, immunocytochemical and immunologic analysis of these ALIPs has demonstrated that it is possible to recognize three types of clusters of immature cells (Mangi & Mufti, 1992): the erythroid, the megakaryocytic and the immature granulocytic and monocytic aggregates ("true ALIPs"). The demonstration of monocytic cells within true ALIPs has identified a group of MDS in which the monocytic component is directly involved in the abnormal proliferation and which perhaps deserves separate evaluation.

Immunophenotype

A great interest was devoted in the last 15 years to the analysis of different classes of surface molecules in MDS. However several methodological considerations should be kept in mind in the evaluation of these results such as the type of cell preparation, the purity of the population, the type of antibody used, and the method of analysis (Elghetany, 1998). CD14 the endotoxin receptor is a GPI-linked molecule expressed at high level of intensity on normal monocytes. This molecule showed a deficient density expression on the monocytes of 32% of MDS patients (Clark et al., 1985). However, in non-CMML patients, nearly 50% of the cases presented an increased percentage of CD14+ cells in bone marrow samples (Hockland et al., 1986; Kristensen et al., 1990), a finding in keeping with histological observations. Conversely CD15, an antigen up-regulated with maturation on neutrophils and monocytes, showed a higher density of expression on MDS monocytes in 42% of the cases (Clark et al., 1985) while an increased percentage of CD15+ cells was found in bone marrow samples in nearly 75% of MDS patients (Guyotat et al., 1990). CD87, the urokinase-type plasminogen activator receptor (u-PAR), a GPI-linked molecule, and CD64, the Fc gamma Receptor I, were found to be over-expressed on both neutrophils and monocytes in high and low risk MDS even though the significance of this observation remains still uncertain (Felzmann et al., 1993). CD116, the GM-CSF receptor, a molecule with a high density of expression on normal blood monocytes, showed a lower antigenic density on the cell surface of MDS monocytes, particularly in high risk cases (Lanza et al., 1997).

Cytogenetics and molecular biology

None of the different MDS categories presents specific cytogenetic abnormalities since most of them are also found in acute leukemias and myeloproliferative disorders (Pedersen-Bjergaard & Rowley, 1994; Heim & Mitelman 1995; de Greef & Hagemeijer, 1996). Nonetheless, for some cytogenetic anomalies, there is a preferential occurrence in the different FAB subtypes. Among MDS with prevalent monocytic disturbances, 12p rearrangements deserve special interest. The short arm of chromosome 12 may be involved not only in deletions, but also in balanced and unbalanced translocations with breakpoints at 12p13 (Sato et al., 1995). A recurrent structural abnormality, t(5;12)(q33;p13), has been described in 10% of CMML (Wessel et al., 1993, Golub et al., 1994) mainly in those patients characterized by dysplastic monocytosis, variable bone marrow fibrosis and progression into acute leukemia. This translocation involves the beta chain receptor gene of the platelet derived growth factor (PDGF), at the 5q33 band, and the ETV6/TEL gene at the 12p13 band. TEL gene is also involved in the variant translocation t(10;12)(q24;p13), which was associated with eosinophilia, hyperleukocytosis, mild monocytosis, and previous exposure to environmental mutagenic substances (Wlodarska et al., 1995). Recently a new translocation, associated with CMML, has been described, t(5;7)(q13;q11.2), involving the receptor gene of PDGF and the Huntingtin Interacting Protein1 (HIP1, Ross et al., 1998). These findings are reminiscent of the picture observed in chronic myeloproliferative diseases.

Molecular biology

Molecular abnormalities have been extensively investigated in MDS (Gallagher et al., 1997). RAS genes, mainly N-RAS, have been found to be mutated in 30-48% of MDS patients (Lyons et al., 1988; Padua et al., 1998). RAS mutations, frequently involving codon 12, have been preferentially observed in CMML, in MDS with monocytosis and in patients with abnormal karyotypes (Yunis et al., 1989). Interestingly RAS genes have also been found mutated with high frequency in M4 and M5 AML FAB subtypes (Vandenberghe et al., 1991). Mutations of the macrophage colony stimulating factor gene, also known as FMS, were observed in 12-20% of MDS patients and were mainly located at codon 969 (Padua at al., 1998; Tobal et al., 1990). FMS mutations were most frequently found in CMML and, as for RAS, in M4 and M5 AML FAB subtypes suggesting a possible role for the FMS gene in the pathogenesis of myeloid disorders expressing an involvement of the monocytic component. From a clinical point of view, patients with RAS and FMS mutations have a higher risk of progression into AML and poorer prognosis (Padua et al., 1998). Amplification of a hemopoietic specific tyrosine phosphatase (HePTP) has been described in hypoplastic MDS with monocytosis. This gene was found to be over-expressed in myelomonocytic cells and, when transferred into cell lines, was capable of inducing alterations in myeloid growth and maturation suggesting a role in normal myelopoiesis (Zanke et al., 1994).

Functional properties

A clear evidence for functional abnormalities of monocytes and macrophages in MDS is still limited. Controversial results have been published concerning phagocytosis, intracellular killing and migration (Hamblin, 1996).

In recent years apoptosis has been extensively investigated in relation to the growth and differentiation impairment which characterizes MDS hemopoiesis (Raza et al., 1995; Parker & Mufti, 1998). It is now quite an accepted contention that cytokines such as TNF-alpha and IFN-gamma play a key role in the suppression of the growth of progenitor cells and induce FAS expression on CD34+ cells (Maciejewski et al., 1995; Gesuk et al., 2000). Elevated TNF-alpha levels have been found in MDS patients (Verhoef et al., 1992) and it has been postulated that peripheral blood monocytes and bone marrow macrophages, which are increased in MDS marrow samples, could represent a probable source of TNF-alpha production (Koike et al., 1995; Kitagawa et al., 1997; Rosenfeld & List, 2000). Elevated serum levels of the M-CSF or point mutations in the c-FMS gene, which encodes the M-CSF receptor, could sustain the increased production of TNF-alpha by monocytic elements. New therapeutic strategies have been developed in order to neutralize TNF-alpha activity. In this regard pentoxifylline, a drug suppressing TNF-alpha m-RNA transcription, in combination with amifostine, ciprofloxacin and dexamethasone has produced hemopoietic responses in selected groups of patients (Raza et al., 2000).

Dendritic cells

A particular functional aspect of monocytes is their ability to differentiate into dendritic cells (DC). DCs are professional antigen presenting cells with an exquisite capacity to initiate and to modulate the immune response. DCs are also believed to be important in the development of specific anti-tumour T-cell responses. In this regard, DCs have been considered an attractive alternative in malignancies that remain incurable by conventional therapies. The possibility to obtain, in vitro, DCs from peripheral blood monocytes in MDS patients has been recently investigated (Rigolin et al., 1999; Vuckovic et al., 1999). In particular it has been demonstrated that, after 10 days of culture in the presence of IL4 and GM-CSF, a reduced number of DCs was obtained in MDS subjects (Figure 1A). When compared to normal subjects, MDS DCs were found to present a significantly lower intensity of expression of CD1a, CD54, CD80, and class II molecules. MDS DCs were able to stimulate an allogeneic mixed luekocyte reaction (MLR) but their ability to stimulate T lymphocytes was less potent than in normal subjects. MDS DCs also showed a reduced receptor-mediated endocytotic capacity, evaluated by FITC-dextran uptake. A simultaneous FISH and immunophenotypic analysis demonstrated that sorted MDS CD1a+/CD14- DCs have the same cytogenetic abnormality as the malignant clone (Rigolin et al., 1999, Figure 1B).

It was therefore possible to conclude that in MDS subjects DCs are part of the malignant clone and present a marked alteration of their function which affects the efficiency of DC generation, the ability to capture and present antigens, and the capability to stimulate T cell responses. From these observations it is possible to speculate that all these abnormalities, in MDS, might contribute to an impaired immunity which results in an increased susceptibility to infectious disease and in a high incidence of autoimmune phenomena and malignant neoplasms especially of lymphoid origin.

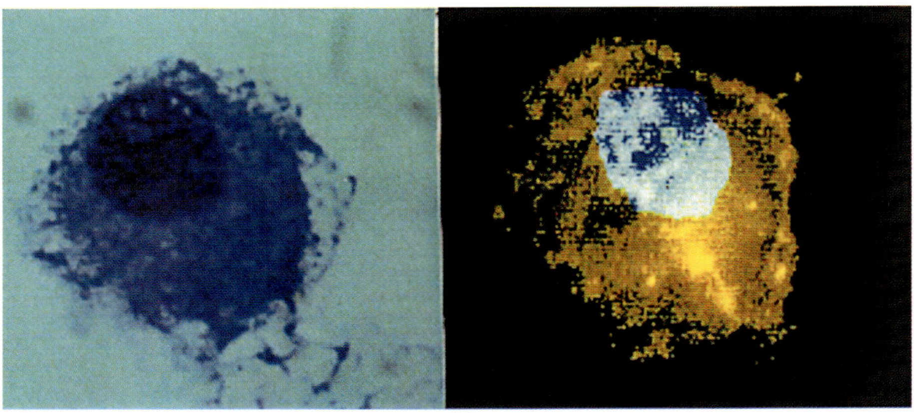

A **B**

Figure 1 (A) Morphology of a DC obtained from peripheral blood moncoytes in a MDS patient after 10 days of culture in the presence of GM-CSF, IL-4 and TNF-alpha.(B) Simultaneous FISH and immunophenotypic analysis in a DC from a MDS patient with trisomy 8. The DC is identified by surface positivity for CD1a.

NEW PERSPECTIVES ON THE CLASSIFICATION OF MDS WITH MONOCYTOSIS

CMML

The FAB classification of MDS in its original proposals (Bennett et al., 1982) has recognized a single subentity in which the monocytic component was markedly involved, namely the CMML. By definition, CMML is characterized by an absolute peripheral blood monocytosis of > 1 x 109/L, a variable degree of dysplasia affecting the three major hematopoietic lineages, and by a percentage of bone marrow blasts below the 20%. The main clinical features of CMML are an increased incidence of splenomegaly and hepatomegaly, rarely observed in other forms of MDS, and a tendency to develop serous effusions in the pleura, pericardium, peritoneum and sinovia, often associated with high peripheral blood monocyte counts. Tissue infiltration, particularly of the skin and gingiva, and an increased incidence of autoimmune phenomena such as polymialgia reumatica and vasculitic rushes, due to circulating immune complexes, have also been reported in a significant number of these patients. The prognosis of CMML patients is variable ranging from 11 to 60 months according to the different series of patients. The percentage of bone marrow blasts and the absolute number of peripheral blood monocytes are perhaps the two most important predictors of survival in CMML.

CMML: a myelodysplastic or a myeloproliferative disorders?

CMML was originally classified among the MDS because of the dysplastic changes characterizing the peripheral and bone marrow hemopoietic cells. However CMML also shares some clinical and hematologic features with the chronic myeloproliferative diseases. In this regard the FAB group (Bennett et al., 1994) proposed to distinguish two forms of CMML depending on the total leukocyte count: a MDS type (MDS-CMML) with a white blood cell count (WBC) below 13 x 10^9/L and a myeloproliferative CMML (MPD-CMML) characterized by a higher number of WBC. More recently the International Scoring System for the evaluation of prognosis in MDS (IPSS, Greenberg et al., 1997), following FAB suggestions, excluded MPD-CMML from its prognostic evaluation even though the cut off value for the WBC, in its analysis, was set at 12 x 10^9/L. However, large retrospective analysis of CMML patients demonstrated that the separation of the two forms provided little prognostic information. In fact even though the two forms were different regarding WBC counts, splenomegaly, LDH and deoxythymidine levels, no differences in terms of overall survival and probability of transformation were observed (Germing et al., 1998; Oscier & Chapman, 1998).

The heterogeneity of CMML pictures at presentation indicates that the discrimination between myelodysplastic and myeloproliferative disorders (MPD) is sometimes difficult. The observation of dysplastic features in MPD with moderate monocytosis is not unsual. In this regard the progression of classical MDS into Ph negative myeloproliferative pictures has been described (Ohyashiki et al., 1993; Verhoef et al., 1994). Among MPD with monocytosis and dysplastic features, the atypical chronic myeloid leukemia (aCML) was recently identified as a new subentity. According to FAB guidelines (Bennett el al., 1994) aCML is characterized by marked myeloid dysplasia, a mild to moderate monocytosis, the presence of a high percentage (>15%) of peripheral immature granulocytes and negativity for BCR rearrangements. The survival of these patients is shorter than that of CMML patients. It is still debated whether or not aCML should be considered a distinct clinical entity. This disoreder, indistinguishable in its early phases from refractory anemia by standard hematological criteria, may represent, as far as the natural history is concerned, an unusual evolution of myelodysplasia with proliferative rather than ineffective myeloid maturation (Oscier, 1996).

The problem of the classification of CMML was specifically considered by the WHO in the Advisory Committee Meeting for the classification of hematologic diseases (Harris et al., 1999). The Committee agreed that CMML is a heterogenous disease that exhibits features of both myelodysplastic and myeloproliferative syndromes. However the Committee observed that no differences have been described between the two types of CMML as far as cytogenetic abnormalities, oncogene mutations, in vitro colony growth patterns and clinical outcome are concerned. It was therefore decided that CMML should be considered as a single entity to be included in a separate category, the myelodysplastic/myeloproliferative diseases, along with juvenile myelomonocytic leukemia and aCML. In the new WHO classification CMML was therefore separated from the other MDS.

MDS With Monocytosis

It is well documented that, in the evaluation of MDS, there is a significant percentage of patients with a monocytic component not exceeding 1×10^9/L monocytes. However, the inclusion of these patients in the existing FAB and WHO categories seems unsatisfactory. The importance of a more definite assessment of the monocytic component in MDS also derives from the observation that a significant percentage of patients with a large number of ALIPs in bone marrow biopsy presents antigens related to monocytic differentiation on immature precursors (Mangi & Mufti, 1992). From a retrospective analysis of nearly 200 consecutive MDS patients, it was found that nearly 20% of non-CMML MDS patients presented, at diagnosis, a monocytosis defined by the presence of more than 10% of blood monocytes. Patients with monocytosis dysplayed a higher incidence of hypercellular bone marrow and were characterized, from a clinical point of view, by a more aggressive course of the disease and worse outcome (Figure 2). These patients presented a higher probability of evolution into high risk MDS or acute myeloid leukemia with monocytic component (M4 and M5). Karyotypic abnormalities and in particular complex karyotypes were more frequently observed among these patients (Rigolin et al., 1997, 1998). In our opinion these observations may support the identification of a subgoup of MDS patients for which the definition of *MDS with monocytosis* might be appropriate.

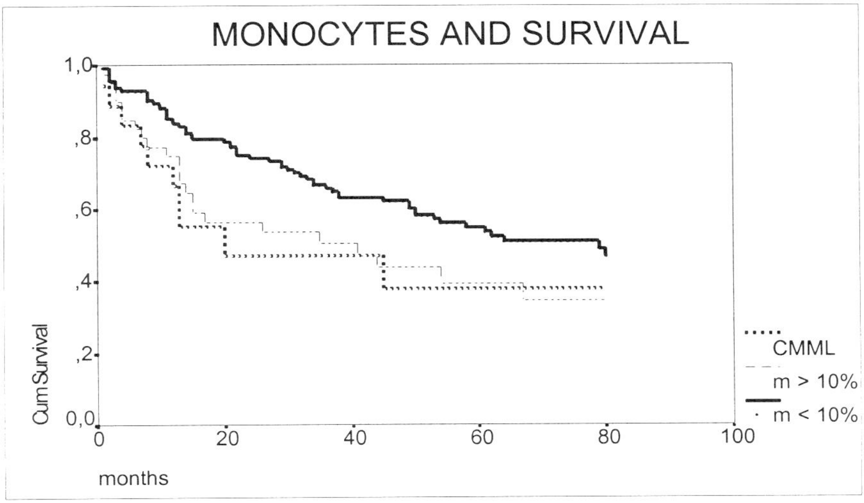

Figure 2 Overall survival of 188 MDS patients according to the presence of monocytosis (CMML= Chronic myelomonocytic leukemia, m = monocytes).

CONCLUSIONS

Morphological, immunological, cytogenetic and molecular data not only demonstrated that, in MDS, the monocytic component is usually part of the abnormal clone, but also support the hypothesis that monocytes could be actively involved in the events contributing to the pathogenesis of the disease. In MDS, the involvement of the monocytic component is more frequently associated with features of chronic MPD supporting the nosographic inclusion of these disorders in the new category of myelodysplastic/myeloproliferative diseases. From a strict biological point of view, these disorders may recognize as for FAB classification of acute myeloid leukemia, two principal subgroups one with myeloid-oriented evolution and the other with prevalent monocytic differentiation frequently originating from MDS with monocytosis.

REFERENCES

Bennett, J.M., Catovsky, D., Daniel, M.T., Flandrin, G., Galton, G., Gralnick, H. & Sultan C. (1982) Proposals for the classification of myelodysplastic syndromes. *British Journal of Haematology*, **51**, 189-199.

Bennett, J.M., Catovsky, D., Daniel, M.T., Flandrin, G., Galton, G., Gralnick, H., Sultan C. & Cox, C. (1994) The chronic myeloid leukemias: guidelines for distinguishing chronic granulocytic, atypical chronic myeloid, and chronic myelomonocytic leukemia. Proposals by the French-American-British cooperative leukemia group. *British Journal of Haematology*, **87,** 746-754.

Castoldi, G. & Cuneo, A. (1996) Special cytological subtypes of acute myeloid leukemias and myelodysplastic syndromes. *Baillière's Clinical Haematology*, **9**, 19-33.

Clark, R.E., Hoy, T.G. & Jacobs, A. (1985) Granulocyte and monocyte surface membrane markers in the myelodysplastic syndromes. *Journal of Clinical Pathology*, **38**, 301-304.

De Greef, G. & Hagemeijer, A. (1996) Molecular and cytogenetic abnormalities in acute myeloid leukemia and myelodysplastic syndromes. *Baillière's Clinical Haematology*, **9**, 1-18.

Elghetany, M.T. (1998) Surface marker abnormalities in myelodysplastic syndromes. *Haematologica*, **83**, 1104-115.

Felzmann, T., Gisslinger, H., Krieger, O., Majadic, O., Ludwig, H. & Koller, U. (1993) Imunophenotypic characterization of myelomonocytic cells in patients with myelodysplastic syndrome. *British Journal of Haematology*, **84**, 428-435.

Gallagher, A., Darley, R.L. & Padua, R.A. (1997) The molecular basis of myelodysplastic syndromes. *Haematologica*, **82**, 191-204.

Germing, U., Gatterman, N., Minning, H., Heyll, A. & Aul, C. (1998) Problems in the classification of CMML – dysplastic versus proliferative type. *Leukemia Research*, **22**, 871-878.

Gersuk, G.M., Beckham, C., Loken, M.R., Kiener, P., Anderson, J.E., Farrand, A., Troutt, A.B., Ledbetter, J.A. & Deeg, H.J. (1998) A role for tumour necrosis factor alpha, FAS and FAS-ligand in marrow failure associated with myelodysplastic syndromes. *British Journal of Haematology*, **103**, 176-188.

Golub, T.R., Bvarker, G.F., Lovett, M., et al. (1994) Fusion of PDGF receptor beta a novel ets-like gene, TEL, in chronic myelomonocytic leukemia with t(5;12) chromosomal translocation. *Cell*, **77**, 307-318.

Greenberg, P., Cox, C., Le Beau, M.M., Fenaux, P., Morel, P., Sanz, G., Sanz, M., Vallespi, T., Hamblin, T., Oscier, D., Ohyashiki, K., Toyama, K., Aul, C., Mufti, G. & Bennett, J. (1997) International scoring system for evaluating prognosis in myelodysplastic syndromes. *Blood*, **89**, 2079-2088.

Guyotat, D., Campos, L., Thomas, X., et al. (1990) Myelodysplastic syndromes : a study of surface markers and in vitro growth patterns. *American Journal of Hematology*, **34**, 26-31.

Hamblin, T.J. (1992) Clinical features of MDS. *Leukemia Research*, **16**, 89-93.

Hamblin, T.J. (1996) Immunological abnormalities in myelodysplastic syndromes. *Seminars in Hematology*, **33**, 150-162.

Harris, M.L., Jaffe, E.S., Diebold, J., Flandrin, G., Muller-Hermelink, K., Vardiman, J., Lister, T.A. & Bloomfield, C.D. (1999) World Health classification of neoplastic diseases of the hematopoitic and lymphoid tissues: report of the clinical advisory committee meeting – Airlie House, Virginia, November 1997. *Journal of Clinical Oncology*, **17**, 3835-3849.

Heim, S. & Mitelman, F. (1995) Cancer Cytogenetics. Second Edition John Wiley & Sons, Inc., New York.

Hockland, P., Kendrup, G., Griffin, J.D. & Ellegaard, J. (1986) Analysis of leukocyte differentiation antigens in blood and bone marrow from preleukemia (refractory anemia) patients using monoclonal antibodies. *Blood*, **67**, 898-902.

Kitagawa, M., Saito, I., Kuwata, T., Yoshida, S., Yamaguchi, S., Takahashi, M., Tanizawa, M., Kamiyama, R. & Hirokawa, K. (1997) Overexpression of tumor necrosis factor (TNF)-alpha and interferon (IFN)-gamma by bone marrow cells from patients with myelodysplastic syndromes. *Leukemia*, **11**, 2049-2054.

Koike, M., Ishiyama, T., Tomoyasu, S. & Tsuruoka, N. (1995) Spontaneous cytokine overproduction by peripheral blood mononuclear cells from patients with myelodysplastic syndromes and aplastic anemia. *Leukemia Research*, **9**, 639-644.

Kouides, P.A. & Bennett, J.M. (1996) Morphology and classification of the myelodysplastic syndromes and their pathologic variants. *Seminars in Hematology*, **33**, 95-110.

Kristensen, J.S. & Hockland, P. (1990) Monoclonal antibody ratios in malignant myeloid diseases: diagnostic and prognostic use in myelodysplastic syndromes. *British Journal of Haematology*, **74**, 270-276.

Lanza, F., Castagnari, B., Rigolin, G., Latorraca, A., Ferrari, L., Bardi, A. & Castoldi, G. (1997) Flow cytometry measurement of GM-CSF receptors in acute leukemic blasts and normal hemopoietic cells. *Leukemia*, **11**, 1700-1710.

Lyons, J., Janssen, J.W., Bartram, C., Layton, M. & Mufti G.J. (1988) Mutations of Ki-ras and N-ras oncogenes in myelodysplastic syndromes. *Blood*, **71**, 1707-1712.

Maciejewski, I., Selleri, C., Anderson, S. & Young, N.S. (1995) Fas antigen expression on CD34+ human marrow cells is induced by interferon gamma and tumor necrosis factor alpha and potentiates cytokine mediated hematopoietic suppression in vitro. *Blood*, **85**, 3183-3190.

Mangi, M.H. & Mufti, G.J. (1992) Primary myelodysplastic syndromes: diagnostic and prognostic significance of immunohistochemical assessment of bone marrow biopsies. *Blood*, **79**, 198-205.

Nilsson, L., Astrand-Grunstrom, I., Arvidsson, I., Jacobsson, B., Hellstrom-Lindberg, E., Hast, R. & Jacobsen, S.E.W. (2000) Isolation and characterization of hematopoietic progenitor/stem cells in 5q-deleted myelodysplastic syndromes: evidence for the involvemenet at he hematopoietic stem cell level. *Blood*, **96**, 212-2021.

Ohyashiki, K., Yokoyama, K., Kimura, Y., Ohyashiki, J.H., Ito, T., Kuratsuji, T., Komatsumoto, S., Nara, M. & Toyama, K. (1993) Myelodysplastic syndrome evolving into a myeloproliferative disorder: one disease or two? *Leukemia*, **7**, 338-340.

Oscier, D.G. (1996) Atypical chronic myeloid leukaemia, a distinct clinical entity related to the myelodysplastic syndrome? *British Journal of Haematology*, **92**, 582-586.

Oscier, D.G. & Chapman, R. (1998) The classification of chronic myelomonocytic leukemia. *Leukemia Research*, **22**, 879-880.

Padua, R.A., Guinn, B.-A., Al-Sabah, A., Smoth, M., Taylor, C., Pettersson, T., Ridge, S., Carter, G., White, D., Oscier, D., Chevret, S. & West, R. (1998) RAS, FMS and P53 mutations and poor clinical outcome in myelodysplasias: a 10-year follow-up. *Leukemia*, **12**, 887-892.

Parker, J.E. & Mufti, G.J. (1998) Ineffective haemopoiesis and apoptosis in myelodysplastic syndromes. *British Journal of Haematology*, **101**, 220-230.

Pedersen-Bjergaard, J. & Rowley, J.D. (1994) The balanced and the unbalanced chromosome aberrations of acute myeloid leukemia may develop in different ways and may contribute differently to malignant transformation. *Blood*, **83**, 2780-2786.

Raza, A., Gezer, S., Mundle, S., Gao, X.-Z., Alvi, S., Borok, R., Rifkin, S., Iftikhar, A., Shetty, V., Parcharidou, A., Loew, J., Marcus, B., Khan, Z., Chaney, C., Showel, J., Gregory, S. & Preisler, H. (1995) Apoptosis in bone marrow biopsy samples involving stromal and hematopoietic cells in 50 patients with myelodysplastic syndromes. *Blood*, **86**, 268-276.

Raza, A., Gawl, H., Lisak, L., Andric, T., Dar, S., Adrews, C., Venugopal, P., Gezer S., Gregory, S., Loew, J., Robin, E., Rifkin, S., Hsu, W.-T-. & Huang R.-W. (2000) Patients with myelodysplastic syndromes benefit from palliative therapy with amifostine, pentoxifylline, and ciprofloxacin with or without dexamethasone. *Blood*, **95**, 1580-1587.

Rigolin, G.M., Cuneo, A., Roberti, M.G., Bardi, A. & Castoldi G. (1997) Myelodysplastic syndromes with monocytic component: hematologic and cytogenetic characterization. *Haematologica*, **82**, 25-30.

Rigolin, G.M., Cuneo, A., Roberti, M.G., Bardi, A., Bigoni, R., Piva, N., Minotto, C., Agostini, P., De Angeli, C., Del Senno, L., Spanedda, R. & Castoldi G.L. (1998) Exposure to myelotoxic agents and myelodysplasia: case-control study and correlation with clinicobiologic findings. *British Journal of Haematology*, **103**, 189-197.

Rigolin, G.M., Howard, J., Buggins, A., Sneddon, C., Castoldi, G., Hirst, W.J.R. & Mufti, G. (1999) Phenotypic and functional characteristics of monocyte-derived dendritic cells from patients with myelodysplastic syndromes. *British Journal of Haematology*, **107**, 844-850.

Rosenfeld, C. & List, A. (2000) A hypothesis for the pathogenesis of myelodysplastic syndromes: implications for new therapies. *Leukemia*, **14**, 2-8.

Ross, T., Bernard, O.A., Berger, R. & Guillard, G.D. (1998) Fusion of Huntingtin interacting protein 1 to platelet derived growth factor beta receptor (PDGFbetaR) in chronic myelomonocytic leukemia wih t(5;7)(q22:q11.2). *Blood*, **91**, 4419-4426.

Saitoh, K., Miura, I., Takahashi, N. & Miura A.B. (1998) Fluorescent in situ hybridisation of progenitor cells obtained by fluorescent-activated cell sorting for the detection of cells affected by chromosome abnormality trisomy 8 in patients with myelodysplastic syndromes. *Blood*, **92**, 2886-2892.

Sato, Y., Suto, Y., Pietenpol, J., et al. (1995) TEL and KIP1 define the smallest region on 12p13 in hematopoietic malignancies. *Blood*, **86**, 1525-1533.

Tobal, K., Pagliuca, A., Bhatt, B., Bailey, N., Layton, M. & Mufti, G.J. (1990) Mutation of the human FMS gene (M-CSF receptor) in myelodysplastic syndromes and acute myeloid leukemia. *Leukemia*, **4**, 486-489.

Tricot, G., De Wolf-Peeters, C., Hendrickx, B. & Verwlghen, R.L. (1984) I. Histological findings in myelodysplastic syndromes and comparison with bone marrow smears. *British Journal of Haematology*, **57**, 423-430.

Vandenberghe, E., Baens, M., Stul, M., et al. (1991) Alterations of N-ras mutations in a patients with AML M4 and trilineage myelodysplasia. *British Journal of Haematology*, **79**, 338-340.

Verhoef, G.E.G., Demuynk, H., Zachee, P. & Boogaerts, M.A. (1994) Myelodysplastic syndrome evolving into a myeloproliferative disorder: one disease or two. *Leukemia*, **8**, 714-715.

Vuckovic, S., Fearnley, D.B., Gunningham, S., Spearing, R.L., Patton, W.N. & Hart, D.N.J. (1999) Dendritic cells in chronic myelomonocytic leukemia. *British Journal of Haematology*, **105**, 974-985.

Wessels, J.W., Fibbe, W.E., Van Der Keur, D., et al. (1993) t(5;12)(q31;p12). A clinical entity with features of both myeloid and chronic myelomonocytic leukemia. *Cancer Genetics and Cytogenetics*, **65**, 7-15.

Wlodarska, I., Mecucci, C., Marynen, P., et al. (1995) TEL gene is involved in myelodysplastic syndromes with either the typical t(5;12)(q33;p13) translocation or its variant t(10;12)(q24;p13). *Blood*, **85**, 2848-2852.

Yunis, J.J., Boot, A.J., Mayer, M.G. & Bos, J.L. (1989) Mechanisms of ras mutations in myelodysplastic syndrome. *Oncogene*, **4**, 609-614.

Zanke, B., Squire, J., Griesser, H., et al. (1994) A hemopoietic protein tyrosine phosphatase (HePTP) gene that is amplified and overexpressed in myeloid malignancies maps to chromosome 1q32.1. *Leukemia*, **8**, 236-244.

6

CYTOKINES AND MDS

Krishnan Allampallam, Vilasini T. Shetty and Azra Raza
MDS Center and Section of Myeloid Diseases, Department of Medicine
Rush University, Chicago, IL

Myelodysplastic syndromes (MDS) are considered to be stem cell disorders. A number of cytogenetic abnormalities have been demonstrated in these patients. In the last decade it has become apparent that besides the cytogenetic and molecular abnormalities at the individual cell level, the global alterations of the bone marrow (BM) microenvironment brought about by shifts in the cytokine milieu may play a crucial role in defining the pathobiology of these disorders. The combination of factors produced by adherent stromal cells and hematopoietic cells constitute the web of cytokines meshing a variety of biological processes including survival, proliferation and differentiation of the hematopoietic cells. Imperatively thus, hematopoiesis in these patients is a result of a critical balance between the stimulatory and inhibitory signals transduced by these cytokines. Primarily effects of these cytokines could be chemotatic, stimulatory or inhibitory to hematopoiesis.

CYTOKINE PROFILE IN THE BONE MARROW

Cytokines in the bone marrow could either come from the stromal cells or the parenchymal cells. The stromal cells are mostly present in bone marrow biopsies where cytokine levels were estimated by immunohistochemical methods while the cytokines expressed by the parenchymal cells were estimated by RT-PCR. Granulocyte Macrophage colony stimulating factor (GM-CSF) and Macrophage CSF (M-CSF) are both hematopoietic growth factors that play a significant role in development of Granulocyte-macrophage and macrophage population respectively. The level of GM-CSF in BM of MDS and normal was the same. In MDS, GM-CSF was localized mainly in the interstitium around the proliferating cells (Shetty et al., 1996). Interestingly, GM-CSF levels negatively correlated with the levels of both Tumor Necrosis Factor (TNF)-α and apoptosis (Shetty et al., 1996). The MDS BM mononuclear cells (BMMNC) express approximately twice the amount of Macrophage-CSF (MCSF) transcript as compared to the normal BM (Allampallam et al., 1999). This increase corresponded to the increase in macrophages, commonly seen in the BM biopsies of MDS patients (Allampallam et al., 2000). Flt3 ligand, a hematopoietic growth factor, supports the maintenance and stimulates early progenitor stem cells (Birg et al., 1994). Its expression in BMMNC was comparable between normal and MDS (Allampallam et al., 1999). IL-1β has a wide range of target cells including hematopoietic cells of lymphoid and myeloid origin and fibroblast (Dinarello CA, 1991). The transcript levels of both IL-1β (two times) and IL-1β ra (1.5 times) in the BMMNC were significantly higher in MDS patients as compared to normal individuals (Allampallam et al., 1999). Two inhibitory cytokines, TNFα and TGFβ, have been studied at length in MDS. Higher than normal levels of both has been reported in the BM of MDS patients (Quadir et al., 1992; Shetty et al., 1996; Kitagawa et al., 1997; Gerzuk et al., 1998; Allampallam et al., 2000). The levels of TGFβ appear to increase with disease progression. On the one hand TGFβ in MDS correlated with macrophage number and TNFα while on the other hand, the number of macrophages correlated with the levels of TNFα and apoptosis in these patients (Allampallam et al., 2000). Further investigations are needed to determine if these events constitute a circuit. Another inhibitory cytokine that is occasionally seen in MDS is interferon gamma (IFN-γ). IFN-γ was expressed by the CD68 positive macrophages (Kitagawa M et al., 1997). Fas antigen, a proapoptotic factor, was found to be up-regulated in BMMNC (Bouscary et al., 1997).

CYTOKINE PROFILE IN PERIPHERAL BLOOD

Serum GM-CSF was rarely detected in MDS patients (Sallerfors et al., 1991). The absence of GM-CSF in the serum may suggest a local production of this cytokine in the BM (Cebon et al., 1990). In contrast, Granulocyte colony stimulating factor (G-CSF) was detectable in the serum of MDS patients and its level were almost 5 times higher in MDS as compared to normal (Verhoef et al., 1992). Intriguingly, high levels of GCSF have been reported in other ineffective hematopoiesis conditions such as, cyclic neutropenia (Misago et al., 1991) and aplastic anemia (Watari et al., 1989). Unlike both these diseases, in MDS however, no correlation between changes in GCSF levels and neutrophil count was found. Therefore, in MDS impairment in the feedback loop of this cytokine has been suspected (Verhoef et al., 1992). Serum MCSF level in MDS patients was 1.8 times higher than normal serum level (unpublished data). Erythropoietin, the principal factor responsible for regulating red blood cell production is also found in increased amounts in MDS patients (Aul et al., 1991; Verhoef et al., 1992). The increased levels negatively correlated with hemoglobin concentration. It has been postulated that the high levels may be a result of a higher production due to decrease in the sensitivity of the erythroid progenitor cells or decreased consumption (Jacobs et al., 1989; Akoi et al., 1992). IL-1β has a wide range of target cells including hematopoietic cells of lymphoid and myeloid origin and fibroblast (Dinarello CA, 1991). IL-1 β was not detected in serum of MDS patients (unpublished data). However, BMMNC cultures from MDS patients were shown to have increased amounts of IL-1 β that positively correlated with the levels of apoptosis in the culture. Interestingly however, blocking IL-1β with IL-1β ra or specific antibodies did not decrease apoptosis. It was also found that interleukin-1β converting enzyme, that converts pro IL-1β to its active form, was involved in apoptosis and increased IL-1β may simply reflect its enhanced activity (Mundle et al., 1996). Another interesting cytokine that is a promoter of hematopoiesis and is found in elevated levels in the serum of MDS patients is interleukin 6 (Herold et al., 1992). RAEB-t patients have significantly higher IL-6 levels than RA, RAEB and CMMoL. No significant difference was seen among the other FAB subtypes. The serum TNFα level was 1.5 times higher in MDS as compared to normal (Allampallam et al., 1997). It was also found that TNFα levels negatively correlated with hemoglobin levels suggesting its relation to the cause of anemia (Verhoef et al., 1992). TNFα mediates its biological effects through its membrane bound receptors TNF-RI (p55) and TNF-RII (p75). The cells shed the extra-cellular domain of both these receptors that bind to the soluble TNF-α, thus inhibiting its action (Jacobsen et al., 1994). In MDS patients, elevated levels of serum TNFα receptors (TNFα RI: 1.5 fold; TNFα RII: 1.4 fold) have been shown. Also, the high-risk group (RAEB/RAEBt/CMMoL) had a significantly higher TNFα receptor levels than the low risk group (RA/RARS) (Allampallam et al., 1997). In MDS, high level of flt3L has been demonstrated in RA while other FAB types show normal levels (Zwierzina et al., 1999). Also, in-vitro culture studies have demonstrated that absence of flt3L correlates with high incidence of apoptosis in MDS patients (Shetty et al., 1998). Moreover, Flt 3 ligand counteracts the TNFα induced apoptosis (Shetty et al., 1997).

ROLE OF CYTOKINE IN DISEASE

Peripheral cytopenia in MDS was thought to be a result of a failing BM. Stimulation of the normal pluripotent stem cells could avert the dysplasia; this is the premise for using growth factors in the treatment of MDS (Ganser et al., 1992). In the recent years, it has been demonstrated not only the proliferation rate of cells in the bone marrow is high but also the rate of apoptosis is very high as compared to normals (Raza et al., 1995a; Raza et al., 1995). An altered cytokine milieu has been suggested to be the cause of both these events. In the bone marrow, IL-1β, TNFα and TGFβ, all proinflammatory and proapoptotic, are expressed in high levels where as the survival factors such as flt3 L and GM-CSF are expressed at low or at levels comparable to normal. This increased presence of proapoptotic factors supports the hypothesis that these cytokines may be responsible for the excessive intramedullary apoptosis.

In the peripheral blood there is increase in the levels of both proapoptotic and stimulatory cytokines while in the bone marrow the increase is seen only in the proapoptotic cytokines. This imbalance may suggest different sources of these cytokines. The origin of these cytokines may thus lie in the bone marrow hematopoietic cells or in accessory cells, or in the other organs of the body. The expression pattern of these cytokines and their receptors in relation to the stage of the disease is also very interesting. For example, flt3 L is present at high levels in the early stages of the disease (RA) but returns to normal level in later stages (RAEB, RAEB-t). The levels of TNFα receptors, TNFαRI and RII, increased as the disease progressed from RA to RAEB-t. Such expression patterns do suggest some clinical role. Flt3 L is a good stimulant for the expansion of potent antigen presenting cells like dendritic cells. Thus, the increase in flt3L might be the response of the immune system to suppress the abnormal clone or any foreign agent that elicited the reaction (Zwierzina et al., 1999). Also, the high level of TNFα receptor released by the cell may be an attempt to neutralize the high levels of TNF α seen in MDS patients. The abnormal cytokine levels might also indicate the functional status of a specific organ. For example, serum flt3L level has been suggested as a sensor for hypoplasia of the bone marrow (Filipowicz et al., 1996). The abnormal cytokine and its receptor levels could also serve as important prognostic markers to measure the progress of the disease and reliable indicators of disease activity in individual patients.

In MDS, increased numbers of activated cytotoxic lymphocytes and circulating immune complexes, increase in natural killer cell activity and T-helper cell lymphopenia are seen, indicating a non-specific immune dysfunction (Colombat et al., 1988; Enright et al., 1995). High levels of macrophages, increase in proinflammatory cytokine levels like TNFα, hypocholesterimia coupled with high MCSF levels, high levels of proliferation and apoptosis in hematopoietic cell in the bone marrow all point towards a hyperactive BM and an inflammatory process. The reaction could be a response to a viral infection. Association of MDS and viruses has been demonstrated on previous occasions (Krueger et al., 1994; Miyahara et al., 1997; Mundle et al., 2001). Based on the above observations it is hypothesized that MDS can begin as a viral disease (Raza, 1998a & b). The chronic inflammatory reaction seen in MDS might be the physiological response the body is mounting to the virus challenge. Over the years this may lead to an abnormal BM microenvironment leading to extensive apoptosis and also favoring the expansion of a defective clone.

In summary, there is increased expression of proapoptotic cytokines in the bone marrow of MDS patients. This seems to be responsible for the excessive apoptosis resulting in peripheral cytopenia. Treatments targeted at neutralizing these proapoptotic forces look very promising.

Table 1. *Comparative study of cytokines in MDS & Normal*

	Normal	**MDS**
Transcripts levels in Parenchymal Cells	**Detected using RT-PCR**	
Flt 3 Ligand	D	Same
Flt3 receptor	D	High
IL-1 ra	D	High
IL-1β	D	High
MCSF	D	High
TNFα	D	Same
BM biopsy (Protein)	**Immunohistochemistry**	
GM-CSF	D	Same
TNFα	D (low)	D (low to high)
TGFβ	D (low)	D (high)
Serum (Protein)	**ELISA**	
GM-CSF	ND	Low
G-CSF	8.14 - 11.4 pg/ml	High
IL-6	ND	High
MCSF	263 - 829 pg/ml	High
Erythropoietin	3.3 - 16.6 mU/ml	High
TNFα	2.89 - 13.76 pg/ml	High
TNFα RI	772 - 1562 pg/ml	High
TNF α RII	1611 - 3244 pg/ml	High
TGFβ	23841 - 63891 pg/ml	Low
IFN α	0 - 130 ng/ml	High
Flt3 ligand	2.2 - 97 pg/ml	High

Legend: 'ND': Not detectable; 'D': Detected

REFERENCES

Allampallam K, Shetty V, Dar S, Hussaini S, Cartilidge J, Broderick E, Townsend W, Qawi H, Mazzoran L, Mahamood W, Mundle S, Reza S, Gundroo A, Yakoob L, Robinson L, Preisler H & Raza A. (1997) Elevated levels of serum tumor necrosis factor receptors in myelodysplastic syndrome, *Blood*, **92**, Abst. # 1743, 422a.

Allampallam K, Shetty V, Hussaini S, Mazzoran L, Zorat F, Huang R & Raza A (1999). Measurement of mRNA expression for a variety of cytokines and its receptors in bone marrows of patients with myelodysplastic syndromes. *Anticancer Research,* **19**,5323-5328.

Allampallam K, Shetty V, Broady Robinson L, Hussaini S., Broderick E, Mundle S, Reddy P, Dar S, Zaidi A, Nascimben F & Raza A (2000). The clinical and biological significance of apoptosis, macrophages and cytokines in 145 patients with myelodysplastic syndromes. *Blood*, **96**,Abst # 1550, 359a.

Akoi I, Higashi K, Homori M, Chikazawa H & Ishikawa K. (1990). Responsiveness of bone marrow erythorpoietic stem cells (CFU-E and BFU-E) to recombinant human erythropoietin (rhEP) in vitro in aplastic anemia and myelodysplastic syndrome. *American Journal Hematology,* **35**, 6-12.

Aul C, Arming M, Runde V & Schneider W (1991) Serum erythropoietin concentrations in patients with myelodysplastic syndromes. *Leukemia Research,* **15**, 571-575.

Birg F, Rosnet O, Carbuccia N & Birnbaum D.(1994). The expression of FMS, Kit and Flt3 in hematopoietic malignancies. *Leukemia and Lymphoma,* **13**, 223-227

Bouscary, D., de Vos, J., Guesnu, M., Jondeau, K., Viguier, F., Melle, J., Picard, F., Dreyfus, F., & Fontenay-Roupie, M. (1997) Fas/Apo-1 (CD95) expression and apoptosis in patients with myelodysplastic syndromes. *Leukemia*, **11**, 839-845..

Cebon JS & Morstyn G (1990). The potential role of granulocyte macrophage colony stimulating factor (GM-CSF) in cancer chemotherapy. Cancer Survey, **9**, 131-155.

Colombat PH, Renouos M, Lamagnere JP & Renous G (1988). Immunologic indices in myelodysplastic syndromes. *Cancer*, **61**, 1075-1081.

Dinarello CA. (1991). Interleukin-1 and interleukin-1 antagonism , *Blood*, **77**,1627-1652.

Enright H, Jacob HS, Vercellotti G, Howe R, Belzer M & Mitter W (1995). Paraneoplastic autoimmune phenomena in patients with myelodysplastic syndromes: response to immunosuppressive therapy. *British Journal of Haematology*, **91**, 403-408.

Filipowicz AW, Lynman SD, Gratwohl A, Tichelli A, Speck B & Nissen C (1996). Flt3 ligand level reflects hematopoietic progenitor cell function in aplastic anemia and chemotherapy-induced bone marrow aplasia. *Blood,***88**,4493-5599.

Gancer A & Hoelzer D (1992). Treatment of myelodysplastic syndromes iwht hematopoietic growth factors. *Hematology Oncology Clinics of North America* , **6**, 633-653.

Gersuk, G.M., Beckham, C., Loken, M.R.Kiener, P., Anderson, J.E., Ferrand, A., Troutt, A.E., Ledbetter, J.A., & Deeg, H.J. (1998) A role for tumor necrosis factor-α, Fas and Fas-ligand in marrow failure associated with myelodysplastic syndrome. *British Journal of Haematology*, **103**, 176-188.

Herold M, Schmalzl R & Swierzina H (1992). Increased serum interleukin 6 levels in patients with myelodysplastic syndrome, Leukemia Research, **16**, 585-588.

Jacobsen SEW, Jacobsen FW, Fahlman C and Rusten LS (1994). TNF-α, the great imitator: role of p55 and p75 TNF receptors in hematopoiesis. *Stem Cells,* **12**, 111-128.

Jacobs A, Janawska-Wieczorek A, Caro J, Bowen DT, Lewis T (1989). Circulating erythropoietin in patients with myelodysplastic syndromes. *British Journal of Haematology*, **73**,36-39.

Kitagawa M, Saito I, Kuwata T, Yoshida S, Yamaguchi S, Takahashi M, Tanizawa T, Kawiyama R, & Hirokawa K. (1997). Overexpression of tumor necrosis factor (TNF)- alpha and interferon gamma by bone marrow cells from patients with myelodysplastic syndromes. *Leukemia,* **11**, 2049-2054.

Krueger GRF, Kudlimay D, Ramon A, Klyepperlbert U & Schumacher K (1994). Demonstration of active and latent Epstein-Barr virus and human herpes virus-6 infections in bone marrow cells of patients with myelodysplastic and chronic myeloproliferative diseases. *In Vivo*, **8**,533-542.

Misago M, Kikuchi M, Tsukada J, Hanamura T, Kamachi S, Eto S. (1991). Serum levels of G-CSF, M-CSF and GM-CSF in a patient with cyclic neutropenia. *American Journal of Hematology* ,**37**, 312-313.

Miyahara M, Shimamoto Y, Yamada H, Shibata K & Matsuzaki K O. (1997) Cytomegalovirus-associated myelodysplasia and thrombocytopenia in an immunocompetent adult. *Annals of Hematology*, **74**, 99-101.

Mundle, S., Venugopal., P., Cartlidge, J., Pandav, D., Broady-Robinson, L., gezer, S., Robin, E., Rifkin, S., Klein, M., Alston, D., Hernandez, B., Rosi, D., Alvi, S., Shetty, V., Gregory, S., & Raza, A. (1996) Indication of an involvement of interleukin-1b converting enzyme-like protease in intramedullary apoptotic cell death in the bone marrow of patients with myelodysplastic syndromes (MDS). *Blood*, **88**, 2640-2647.

Mundle S, Allampallam K, Rashid KA, Dangerfield B, Cartlidge J, Zeitler D, Afenya E, Alvi S, Shetty V, Venugopal P & Raza A. (2001) Presence of activation-related m-RNA for EBV and CMV in the bone marrow of patients with myelodysplastic syndromes *Cancer Letters*, **164**, 197-205.

Qadir K, Bokhari SAJ, Miller MA, Siegrist C, Bismayer J & Raza A. (1992) In situ localization of Transforming growth factor beta and S-phase cells in patients with acute myeloid leukemia and myelodysplastic syndrome. *AntiCancer Research,* **12**,403-408.

Raza A, Gezer S, Mundle S, Gao X-Z, Alvi S, Borok R, Rifkin S, Iftikhar A, Shetty V, Parcharidou A, Loew J, Marcus B, Khan Z, Chaney C, Showel J, Gregory S & Preisler H.(1995a). Apoptosis in bone marrow biopsy samples involving stromal and hematopoietic cells in 50 patients with myelodysplastic syndromes. *Blood*, **86**, 268-276.

Raza A, Mundle S, Iftikhar A, Gregory S, Marcus B, Khan Z, Alvi S, Dameron S, Wright V, Adler S, Loew J, Schoot S, Ali N & Preisler H. (1995) Simultaneous assessment of cell kinetics and programmed cell death in bone marrow biopsies of myelodysplastic reveals extensive apoptosis as the probable basis for ineffective hematopoiesis. *American Journal of Hematology*, **48**,143-154.

Raza A (1998a) Hypothesis: myelodysplastic syndromes may have a viral etiology. *International Journal of Hematology*, **68**, 245-256.

Raza A (1998b) Initial transforming even in myelodysplastic syndromes may be viral: case for cytomegalovirus. *Medical Oncology*, **15**, 166-173.

Sallerfors B & Olofsson T (1991). Granulocyte-macrophave colony stimulating factor (GM-CSF) and granulocyte colony-stimulating factor (G-CSF) in serum during induction treatment of acute leukaemia. *British Journal of Haematology* , **78**, 343-351.

Shetty V, Allampllam K, Hussaini S, Ali A, Mundle S, Akhtar A, Cartlidge J, Mativi B, Qawi H, Venugopal P & Raza A (1998). Absence of flt3 ligand correlates with high incidence of apoptosis in myelodysplastic syndrome (MDS) *Proceedings of American Association of Cancer Research*, **39**, 142-143, abstr# 973.

Shetty V. , Hussaini S, .Borady-Robinson L, Gao X, Dar S, Mundle S, Cartlidge J, Bagai K, Showel M, Andrews C, Akhtar A, Ali A, Mativi BY, Venugopal P, Chopra H, Bi S, Gregory SA, Preisler H and Raza A. (1997) Suppression of tumor necrosis factor – alpha (TNF-α) induced apoptosis by Flt-3 ligand in myelodysplastic syndromes (MDS) and HL-60 cells. *Blood,* **90**, 203a, abstr # 894.

Shetty, V., Mundle, S., Alvi, S., Showel, M., Broady-Robinson, L., Dar, S., Borok, R., Showel, J., Gregory, S., Rifkin, S., Gezer, S., Parcharidou, A., Venugopal, P., Shah, R., Hernandez, B., Klein, M., Alston, D., Robin, E., Dominguez, C. & Raza, A. (1996) Measurement of apoptosis, proliferation and three cytokines in 46 patients with myelodysplastic syndromes. *Leukemia Research,* **20**, 891-900.

Verhoef GEG, Schowwer DP, Ceuppens JL, Damme JV, Goossens W & Boogaerts MA (1992). Measurement of serum cytokine levels in patients with myelodysplastic syndromes. *Leukemia,* **6**,1268-1272.

Watari K, Asano S, Shirafuiji J, Kodo H, Ozawa K, Takaku F. & Kamanchi S, (1989). Serum granulocyte colony stimulating factor levels in healthy volunteers and patients with various disorders as estimated by enzyme immunoassay. *Blood*, **73**,117-122.

Zwierzina H, Anderson JE< Holzinger RI, Storb TB, Nuessler V & Lyman SD (1999). Endogenous Flt-3 ligand serum levels are associated with disease stage in patients with myelodysplastic syndromes. *Leukemia* , **13**, 553-557.

7

APOPTOSIS IN MDS: A NEW PERSPECTIVE

Suneel D. Mundle
MDS Center and Section of Myeloid Diseases, Department of Medicine
Rush University, Chicago, IL

As described in many chapters in this volume it is evident that excessive intramedullary apoptosis constitutes a salient feature of the pathobiology of myelodysplastic syndromes (MDS). Since the first indication of increased apoptosis upon examining the bone marrow (BM) histology in 1990 by Clark and Lampert, followed by histochemical demonstration by our group in 1994-95 (Mundle et al., 1994a and b; Raza et al., 1995a and b), a number of studies using a variety of techniques in independent demographic populations around the globe have repeatedly confirmed this finding (Yoshida & Mufti, 1999). In spite of such an endorsement, it must be acknowledged that as pointed out by Dar et al. (1999), exceptions to this rule showing undetectable apoptosis are also commonly found in MDS. In cases with high apoptosis, the most striking feature is the engagement of all types of hematopoietic and stromal cells in the apoptotic death process. As a result the presence of an apoptosis-inducing microenvironmental factor(s) with a wide range of target cells was suspected. Different studies have revealed exceedingly high levels of proinflammatory factors like tumor necrosis factor alpha (TNFα), interferon gamma (IFN γ), interleukin (IL) 1 and 6, etc. (Mundle et al., 1996; Shetty et al., 1996; Kitagawa et al., 1997; Gersuk et al., 1998; Deeg et al., 2000). Subsequent studies highlighted TNFα as probably the most apical trigger of apoptosis in MDS (Mundle et al., 1999 a and b).

TNFα: THE DEATH SWITCH IN MDS

TNF α is known to induce apoptosis in a wide variety of parenchymal and mesenchymal cells and as mentioned above, has been shown to be present in exceedingly high amounts in the BM interstitium as well as in the peripheral blood of MDS patients (Shetty et al., 1996; Gersuk et al., 1998). The exact cell of origin of TNFα is still not clearly demonstrated, but recent studies indicate that it may come from the cell type belonging to the mononuclear cell fraction of the BM aspirate (BMMNC) of these patients (Gupta et al., 1999; Deeg et al., 2000). The amounts of TNFα secreted by BMMNC are significantly higher than the normal BMMNC and rather mimic those secreted by the latter after stimulation with monoclonal antibody ligation of HLA-DR antigen (Deeg et al., 2000). The apoptotic signaling by TNFα may occur via a secondary signaling system, viz. Fas/Fas-ligand (Fas L). This is why perhaps neutralization of only TNFα does not successfully alleviate growth inhibitory effect seen in MDS marrows (Gupta et al., 1999). TNFα and IFNγ are known to enhance the expression of Fas and Fas-L on the surface of a variety of cells (Dai et al., 1998; Bretz et al., 1999; Moulian et al., 1999). Additionally as we reported in HL60 promyelocytic cells, TNFα downregulates the negative regulator of Fas called Fas-associated phosphatase 1 (Fap-1) (Mundle et al., 1999a). In many MDS patients on one hand Fas and Fas-L are reportedly present in high amounts in the BM (Gersuk et al., 1996; Bouscary et al., 1997; Kitagawa et al., 1998; Fontenay-Roupie et al., 1999; Gupta et al., 1999) and on the other hand Fap-1 is either undetectable (Gersuk et al., 1998) or shows rapid turnover (Mundle et al., 1999a). The abrogation of Fap-1 regulation may set in the Fas mediated signal causing subsequent activation of the apoptosis-executing machinery of proteolytic enzymes called Caspases (Cysteine aspartases). Our group and others have demonstrated participation of at least 2 caspases in the process of apoptosis in MDS (Mundle et al., 1996; Ali et al., 1999; Mundle et al., 1999b; Bouscary et al., 2000; Matthes et al., 2000). Interestingly, these 2 caspases appear to be activated sequentially, where caspase 1-activity (or IL1β converting enzyme/ICE) peaks first followed by the increase in caspase 3 (apopain/Yama) enzyme activity with a definite time interval between the two peaks (Ali et al., 1999). The increased levels of TNFα, Fas/Fas-L, Caspases, and apoptosis, and lowered Fap-1 levels have been shown to be significantly correlated and interlinked in the above-mentioned studies. Intervention of this pathway by blocking Fas, Fas-L with specific antagonistic antibodies or recombinant FasFc protein, or by inhibiting caspase activity with specific tetrapeptide inhibitors of Caspase 1 and 3, led to suppression of apoptosis and improvement in the growth characteristics of the BMMNC in MDS marrows (Mundle et al., 1996; Gersuk et al., 1998; Ali et al., 1999; Gupta et al., 1999; Mundle et al., 1999a). These observations thus confirmed the involvement of TNFα induced Fas/Fas-L mediated pathway of apoptosis in MDS that is triggered by abrogation of Fap-1 regulation and executed by Caspase activation.

Apoptosis in most MDS patients seems to be cell cycle-independent. Our group demonstrated that in some patients however, the proportion of S-phase cells engaged in apoptosis is substantially increased (Mundle et al., 1994a and b; Raza et al., 1995a and b) and this phenomenon called "Signal Antonymy," appears to be characteristically found in MDS (Mundle et al., 2000). Interestingly, preliminary studies have revealed a novel molecular abnormality, viz. altered expression of a transcription factor E2F1, linked with Signal Antonymy in MDS (Mundle et al., 2000).

APOPTOSIS IN RELATION TO DIFFERENTIATION STATUS AND DISEASE PROGRESSION

MDS is considered to be a stem cell disorder and hence attempts have been made by different groups to estimate the rates of apoptosis in immature progenitor cells and in cells with different differentiation markers. Owing to high apoptosis in general and poor yield of CD34+ cells from BMMNC of MDS patients, studies on separated subfractions of CD34+ cells are extremely rare. Flow cytometric studies detecting different parameters of apoptosis simultaneously with localization of CD34+ phenotype have demonstrated varying degree of apoptosis (Rajapaksa et al., 1996; Mundle et al., 1999c, Parker et al., 1998 and 2000) with a median comparable to that observed in maturing/matured CD34- cells. Furthermore, in some of these studies, a significant reduction in the rates of apoptosis in the CD34+ population has been noted in patients in transformation to acute myelogenous leukemia (AML; Parker et al., 2000). On the other hand, when separated CD34+ cells were assessed in isolation from CD34- cells, the propensity to undergo apoptosis was negligible in the former and retained higher in the latter (Anzai et al,, 1997; Mundle et al,, 1999c). Corroborating with these results, when colony formation was assessed in BMMNC vs. CD34+ cells or its subfractions, while BMMNC consistently failed, the purified progenitors showed significant growth (Hoffman et al, 1998). On the other hand, Brada et al. (1998) have reported that sorted CD34+/CD36- cells from MDS patients demonstrated only a limited clonogenic potential in response to erythropoietin and mast cell growth factor. It thus appears that in early MDS (stages prior to finding excess blasts in transformation) the susceptibility to undergo apoptosis may vary in immature CD34+ progeny of the MDS stem cell(s), but clearly the maturing CD34- cells and more importantly high density BM aspirate cells constituting matured fraction show significant proclivity to apoptotic death (Lepelley et al., 1996; Mundle et al., 1999c; Shetty et al., 2000). With the progression of the disease towards transformation an increase in the numbers of apoptosis resistant CD34+ cells is noted (Rajapaksa et al., 1996;Parker et al., 1998 and 2000), while the maturing and matured cells continue to demonstrate increased apoptosis (Raza et al., 1995a and b). In MDS differentiated cells are seen at all stages and as Horikawa et al. (1997) showed such cells in the peripheral blood are resistant to apoptosis especially induced by Fas. It is possible that the lack of susceptibility to apoptosis in these cells be an inherent property and these cells may represent the progeny of the early progenitor CD34+ cells that are non-responsive to Fas apoptotic stimulus in the BM (Horikawa et al., 1997). Thus the CD34+ subclones of the original MDS stem cell may reveal a spectrum of susceptibility to apoptosis.

KINETICS OF PRO- AND ANTI-APOPTOTIC FACTORS IN THE COURSE OF MDS

The mechanism of apoptosis in MDS is bipartite and depends on one hand on the availability of the extracellular stimuli and on the other hand relies on the stoichiometry of the intracellular susceptibility-determinants. As shown by many studies TNFα and Fas-L may serve as the primary stimuli, which may plausibly come from BMMNC (Bouscary et al., 1997; Gersuk et al., 1998; Gupta et al., 1999; Deeg et al., 2000). The possibility of adherent stromal origin of these stimuli appears to be remote at this point (Deeg et al., 2000). Of the determinants of susceptibility, density of Fas expression on the surface of different cells seems to vary and would largely be modulated by the microenvironmental factors like TNFα, IFNγ and IL1β (Dai et al., 1998). The degree of Fas expression on CD34+ cells correlated positively with the levels of apoptosis in the study by Fontenay-Roupie,et al. (1999). At the next step of Fas signaling lies the major susceptibility determinant, Fap-1; a negative regulator of Fas. Again, the levels of Fap-1 and its turnover rate would contribute immensely to the relative propensity of individual cells to undergo apoptosis (Gersuk et al., 1998; Mundle et al., 1999a). Stable high levels of Fap-1 have been reported following transformation correlating with dismal apoptosis shown by the leukemic BMMNC (Mundle et al., 1999a). Two other downstream regulators of apoptosis thus far identified in MDS are bcl-2 and p53 (Davis and Greenberg, 1998; Kurotaki et al., 1999; Parker et al., 2000). Interestingly, cytoplasmic bcl-2 was primarily detected in immature myeloid cells and was undetectable in matured granulocytes and monocytes (Kurotaki et al., 1999). The levels of bcl-2 expression appear to increase with the increased blast count at the advanced stages of the disease (Davis and Greenberg, 1998; Kurotaki et al., 1999; Parker et al., 2000). Similarly Kurotaki et al.'s studies also demonstrated that detectibility of p53 protein icnreased with disease progression which is in line with the increased rates of p53 mutations at advanced stages discussed by A. McGlynn, H. McGlynn and R.A. Padua in this book.

The rate of proliferation does not seem to change much over the course of MDS and perhaps slightly decreases at and upon transformation (Raza et al., 1992; Parker et al., 2000). In contrast, a change in the ability to differentiate seems highly likely. The BMMNC of MDS cells appear to retain the ability to differentiate by virtue of the intact erythropoietin responsive STAT-5 activation (Fontenay-Roupie et al., 1999). Thus in the initial phases of MDS if the cells escape infliction of apoptosis, can differentiate and enter circulation (Horikawa et al., 1997). At transforamtion of MDS to AML, the increase in the number of CD34+ cells showing low Fas expression, high bcl-2 levels (and/or Fap-1, etc.) and, resultantly low propensity for apoptosis, as noted in different above-mentioned investigations, may indicate a block in differentiation occurring as a secondary major event(s) on the background of low susceptibility to apoptosis.

It thus appears that pro-apoptotic stimuli dominate the scene at the early stages of MDS, but the survival advantage provided by the determinants of susceptibility to apoptotic death provide grounds for clonal expansion, accumulation of additional abnormalities and eventual leukemic transformation.

POSTULATE FOR THE ROLE OF APOPTOSIS IN MDS AND MDS-DERIVED AML

The varying incidence of apoptosis in CD34+ subclones of the original MDS stem cell in the BM of MDS patients reported by different investigators may likely imply an existence of a spectrum of susceptibility to apoptosis in these cells constituting a combination of suboptimal and abnormal hematopoiesis in these patients. The BM microenvironment in MDS patients shows increased numbers of different immune cells like macrophages and mast cells, NK cells, subsets of T cells, B cell aggregates, etc., and their inflammatory cytokines like TNFα, IFNγ, IL1β, IL6, TGFβ, etc (Ganser A., 1999). It appears that the apoptosis inducing activity may reside in the BMMNC and more likely in the CD34- maturing/matured fraction of BMMNC. Although the exact cell of origin of the apoptosis inducing activity still awaits confirmation, the final pathway appears to involve TNFα initiated, Fas/Fas-L-mediated signal that is transduced intracellularly as a result of either rapid turnover or a lack of the negative regulator; Fas associated phosphatase-1 (Fap-1) and eventually via sequential activation of Caspases. An additional abnormality in a transcription factor; E2F1 could shift the otherwise cell-cycle independent apoptosis to S-phase (Signal Antonymy). Differential susceptibility to apoptosis of the MDS subclones may be related to varying stoichiometry of the antiapoptotic proteins like Fap-1, bcl-2, etc.

The relatively non-susceptible cells seem to differentiate and contribute to the peripheral blood cell pool. It is possible that the leukemic transformation would occur due to a secondary event(s) blocking differentiation on the background of non-susceptibility to apoptosis (Figure 1).

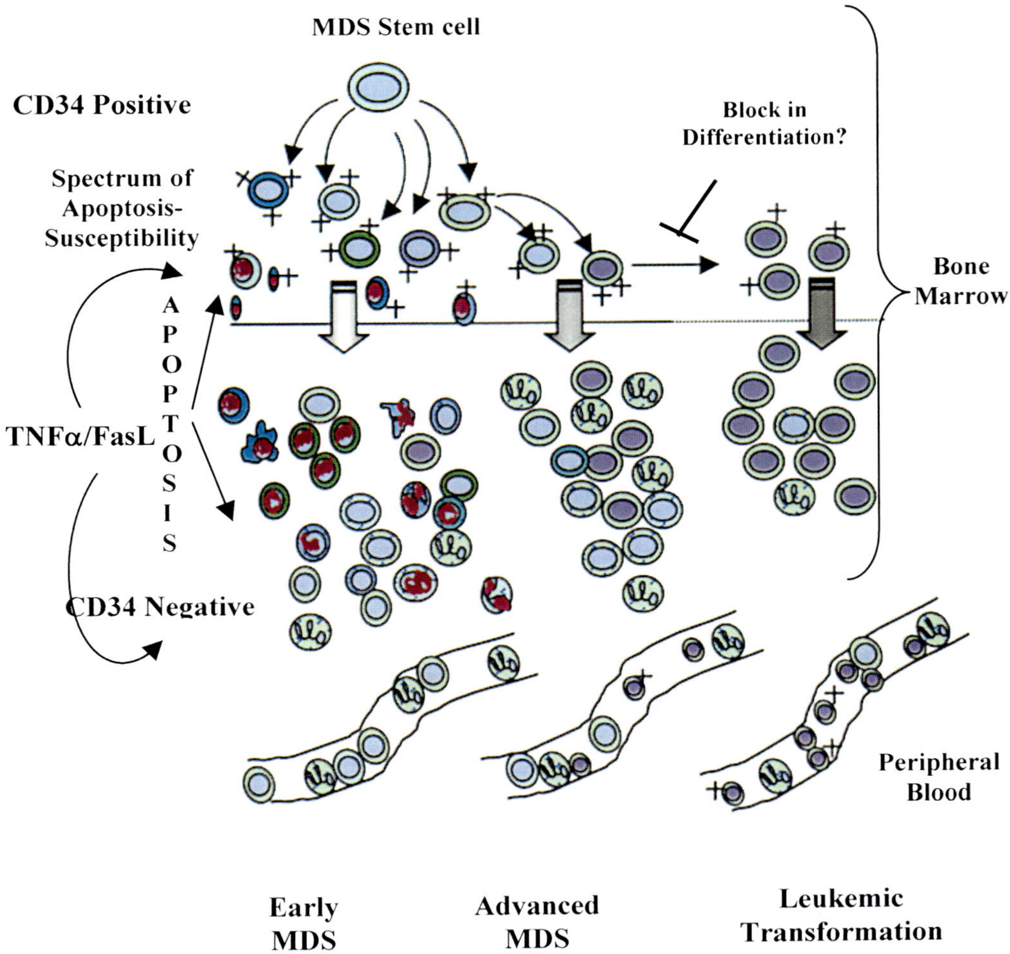

Figure 1. Combined role of apoptosis-effectors and susceptibility determinants in the pathobiology of MDS. The apoptotic signals like TNFα and FasL may come from BMMNC (CD34-). The CD34+ subclones of the parent MDS stem cell may show a spectrum of apoptosis-susceptibility (Different cytoplasmic colors indicative of varying stoichiometry of antiapoptotic proteins-green being the least susceptible to apoptosis). Dark brown nuclei indicate apoptotic death. Secondary event may block differentiation (dark purple nucleus and green cytoplasm) and subsequent expansion of this clone may mark leukemic transformation.

The real therapeutically relevant challenge in the arena of apoptosis in MDS thus lies in unraveling the origin and bases for TNFα/Fas mediated cytopathic effects and, also in delineating the bases for and types of determinants of differential susceptibility to apoptosis in MDS subclones.

REFERENCES

Ali, A., Mundle, S.D., Ragasa, D., Reza, S., Shetty, V., Mativi, B.Y., Cartlidge, J.D., Azharuddin, M., Qawi, H., Dar, S., & Raza, A. (1999) Sequential activation of Caspase-1 and Caspase-3-like proteases during apoptosis in myelodysplastic syndromes. *Journal of Hematotherapy & Stem Cell research*, **8**, 343-356.

Anzai, N., Kawabata, H., Hishita, T., Yoshida, Y., Ueda, Y., & Okuma, M. (1997) Ca^{2+}/Mg^{2+}-dependent endonuclease in marrow CD34 positive and erythroid cells in myelodysplasia. *Leukemia Research*, **21**, 731-734.

Bouscary, D., de Vos, J., Guesnu, M., Jondeau, K., Viguier, F., Melle, J., Picard, F., Dreyfus, F., & Fontenay-Roupie, M. (1997) Fas/Apo-1 (CD95) expression and apoptosis in patients with myelodysplastic syndromes. *Leukemia*, **11**, 839-845.

Bouscary, D., Chen, Y.L., Guesnu, M., Picard, F., Viguier, F., Lacombe, C., Dreyfus, F. & Fontenay-Roupie, M. (2000) Activity of the caspase-3/CPP32 enzyme is increased in "early stage" myelodysplastic syndromes with excessive apoptosis, but caspase inhibition does not enhance colony formation in vitro. *Experimental Hematology*, **28**, 784-791.

Brada, S.J.L., de Wolf, J.Th.W., hendriks, D.W., Smit, J.W. & Vellenga, E. (1998) $CD34^{+}/CD36^{-}$ cells from myelodysplasia patients have a limited capacity to proliferate but can differentiate in response to Epo and MGF stimulation. *Leukemia*, **12**, 882-886.

Bretz, J.D., Arscott, P.L., Myc, A., & Baker, J.R. Jr. (1999) Inflammatory cytokine regulation of Fas-mediated apoptosis in thyroid follicular cells. *Journal of Biological Chemistry*, **274**, 25433-25438.

Clark, D.M. & Lampert, I.A. (1990) Apoptosis is a common histopathological finding in myelodysplsia: the correlate of ineffective hematopoiesis. *Leukemia and Lymphoma*, **2**, 415-418.

Dai, C-H., Price, J.O., Brunner, T., & Krantz, S.B. (1998) Fas ligand is present in human erythroid colony-forming cells and interacts with Fas induced by interferon γ to produce erythroid cell apoptosis. *Blood*, **91**, 1235-1242.

Dar, S. Mundle, S., Andric, T., Qawi, H., Shetty, V., Reza, S., Mativi, B.Y., Allampallam, K., Ali, A., Venugopal, P., Gezer, S., Broady-Robinson, L., Cartlidge J.D., Showel, M., Hussaini, S., Ragasa, D., Ali, I., Chaudhary, A., Waggoner, S., Lisak, L., Huang, R.W., & Raza, A. (1999) Biological characteristics of myelodysplastic syndrome patients who demonstrate high versus no intramedullary apoptosis. *European Journal of Haematology*, **62**, 90-94.

Davis, R.E. & Greenberg, P.L. (1998) Bcl-2 expression by myeloid precursors in myelodysplastic syndromes: relation to disease progression. *Leukemia Research*, **22**, 767-777.

Deeg, H.J., Beckham, C., Loken, M.R., Bryant, E., Lesnikova, M., Shulman, H.M., & Gooley, T. (2000) Negative regulators of hemopoiesis and stroma function in patients with myelodysplastic syndromes. *Leukemia and Lymphoma*, **37**, 405-414.

Fontenay-Roupie, M., Bouscary, D., Guesnu, M., Picard, F., Melle, J., Lacombe, C., Gisselbrecht, S., Mayeux, M., & Dreyfus, F. (1999) Ineffective erythropoiesis in myelodysplastic syndromes: correlation with Fas expression but not with lack of erythropoietin receptor signal transduction. *British Journal of Haematology*, **106**, 464-473.

Ganser, A. (1999) Finally progress in the understanding of myelodysplastic syndromes? *Wiener klinische wochenschrift (the middle european journal of medicine)*, **111/19**, 781-783.

Gersuk, G.M., Lee, L.W., Beckham, C.A., Anderson, J., & Deeg, H.J. (1996) Fas (CD95) receptor and Fas-ligand expression in bone marrow cells from patients with myelodysplastic syndrome [letter]. *Blood*, **88**, 1122-1123.

Gersuk, G.M., Beckham, C., Loken, M.R., Kiener, P., Anderson, J.E., Ferrand, A., Troutt, A.E., Ledbetter, J.A., & Deeg, H.J. (1998) A role for tumor necrosis factor-α, Fas and Fas-ligand in marrow failure associated with myelodysplastic syndrome. *British Journal of Haematology*, **103**, 176-188.

Gupta, P, Niehans, G.A., LeRoy, S.C., Gupta, K., Morrison, V.A., Schultz, C., Knapp, D.J., & Kratzke, R.A. (1999) Fas ligand expression in the bone marrow in myelodysplastic syndromes correlates with FAB subtype and anemia, and predicts survival. *Leukemia*, **13**, 44-53.

Hoffman, R., Fitting, P., Preisler, H., Raza, A., Chyna, B., Horrigan, S., & Westbrook, C. (1998) Analysis of primitive hematopoietic progenitor cells in myelodysplastic syndromes. *Blood*, **92**, sppl.1, 417a; abstract # 1724

Horikawa, K., Nakakuma, H., Kawaguchi, T., iwamoto, N., Nagakura, S., Kagimoto, T., & Taktsuki, K. (1997) Apoptosis resistance of blood cells from patients with Paroxysmal Nocturnal Hemoglobinuria, Aplastic Anemia, and Myelodysplastic syndrome. *Blood*, **90**, 2716-2722.

Kitagawa, M., Saito, I., Kuwata, T., Yoshida, S., Yamaguchi, S., Takahashi, M., Tanizawa, T., Kamiyama, R., & Hirokawa, K. (1997) Overexpression of tumor necrosis factor (TNF)-alpha and interferon (IFN)-gamma by bone marrow cells from patients with myelodysplastic syndromes. *Leukemia*, **11**, 2049-2054.

Kitagawa, M., Yamaguchi, S., Takahashi, M., Tanizawa, T., Hirokawa, K., & Kamiyama, R. (1998) Localization of Fas and Fas ligand in bone marrow cells demonstrating myelodysplasia. *Leukemia*, **12**, 486-492.

Kurotaki, H., Tsushima, Y., Nagai, K., & Yagihashi, S. (1999) Apoptosis, bcl-2 expression and p53 accumulation in myelodysplastic syndrome, myelodysplastic syndrome-derived acute myelogenous leukemia and de novo acute myelogenous leukemia. *Acta Haematologica*, **102**, 115-123.

Lepelley, P, Campergue, L., Grardel, N., Preudhomme, C., Cosson, A., & Fenaux, P. (1996) Is apoptosis a massive process in myelodysplastic syndromes? *British Journal of Haematology*, **95**, 368-371.

Matthes, T.W., Meyer, G., Samii, K., & Beris, P. (2000) Increased apoptosis in acquired sideroblastic anaemia. *British Journal of Haematology*, **111**, 843-852.

Moulian, N., Renovoize, C., Desodt, C., Serraf, A., & Berrih-Aknin, S. (1999) Functional Fas expression in human thymic epithelial cells. *Blood*, **93**, 2660-2670.

Mundle, S., Iftikhar, A., Shetty V., Alvi, S., Dameron, S., Gregory, S., Marcus, B., Khan, S. & Raza, A. (1994a) In situ end labeling of DNA to detect apoptotic cell death in a variety of human tumors. *Cell Death & Differentiation*, **1**, 117-122.

Mundle, S., Iftikhar, A., Shetty V., Dameron, S., Wright-Quinones, V., Marcus, B., Loew, J., Gregory., S., & Raza, A. (1994b) Novel in situ double-labeling for simultaneous detection of proliferation and apoptosis. *Journal of Histochemistry and Cytochemistry*, **42**, 1533-1537.

Mundle, S., Venugopal, P., Cartlidge, J., Pandav, D., Broady-Robinson, L., Gezer, S., Robin, E., Rifkin, S., Klein, M., Alston, D., Hernandez, B., Rosi, D., Alvi, S., Shetty, V., Gregory, S., & Raza, A. (1996) Indication of an involvement of interleukin-1β converting enzyme-like protease in intramedullary apoptotic cell death in the bone marrow of patients with myelodysplastic syndromes (MDS). *Blood*, **88**, 2640-2647.

Mundle, S., Mativi, B.Y., Bagai, K., Feldman, G., Cheema, P., Gautam, U., Reza, S., Cartlidge, J., Venugopal, P., Shetty, V., Gregory S.A., Robin, E., Rifkin, S., Shah, R. & Raza, A. (1999a) Spontaneous down-regulation of Fas-associated phosphatase-1 (Fap-1) may contribute to the excessive apoptosis in myelodysplastic marrows. *International Journal of Hematology*, **70**, 83-90.

Mundle, S., Reza, S., Ali, A., Mativi, B.Y., Shetty, V., Venugopal, P., Gregory, S.A., & Raza, A. (1999b) Correlation of tumor necrosis factor α (TNFα) with high Caspase-3-like activity in myelodysplastic syndromes. *Cancer Letters*, **140**, 201-207.

Mundle, S. Venugopal, P., Shetty, V., Ali., A., Chopra, H., Rose, S., Mativi, B.Y., Gregory, S., Preisler, H. & Raza, A. (1999c) The relative extent and propensity of $CD34^+$ vs. $Cd34^-$ cells to undergo apoptosis in myelodysplastic marrows. *International Journal of Hematology*, **69**, 152-159.

Mundle, S., Mativi, B.Y., Cartlidge, J., Dangerfield, B., Broady-Robinson, L., Li, B., Shetty, V., Venugopal, P., Gregory, S.A., Preisler, H.D. & Raza, A. (2000) Signal antonymy unique to meylodysplastic marrows correlates with altered expression of E2F1. *British Journal of Haematology*, **109**, 376-381.

Parker, J.E., Fishlock, K.L., Czepulkowski, B., Mijovic, a., Pagliuca, A., & Mufti, G.J. (1998) 'Low Risk' myelodysplastic syndrome (MDS) is associated with excessive apoptosis and increased ratio of pro-versus anti-apoptosis bcl-2 related proteins. *British Journal of Haematology*, **103**, 1075-1082.

Parker, J.E., Mufti, G.J., Rasool, F., Mijovic, A., Devereux, S., & Pagliuca, A. (2000) The role of apoptosis, proliferation, and the bcl-2-related proteins in the myelodyspalstic syndromes and acute myeloid leukemia secondary to MDS. *Blood*, **96**, 3932-3938.

Rajapaksa, R., Ginzton, N.,Rott, L.S. & Greenberg, P.L. (1996) Altered oncoprotein expression and apoptosis in myelodysplastic syndrome marrow cells. *Blood*, **88**, 4275-4287.

Raza, A., Yousuf, N., Bohkari, S.A.J., Sheikh, Y., Akhtar, S., Chughtai, S., Umerani, A., Mehdi, S.A., Miller, M.A., Masterson, M., & Lampkin, B. (1992) In situ cell cycle kinetics in bone marrow biopsies following sequential infusions of IUdR/BrdU in patients with hematopoietic malignancies. *Leukemia Research*, **16**, 299-306.

Raza A., Mundle, S., Iftikhar, A., Gregory, S., Marcus, B., Khan, Z., Alvi, S., Shetty, V., Dameron, S., Wright, V., Adler, S., Loew, J., Shott, S., Ali, N., & Preisler, H.D. (1995a) Simultaneous assessment of cell kinetics and programmed cells death in bone marrow biopsies of myelodysplastics reveals extensive apoptosis as the probable basis for ineffective hematopoiesis. *American Journal of Hematology*, **48**,143-154.

Raza, A., Gezer, S., Mundle, S., Borok, R., Rifkin, S., Iftikhar, A., Shetty, V., Parcharidou, A., Loew, J., Alvi, S., Chaney, C., Showel, J., Gregory, S., & Preisler, H.D. (1995b) Apoptosis in bone marrow biopsies involving stromal and hematopoietic cells in 45 patients with myelodysplastic syndromes. *Blood*, **86**, 268-276.

Shetty, V., Mundle, S., Alvi, S., Showel, M., Broady-Robinson, L., Dar, S., Borok, R., Showel, J., Gregory, S., Rifkin, S., Gezer, S., Parcharidou, A., Venugopal, P., Shah, R., Hernandez, B., Klein, M., Alston, D., Robin, E., Dominguez, C. & Raza, A. (1996) Measurement of apoptosis, proliferation and three cytokines in 46 patients with myelodysplastic syndromes. *Leukemia Research*, **20**, 891-900.

Shetty, V., Hussaini, S., Broady-Robinson, L., Allampallam, K., Mundle, S., Borok, R., Cartlidge, J., Broderick, E., Mazzoran, L., Zorat, F., & Raza, A. (2000) Intramedullary apoptosis of hematopietic cells in myelodysplastic syndrome patients can be massive: apoptotic cells recovered from high density fraction of bone marrow aspirates. *Blood*, **96**, 1388-1392.

Yoshida, Y. & Mufti, G.J. (1999) Apoptosis and its significance in MDS: controversies revisited. *Leukemia Research*, **23**, 777-785.

8

MOLECULAR, CYTOGENETIC AND GENETIC ABNORMALITIES IN MDS AND SECONDARY AML

Rose Ann Padua[1], Angela McGlynn[2] and Hugh McGlynn[2],
[1]*Hematology Department, University of Wales College of Medicine, Cardiff , UK*
[2]*Cancer and Ageing Research Group, School of Biomedical Sciences, University of Ulster at Coleraine, UK,*

ABSTRACT

Myelodysplasia (MDS) is a clonal disease, which increases with age, suggesting that multiple steps are required for the evolution of the condition. Approximately 30% of MDS evolve into acute myelogenous leukemia (AML). In this review, we intend to delineate the genetic events, which may drive this sequence and therefore we will focus primarily on cytogenetic abnormalities where the genes have been identified and oncogenes and suppressor genes that have been implicated. In terms of the biological mechanisms, which characterise this process, it is generally thought that the MDS cell has impaired differentiation, and has increased apoptosis. As the disease progresses in addition, the cells have increased proliferation. As the disease evolves, the population of cells, which predominate remain immature, have decreased apoptosis and in many cases, upregulate anti-apoptotic genes and have deregulated proliferation as the number of blast cells increase. Etiological factors, which contribute to the development of leukemia, include therapeutic agents administered for a primary malignancy. The cytogenetic abnormalities, predisposition factors and genes involved in secondary leukemia will also be reviewed.

INTRODUCTION

The biology of MDS suggests that the abnormalities lie in the very primitive progenitors, possibly in a stem cell (see Figure 1 for model). It is thought that an initiating event occurs in such a cell, giving rise to an abnormal clone, which has a selective advantage and expands. This is the stage that is clinically described as MDS or preleukemia. In some cases, given time, progression occurs, which allows a leukemic clone to evolve and give rise to AML. MDS is usually diagnosed in older patients (greater than 60 years) but primary MDS has been reported with increasing frequency in younger patients especially children. Congenital MDS has been reported in a single case with abnormalities in at least two hematological cell lineages (reviewed by Gallagher et al., 1997). Therapy-related MDS and AML following radiotherapy or cytotoxic drug therapy have been reported in all age groups. The etiology of secondary leukemia has been reviewed by Smith et al., (1996). Secondary or therapy-related AML (t-AML) is considered to be a distinct entity from *de novo* AML, accounting for around 10% of AML. Certain therapeutic agents such as those which target topoisomerases are well documented as contributing factors to t-AML (reviewed in Felix, 1998). Although there are changes proposed in the classification of MDS, and the formal definition of AML is now those with >20% blasts as recommended by the World Health Organization (WHO), for the purposes of this review we shall retain the FAB classification when referring to MDS.

CYTOGENETIC ABNORMALITIES

Some 50% of MDS patients have karyotypic non-random abnormalities with frequency increasing with higher risk disease (White et al., 1994; Greenberg et al., 1997). The most common karyotypic lesions involve 5 (loss/deletion), chromosomes 8 (gain), and 7 (loss/deletion), but translocations are rare. Survival of patients with abnormalities involving chromosomes 5, 7, and 8 has been shown to be significantly reduced compared with patients with normal karyotypes (Greenberg et al., 1997; White et al., 1994; Suciu et al.,1990). With the exception of 5q- as a sole abnormality, those with cytogenetic abnormalities have a poor prognosis compared to cytogenetically normal patients. Furthermore, patients with evolving karyotypes have poor outcome compared with those with stable abnormalities (White et al, 1994). It is hardly surprising that patients in the poor prognostic groups of refractory anemia with excess blast (RAEB) and RAEB in transformation (RAEB-t) have a greater number of karyotypic abnormalities than the refractory anemia

(RA) and RA with ringed sideroblasts (RARS) FAB subtypes or chronic myelomonocytic leukemia (CMML). Cytogenetic status is now part of the diagnostic profile of MDS patients and has been incorporated in a number of scoring systems, including the international prognostic scoring systems (IPSS)(Greenberg et al, 1997).

The etiological insults leading to the development of primary MDS and the latency period between the initial genomic insult and disease manifestation are not yet well understood. The best-defined xenobiotic insult in the disease's development is that which follows cytotoxic chemotherapy for cancer with alkylating agents in secondary MDS/AML. Therapy-related MDS (t-MDS) and t-AML is associated with a higher frequency of karyotypic abnormalities than *de novo* MDS/AML (Larson et al 1996; Vanleeuwen, 1996). The majority of these abnormalities involve chromosomes 5 and/or 7, suggesting that these chromosomes are particularly susceptible to genomic damage and that this leads to proliferative advantage. Post-chemotherapy patients do not however, show increased chromosome aberration frequencies compared to normal subjects. Patients who received multiple compared with single courses of therapy, exhibit a higher frequency of exchanges and a lower frequency of gaps (White et al., 1992).

A number of studies have reported associations between histories of exposures to certain organic chemicals, notably benzene and benzene-related solvents, pesticides, and radiation and MDS (West et al., 1995; Nisse et al.,1995; Yin et al., 1996). Benzene has been most consistently implicated in the etiology (Aul et al., 1998; Yin et al., 1996). *In vitro* benzene metabolites induce peripheral blood lymphocyte chromosome 5 and 7 loss and long arm deletion (Zhang et al., 1998) and specifically 5q31 deletion and -7 in CD34+ bone marrow cells (Stillman et al., 2000). Exposure to pesticides and organic solvents have been associated with aberrations in chromosomes 5 and 7 in both AML and MDS (Mitelman et al., 1978; Golomb et al., 1982; Rowley & Golomb, 1984; Fagioli et al., 1992; Crane et al., 1996; Narod & Dube, 1989; Rigolin et al., 1998). Semi-metals particularly arsenic and metals in their chemically reactive states have also been implicated in karotypically abnormal MDS (West et al.,2000).

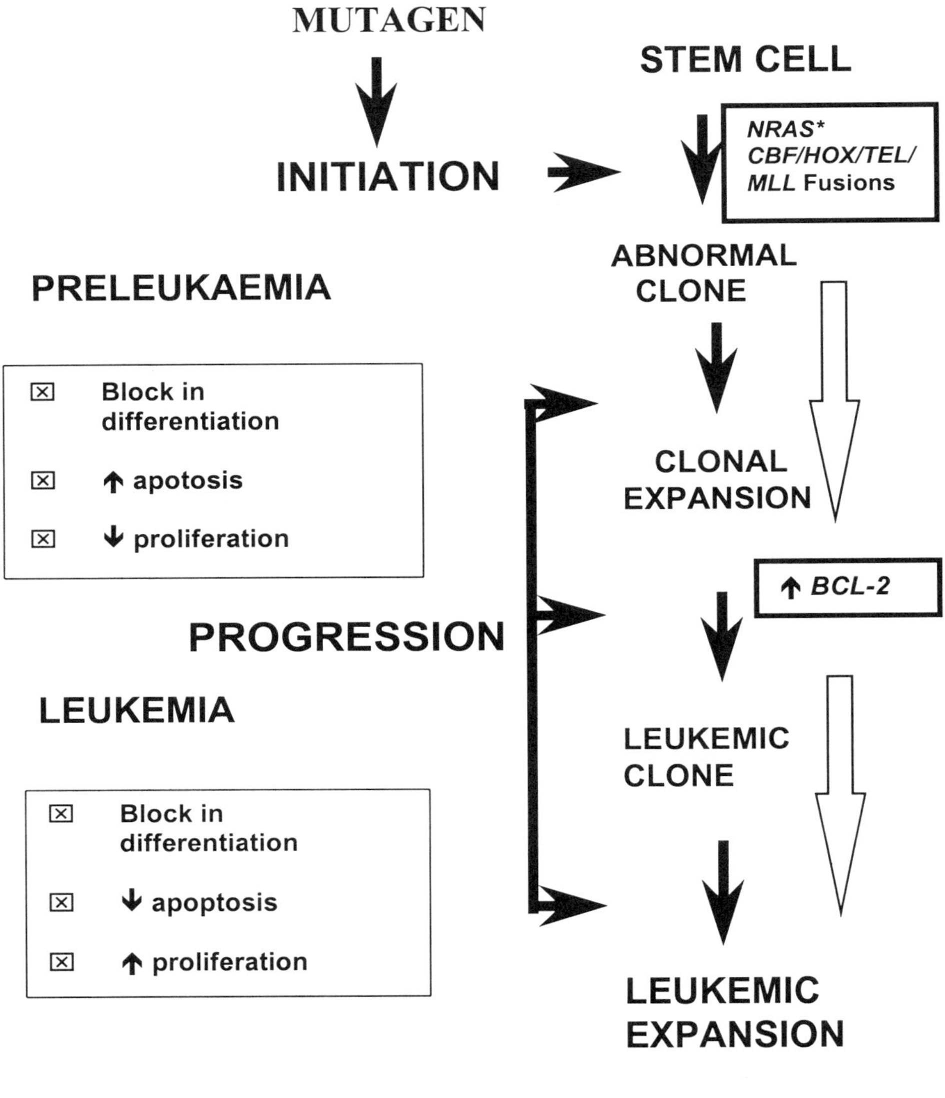

Figure 1. *Model for development of MDS and progression to AML.*

Del(5q)

The 5q- syndrome represents an MDS characterised by interstitial deletions of the long arm of chromosome 5. Clinically RA with a hypercellular marrow with erythroid hypoplasia characterizes this disorder. A high degree of heterogeneity of 5q- occurrence in MDS bone marrow (BM) cells has been reported recently when a combination of loss of heterozygosity (LOH) and fluorescence *in situ* hybridisation (FISH) analysis was used, with not all cells harbouring the lesion (Westbrook et al., 2000a). Combined immunophenotyping and FISH analysis has identified the involvement of B cells in this syndrome (Jaju et al., 2000). Although the limits of the deletions vary among patients, there is a critical region of overlap at 5q31 that is deleted in most cases (review in Gallagher et al., 1997). The frequent (25%) involvement of chromosome 5q in MDS has aroused considerable interest in the mechanism of the involvement of this chromosome in abnormal growth and differentiation underlying leukemogenesis. The 5q- syndrome MDS patients normally have a del(5q) as their sole abnormality, although a novel translocation t(5;11)(q35;p15.5) was shown to be associated with del(5q) in childhood AML, but not MDS (Jaju et al., 1999). In addition, the association of del(5q13.3-qter) and 17p loci in a single patient diagnosed with secondary MDS, suggests a functional co-operation between a putative tumour suppressor gene at 5q13.3, that contributes towards the progression of early stage MDS and upon p53 mutation, causes transformation to AML (Castro et al., 2000). Horrigan et al., (2000), have used LOH analysis to define a minimal deletion interval for this candidate tumour supressor gene, candidates for which were named as *CDC25, HSPA9, EGR1, CTNNA1* and in a separate report, 5qNCA (Westbrook et al., 2000b). Another critical region has been mapped within 5q32 associated with the 5q- syndrome (Jaju et al., 1998, Figure 2) and candidate genes have also been isolated (Boultwood et al., 2000a,b). The *HAH1*, a candidate gene plays a role in antioxidant defence. Antioxidant levels are low in most cancers. Another candidate gene encodes an ATP or GTP-binding protein. 7 other candidate genes, expressed in bone marrow, may also be potential candidates for the 5q- syndrome.

A large number of hematopoietic growth factor and receptor genes are located on the long arm of chromosome 5, for example, IL-3, IL-4, IL-9 and GM-CSF are clustered at the critical region. A list of genes encoded by the region 5q13-q33, is given in Table 1. *SMAD*s are evolutionarily conserved transducers of the differentiation and growth arrest signals from the transforming growth factor BMP (TGF/BMP) family of ligands. Frequent inactivating mutations of *SMAD*4 and *SMAD*2 in solid tumours suggest these genes have a supressor function. *SMAD*5 localizes to the critical region of loss in chromosome 5q31.1 in MDS and AML. The levels of transcript of a novel *SMAD*5beta isoform has been implicated in stem cell homeostasis and has been suggested as a novel mechanism to protect pluripotent stem cells and malignant cells from growth inhibitory and differentiation signals of BMP (Jiang et al., 2000).

Table 1. *Genes localized to chromosome region 5q13-q33.*

Symbol	Gene name
HEXB	Hexosaminidase β
DHFR	Dihydrofolate reductase
GAP	GTPase activating protein for p21RAS
FER	FER (FPS/FES-related) tyrosine kinase
APC	Adenomatous polyposis coli
MCC	Mutated in colorectal cancer
IL-4	Interleukin-4
IL-5	Interleukin-5
IRF-1	Interleukin regulatory factor 1
IL-3	Interleukin-3
CSF-2	Colony stmulating factor-2 (GM-CSF)
TCF7	T-cell-specific transcription factor 7
IL-9	Interleukin-9
EGR-1	Early growth response 1
CD14	Myeloid antigen 14
FGFA	Fibroblast growth factor, acidic
GR	Glucocorticoid receptor
ADRB2	Adrenergic, β2 receptor, surface
CSF 1R	CSF1 receptor (FMS)
SPARC	Secreted protein, acidic, cysteine-rich (osteonectin)
GLUHI	Glutamate receptor
NKSF1	Subunit of Interleukin 12
GABRA1	Aminobutyric acid (GABA) A receptor
5qNCA	5q nuclear receptor coactivator

+8

Trisomy 8 has been found in MDS patients at a frequency of up to 20%. The detection of trisomy 8 by FISH techniques in bone marrow smears prior to the appearance of marked myelodysplastic changes, suggest that this analysis may prove useful in the diagnosis of MDS. Genes mapped to chromosome 8 include *MYC, MOS* and *LYN*, a member of the c-*SRC* gene family and the tumour virus integration site (reviewed by Gallagher et al., 1997).

-7

The loss of chromosome 7 (monosomy 7 and del7q) is a recurring aberration in MDS and AML with frequencies of approximately 15% and 4% respectively. Monosomy 7 syndrome is particularly associated with childhood leukemia. 7q- is also frequently associated with secondary MDS and AML (reviewed by Gallagher et al., 1997). The deletions in chromosome 7 extend from q11 to q36, with the critical region encompassing q32 to 34. Genes deleted in this syndrome include the *MET* proto-oncogene, mapped to 7q31. Other genes localized to chromosome 7q encode the multi-drug resistance protein, p-glycoprotein and erythropoietin.

11q

Chromosome 11 abnormalities in MDS account for 7% of patients with chromosomal abnormalities: (inv (11)(p15q23), del (11q), t(2;11) and t(11;21). In one study the H-*RAS* 1 gene locus, located at chromosome 11p15, was shown to be translocated to the long arm of the rearranged chromosome 11 in one MDS patient, whilst the H-*RAS* gene was deleted in the rearranged chromosome in another patient. The *ETS*-1 gene, mapped to 11q23, was demonstrated to have translocated to the short arm in the rearranged chromosome 11 in both of these patients (reviewed by Gallagher et al., 1997). More recently, structural aberration of chromosome band 11q23 has been associated with over-expression or amplification of the *MLL* (mixed lineage leukemia) gene and is coincident with a poor prognosis in elderly patients with dysplastic bone marrow or with complex karyotypic aberrations, suggestive of genotoxic exposure (Michaux et al., 2000). Tandem duplications of MLL have been found in AML of different FAB types and in secondary AML associated with a poor prognosis (Schnittger et al., 2000). Furthermore, the translocation t(11;16)q23;p13.3) resulting in the fusion of *MLL* and CBP (CREB binding protein), has been reported to occur almost exclusively in acute leukemia and MDS secondary to therapy with DNA topoisomerase targeting drugs (reviewed in Felix, 1998). *MLL* is thought to regulate homeobox (HOX) genes, which are required for development (discussed below). Over 40 translocation sites have been identified so far for *MLL* and over 20 fusion partners have been cloned.

MLL deficient mice are embryonically lethal with skeletal and hematopoietic abnormalities (Yu et al., 1998). In a mouse model of the t(11;16) translocation fusing the DNA binding domain of *MLL* gene to the bromodomain, histone acetyl transferase domain, E1A binding domain and the steroid-receptor co-activator binding domains of CBP (suggestive of chromatin association), myeloid leukemia was obtained preceded by a long preleukaemic or MDS phase (Lavau et al., 2000). In another animal model, the MLL-AF9 fusion associated with the translocation t(9;11) gave rise to AML, which evolved from a myeloproliferative phase (Dobson et al., 1999).

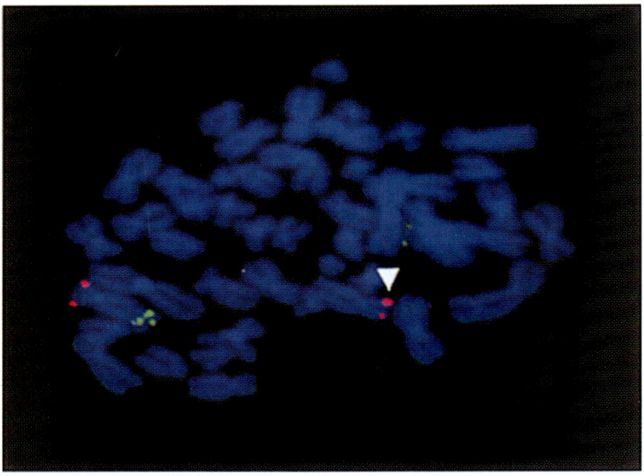

Figure 2. *FISH to leukemic metaphase from a 5q- syndrome patient. The control 5p probe (in red) and the locus specific 5q probe from the common deleted region (in green) are seen present on the normal chromosome 5; the del(5q) shows only signals corresponding to the 5p probe (arrowhead). (From Jaju et al 1998).Courtesy of Jaju, Kearney & Wainscoat, Oxford. Reproduced with permission from John Wiley & Sons.*

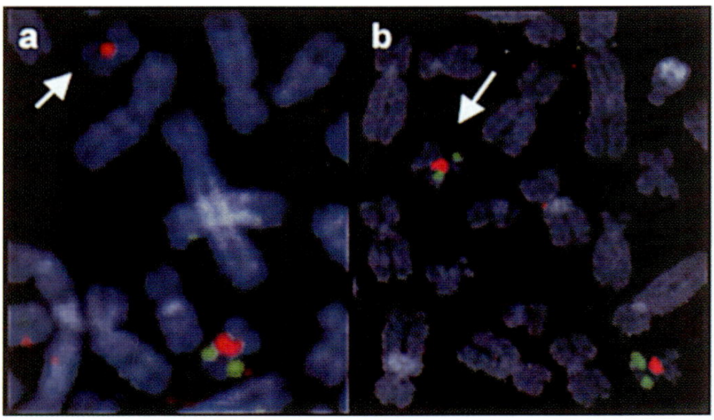

Figure 3. *Deletions of 20q in myeloproliferative disease (MPD) identified by FISH mapping.*
a. *Part of a metaphase cell with typical FISH signal pattern showing deletion of markers from the commonly deleted region; normal chromosome 20 with a centromere (in red) and locus specific probe (in green); the del (20)q homologue carries only the centromere probe (arrow).*
b. *Part of a metaphase cell with FISH signals from centromere 20 probe (red) and a locus specific probe (green) present in both the normal 20 and del (20)q marker (arrow).*
(From Bench et al., 2000). Courtesy of Nacheva & Green, Cambridge. Reproduced with permission from Macmillan Press

20q-

Deletions of the long arm of chromosome 20 have been identified in approximately 5% of patients with MDS. FISH studies have identified a commonly deleted region from 20q11.2 to q12. Genes that have been mapped to this region include *HCK* (hematopoietic cell kinase) that encodes a protein tyrosine kinase expressed in hematopoietic cells, phospholipase C gene, topoisomerase 1 and phosphotyrosyl phosphatase 1B, all of which have roles in the regulation of cell growth (reviewed by Gallagher et al., 1997). FISH or microsatellite PCR analysis has enabled the detection of a new MDS commonly deleted region (CDR) and the assignment of genes, which are both positional, and expression candidates for the target gene(s) on 20q. The deleted region has now been further mapped to a common deleted region of 2.6Mb and 16 expressed candidate genes are currently being analyzed. Of these, 5 are expressed in both normal marrow and purified CD34 positive cells (Bench et al., 2000) (Figure 3). These include *SFRS6*, which encodes a protein important in the regulation of mRNA alternative splicing, and b-*MYB*, a member of the *MYB* family of transcription factors and believed to play a role in cell cycle control.

Translocations

Other chromosomal translocations have been described in MDS and t-AML (Table 2). As individual translocations occur relatively rarely in MDS this review will be restricted to include translocations where the genes have been cloned. These translocations can be broadly grouped into core binding factors (CBF), HOX family members, ETS family members and others involving transcriptional regulatory proteins. They all tend to be transcription factors or target the transcriptional apparatus resulting in abnormal differentiation, proliferation and/or apoptosis (Figure 4). They also are generally associated with therapy-related MDS/AML and affect all age groups.

Core Binding Factors

CBFs are required for definitive hematopoiesis as evidenced by the disruption of these genes, which are lethal in mice (Yergeau et al, 1997; Castilla et al, 1996). Fusion genes generated by the t(8;21) translocation and inversion 16 result in fusions of AML1/ETO and *CBFβ-MYH11* transcription factors respectively (Table 2). The AML1/ETO fusion is normally associated with AML (FAB type M2). The inv16 fusion is associated with AML (subtype M4Eo). Both fusions have been reported in a small number of MDS. These abnormal fusions act as dominant negatives, suppressing the function of their respective wild type genes resulting in a block in differentiation (reviewed in Friedman, 1999). AML/ETO has been found to bind proteins like the promyleocytic leukemia Zinc finger (PLZF), which in turn binds the nuclear co-repressor (NCOR), which binds histone deacetylase (HD) (Melnick et al., 2000, reviewed in Redner et al., 1999) and may involve the modification of chromatin. The human AML1/MDS1/EVI1 fusion associated with t(3;12) in secondary leukemia (Nucifora et al., 1994; Roulston et al., 1998) was found to give rise to AML in a retroviral transduction mouse model (Cuenco et al., 2000)

HOX family

In addition to their role in development, HOX genes are important in hemopoiesis and their disruption results in the development of leukemia (reviewed by Buske & Humphries, 2000). The nucleoporin NUP98 is a transactivator. In the NUP98/HOXA9 fusion, the domain in NUP98 required for its interaction with the transcriptional co-activator CBP/p300, the FXFG repeats from the RNA binding domain, is deleted. Therefore deregulation of the HOX genes and their partners will affect transcription of target genes resulting in impaired differentiation. There is a possibility that fusions involving NUP98 results in aberrant nucleoplasmic transport. One of its partners is a putative RNA helicase, DDX10, which may be involved in ribosome assembly, predicted to result in altered transcriptional regulation (Arai et al 1997; Ikeda et al., 1999; Nakao et al., 2000).

ETS family

The molecular consequence of a t(5;12) is a fusion between the transmembrane and tyrosine kinase domains of *PDGF* receptor beta gene on chromosome 5 and a novel *TEL* gene. *TEL* is a member of the *ETS* gene family (reviewed in Golub et al., 1994). The common features of MDS with translocations involving the *TEL* gene were shown to include monocytosis and eosinophilia. An MDS patient harbouring the translocation t(5;12)(q31;p12) demonstrated over-expression of the K-*RAS* 2 gene, which maps at 12p12 (reviewed by Gallagher et al., 1997). TEL/PDGFβR phosphorylates STAT5, which may contribute to transformation by promoting proliferation (Wilbanks et al., 2000). Since its isolation, *TEL* has been found to be involved in many other translocations with a variety of different phenotypes, depending on the partner gene. So far 35 chromosomal regions have been described with *TEL* as one of the partners, of which 12 other partner genes have been identified including EVI1 (Golub et al 1997; Tosi et al., 2000) and associated with therapy-related events (Shimada et al., 2000; Vieira et al., 2000).

Deregulation of other transcriptional regulators, result in the inhibition of normal function of their wild type counterparts. These abnormalities tend to be associated with secondary leukemia or those patients of poor prognostic groups such as RAEB-t and CMML. CBP and the *MLL* genes fall in this class and have been discussed above. The DEK-CAN fusion is likely to be involved in nucleocytoplasmic transport and cell cycle progression (Fornerod et al., 1996; Boer et al., 1998).

Telomerase

Telomeres are essential for function and stability of chromosomes. Telomerase activity has been found to be higher in MDS and higher still in AML compared to normal (Counter et al.,1995). This increased telomerase activity occurs as the cells acquire increased proliferative potential (Li et al., 2000). Although telomere length varies in MDS 60% have been found with elevated levels and telomere is significantly shortened in high risk groups and correlated with a poor prognosis (Ohyashiki et al., 1999). With a background of genomic instability, other genetic events are more likely to occur resulting in disease progression.

ONCOGENES

Most oncogenes have gain of function effects. Some, like mutant *RAS* result in a differentiation block, which if activated later, accelerate differentiation. Therefore the effect of a deregulated or abnormal gene is context-dependent both in compartment and in the genetic environment. Cellular proto-oncogenes can acquire oncogenic potential usually by DNA point mutations as in *RAS* genes, or by gene deletions as in *SRC* and *ERB* (reviewed by Gallagher et al., 1997).

Table 2. *Chromosomal translocations in MDS and secondary AML*

Translocation	Fusion Gene	FAB type	Reference
Core binding factors			
t(3;21)(q26;q22)	*AML1/MDS1/EVI1*	t-AML	Nucifora (1994)
t(8;21)(q22;q22)	*AML1/ETO*	t-MDS/AML	Fujisawa (1999)
t(16;21)(q24;q22)	*AML1/MTG16*	t-MDS/AML	Gamou (1998)
Inv16(p11;q22)	*CBFβ/MYH11*	t-MDS/AML	Dissing (1998)
HOX family			
t(2:11)9q31;p15)	*NUP98/HOXD13*	t-MDS/AML	Shimada (2000)
t(7;11)(p15;p15)	*NUP98/HOXA9*	t-MDS/AML, RAEB-t/CMML	Hatano (1999)
t(11;12)(p15;q13)	*NUP98/HOXC*	t-MDS/AML	Nishiyama (1999)
ETS family			
t(3;12)(q26;p13)	*TEL/MDS1/EVI1*	MDS/AML	Peeters (1997)
t(5;12)(q33;p13)	*TEL/PDGFRβ*	CMML	Golub (1994)
t(5;12)(q31;p13)	*TEL/ACS2*	RAEB	Yagasaki (1999)
t(12;22)(p13;q11)	*MN1/TEL*	t-MDS	Buijs (2000)
Other Transcription regulators			
t(3;5)(q25.1;q34)	*NPM/MLF1*	RAEB-(t)	Matsumoto (2000)
t(4;11)(q21;q23)	*MLL/AF4*	t-AML	Blutters (1995)
t(5;11)(q31;q23)	*GRAF/MLL*	JCMML	Borkhardt (2000)
t(9;11)(p22;q23)	*MLL-AF9*	t-AML	Atlas (1998)
t(10;11)(p13;q14)	*MLL or CALM/AF10*	t-AML	Dreyling (1998)
t(11;16)(q23;p13.3)	*MLL/CBP*	t-CMML/AML	Rowley (1997)
t(11;20)(p15;q11)	*NUP98/TOP1*	t-MDS/AML	Ahuja (1999)
inv11(p15;q22)	*NUP98/DDX10*	t-MDS	Nakao (2000)
t(6;9)(p23;q34)	*DEK-CAN*	RAEB-t	Soekarman (1992)

RAS

Clinical studies

Oncogenic activation of one or more of the three *RAS* genes has been observed in a variety of malignancies (Table 3) and has been reported at high frequency in a number of hematological malignancies. *RAS* mutations occur at an approximate frequency of 25% in acute myeloid leukemia, 30% in myeloma and 6-20% in acute lymphoblastic leukemia. The highest incidence reported, however, is from studies on the myelodysplastic syndromes, with an incidence of approximately 30-40% (Padua et al., 1998; reviewed by Gallagher et al., 1997)) with the proportion of mutations occurring highest in the poorer prognostic groups of CMML and RAEB compared to RA and RARS. Most studies agree that mutations of N-*RAS* gene are the most common and that in the larger studies, *RAS* mutations are preferentially found in either CMML or other groups demonstrating monocytosis (Yunis et al.,

1989). This mirrors the high frequency of *RAS* mutations found in AML FAB type M4 (reviewed by Gallagher et al., 1997).

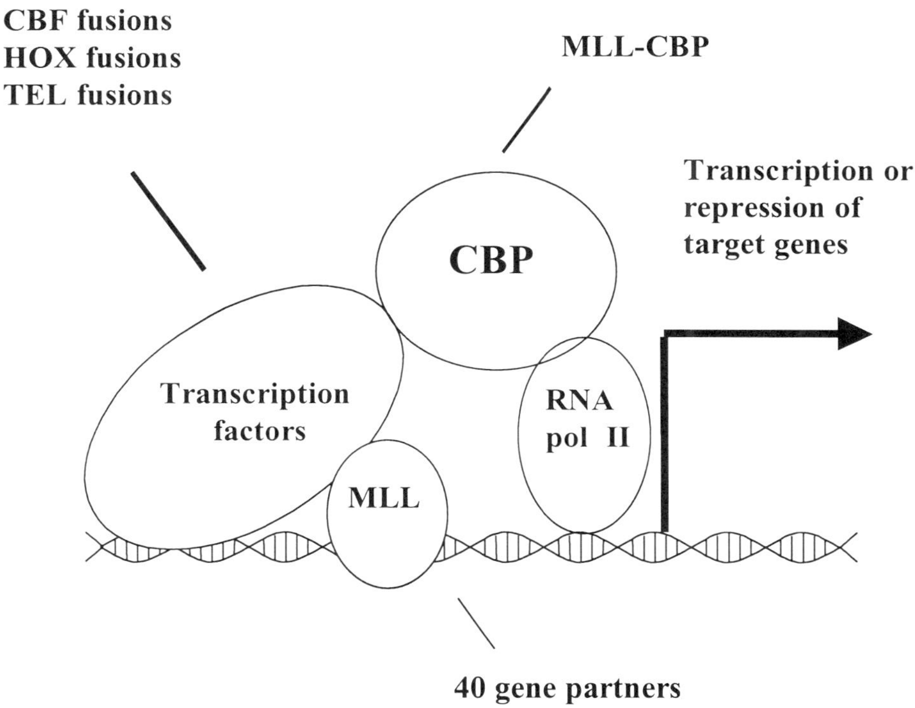

Figure 4. *Chromosomal translocations in MDS target the transcriptional apparatus in hematopoietic cells. Over 40 proteins are implicated in the basal transcriptional machinery (referred schematically as RNA polII).*

The association of *RAS* mutations with the preleukaemic state in MDS infers a role early in leukemogenesis. Within individual MDS patients *RAS* mutations have been reported in a multipotent stem cell where the mutation is associated with all cell lineages, thus inferring an initiating role in the disease. A positive correlation between the presence of *RAS* mutations and acute leukaemic transformation has been reported (Padua et al., 1998; reviewed by Gallagher et al., 1997). The results of a larger study (Paquette et al., 1993), showed this correlation to hold even after the stratification on percentage blasts in the bone marrow. More recently, in a study of 75 MDS patients who were followed up for 10 years, patients with *RAS* mutations had a poor outcome with a median survival of 13 months, compared to those without mutations who survived on average for 30 months, independent of FAB or other scoring systems, including the IPSS (Greenberg et al., 1997; Padua et al 1998; Padua & West, 2000).

The association between *RAS* mutations and abnormal karyotypes in MDS has been noted by other investigators: an increased incidence of mutant *RAS* was found in patients demonstrating abnormal karyotypes compared with others with normal karyotypes; a positive correlation of the incidence of *RAS* mutations with leukaemic transformation was revealed only when these data were combined with chromosomal abnormality details. These data could suggest that acquisition of *RAS* mutation alone is not sufficient to induce clinical preleukemia but rather requires accumulation of other molecular abnormalities. The finding of mutated *RAS* in hematologically normal individuals and in individuals in remission at risk of developing secondary therapy related leukemia, supports this view (Taylor et al., 1995a, b & 2000; Carter et al., 1990; Jacobs, 1991). In addition, non-dysplastic myelodysplasia has been observed in a patient in remission from Hodgkin's disease (Cachia et al., 1994). This patient harboured an activated *N RAS*, 7q- deletion in a minority of metaphases and abnormal colony growth, characteristic of MDS but remained hematologically normal for four years after combination therapy. It must be added, however, that dysplastic changes may not be seen if these abnormalities are only present in a minor clone.

The simultaneous activation of different *RAS* or of *RAS* with the tumour supressor gene, *p53*, has been described, which further suggests that activation of single *RAS* genes are not always sufficient for complete pre-neoplastic or neoplastic transformation *in vivo*. It must be added, however, that simultaneous activation of both *RAS* and p53 genes is a rare event (reviewed by Gallagher et al., 1997; Padua et al., 1998). It is clear that activation of *RAS* genes has a fundamental role to play in hematological malignancy, and in MDS in particular.

In vitro studies

In vitro, the effect of mutant *RAS* in hematopoietic cells has been shown to be context dependent. Many studies have been undertaken *in vitro* whereby both cell lines (Maher et al., 1996; Baker et al., 1994) and primary hematopoietic cells (Darley et al., 1997; Maher et al., 1994) have been infected with an activated *RAS* gene. In these experiments, both growth-promoting and maturation-inducing effects of activated *RAS* were observed in a cell specific manner (Maher et al., 1996). In addition, functional disparity was observed with greatest transforming ability upon infection with *H RAS* in fibroblasts; in the hematopoietic cell line, TF-1, activated *NRAS* demonstrated greatest activity (Maher et al., 1995). In an AML immortal cell line, P39, derived from a patient with preceding MDS, it has been shown that mutant *HRAS* accelerates the differentiation mediated by all-trans retinoic acid (ATRA) (Gallagher et al., 1998). Conversely, in the murine hematopoietic cell line FDCP-1, which is not malignant, mutant *NRAS* induces proliferation and reduces growth factor dependence (McGlynn et al., 2000). Although these cell line studies have provided a valuable contribution towards the understanding of RAS in cell function, the interpretation of results is limited by the already transformed nature of the majority of cell lines with unknown genetic lesions. Retroviral infection of *NRAS* into human primary cells using cord blood progenitors (CD34+ cells) resulted in abnormalities of the erythroid lineage, reminiscent of MDS, including impairment of proliferation, increased cell cycle time and impaired erythroid colony formation (Darley et al., 1997). More recent work using the same model, has shown that this oncogene promotes amplification of early erythroid progenitors at the expense of their proliferative capacity during the EPO-dependent stages of development (R.L. Darley, personal communication). This is the clearest experimental evidence in the hematopoietic system that mutant *RAS* may be an initiating event, giving rise to biological features of MDS (Figure 5).

Animal Models

Animal models of myeloid leukemia using mutant *RAS* have also generated varying results. In some cases, lymphoid rather than myeloid disease has been observed, possibly due to inappropriate choice of promoters (Adams & Cory 1992; Haupt et al., 1992) and/or the use of mutant *HRAS* (Dunbar et al 1991; Hawley et al.,1995), rather than *NRAS*. The latter is more frequently found in myeloid leukemia and *H* and *N RAS* have been shown to have different patterns of expression and different transformation capacities in hematopoietic cells (Maher et al., 1995). However, even transgenic mice with mutant *NRAS* did not recapitulate the phenotype of MDS and did not develop leukemia (Kogan et al., 1998), though in this case a likely explanation was the use of the MRP8 promoter which drives expression at a "late" stage in the neutrophilic lineage. The closest phenotypes to human MDS have been obtained using a retroviral approach in which bone marrow cells transduced with mutant *NRAS*, driven by a non tissue-specific promoter (Moloney murine leukemia virus LTR) and then transplanted into lethally irradiated mice. This generated a heterogeneous range of hematopoietic disorders including AML (Mackenzie et al 1999).

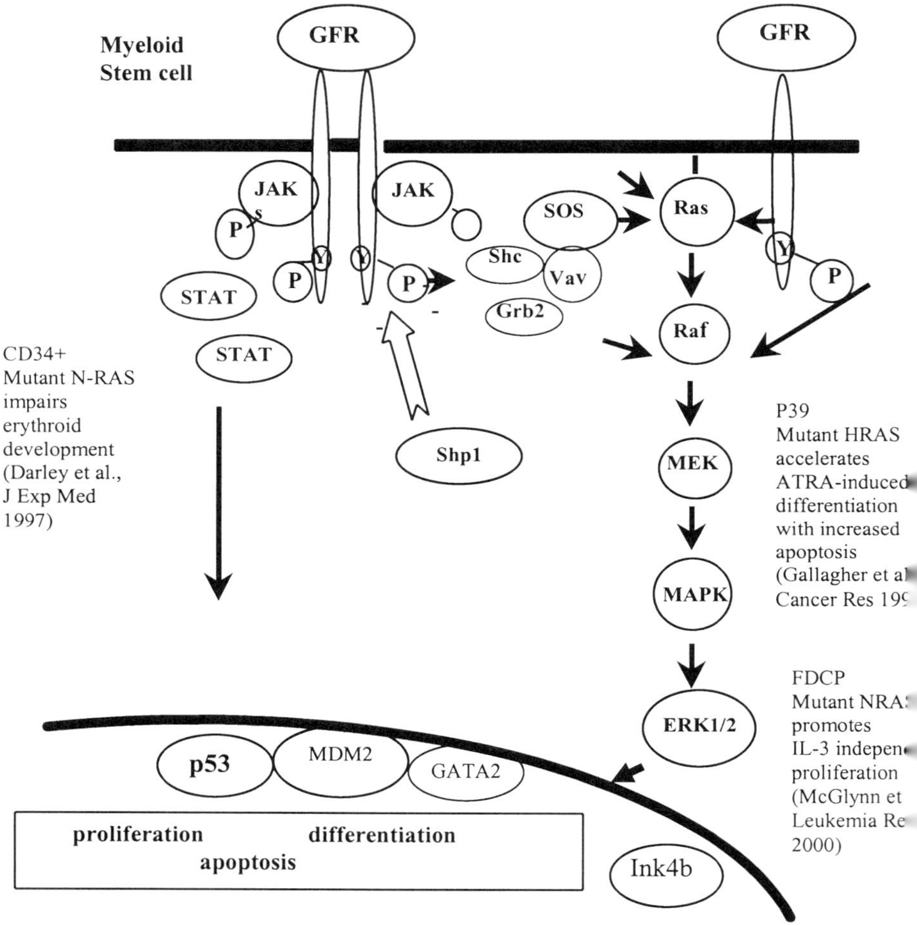

Figure 5. Signal transduction pathways that are mediated by RAS control cell growth a differentiation. Binding of a growth factor to its receptor causes autophosphorylation tyrosine residues on the cytoplasmic domain of the receptor. The phosphorylated recept activates various signal transduction pathways, includingthe MAPK pathway. In the MAI pathway, adaptor molecules such as GRB2 bind to the phosphorylated receptor and activc RAS. This leads to the activation of RAF-1which triggers a phosphorylation casca involving MAPK and its kinase, MEK-1. This results in the activation of transcription factc that lead to the regulation of proliferation, differentiation and apoptosis in hematopoie cells.

Table 3. *The incidence of RAS gene mutations in MDS*

Reference	*RAS* +/Total [(a)]	RAS+/RAS- [(b)] Transformed --> AML	Mutation [(c)]
Lyons (1988)	3/34 (8%)	0/4	K *RAS* 12 N *RAS* 12
Padua (1998)	36/75 (48%)	14/6	H,K,N *RAS* 12, 13, 61
Yunis (1989)	11/27 (40%)	8/3	N*RAS* 12, 13 K *RAS* 12
Lubbert (1992)	3/9 (33%)	3/1	N *RAS* 12
Van Kamp (1992)	3/90 (3%)	2/15	N *RAS* 12
Paquette (1993)	20/220 (9%)	NR	N *RAS* 12
Horiike (1994)	6/35 (17%)	4/8	N *RAS* 12, 13
Sheng (1997)	1/29 (3%)	NR	N *RAS* 12, 13, 61
de Souza Fernandez (1998)	21/50 (42%)	6/2	N *RAS* 12

(a) The number of analyzed patients with RAS gene mutations/ the total number of patients analyzed.
(b) Transformation to acute leukemia in patients followed: number who harbored a RAS gene mutation / number without a RAS mutation.
(c) The specific RAS gene mutated and the codon(s) demonstrating mutations.
NR not recorded

FMS

The macrophage colony-stimulating factor gene, *FMS*/CSF-1 receptor localizes to 5q31-33 and is a member of the family of growth factor receptors exhibiting ligand-induced tyrosine kinase activity. Two mutations of the *FMS* gene have been identified at codons 969 and 301 in both MDS and AML at frequencies 13-20% and 10-25% respectively (reviewed by Gallagher et al., 1997). Mutation at codon 301 produces a receptor with tyrosine kinase activity and transforming ability while alterations at codon 969 enhance transformation in the presence of CSF-1 ligand. Despite this, the most common mutation found in these studies was at codon 969 with gene product replacement of tyrosine with cysteine. *FMS* mutations were most commonly detected in CMML in MDS and AML M4 and M5 sub-types, each of which demonstrates a monocytic phenotype. This finding suggests that activation of the *FMS* gene may play a role in the pathogenesis of these conditions. In a model cell line, FDC-P1, the biological consequences of this mutation have been discerned where a *FMS* 969 mutation conferred growth factor independence, in a manner similar to transfection with v-*fms* (McGlynn et al., 1998). As well as mutation, some patients have demonstrated homozygous or heterozygous loss of the *FMS* gene (reviewed by Gallagher et al., 1997; McGlynn et al., 1997; Baker et al., 1995). No synergy between *FMS* gene deletion and codon 969 point mutation of the remaining allele was observed when examined by Jaquet et al. (1993). It has been speculated that hemi- or homozygous loss of *FMS* sequences on chromosome 5 may point to the loss of a proximal tumour supressor gene. The possibility still exists, that alteration of the *FMS* gene could enhance response to colony stimulating factor and hence contribute to clonal outgrowth in MDS.

TUMOUR SUPPRESSOR GENES

Tumour suppressor genes are mostly involved in solid tumours, however p53 and neurofibromatosis type 1 (NF-1) has been implicated in the pathogenesis of MDS. The *NF*-1 gene is activated through rearrangements and/or mutation in the genetic disorder Von Recklinghausen's neurofibromatosis (NF-1 disease). Rearrangements and mutations of the *NF*-1 gene have been reported in cases of sporadic tumours in some cases of MDS, either point mutation or allelic loss in childhood MDS (reviewed by Gallagher et al., 1997)

The *IRF*-1 gene, encoding interferon regulatory factor-1, maps to 5q3.1 and its gene product has anti-oncogenic potential. Loss of *IRF*-1 gene at one or both alleles has been demonstrated in MDS and AML. The retinoblastoma-susceptibility (Rb) gene is an anti-oncogene that frequently harbours alterations in retinoblastomas, sarcomas and some epithelial tumours. Although abnormal expression of the RB protein has been found in 20-30% of AML cases, structural alterations of the gene or abnormal expression of the protein appears to be rare in MDS.

The tumour suppressor gene, *p53*, maps to chromosome 17p and is often inactivated through deletion in solid tumours and to a lesser extent in hematopoietic malignancies. In hematopoietic malignancies including therapy-related MDS (Merlat et al., 1999) and MDS, 17p deletion is not uncommon and is associated with more mature granulocytes although patients with 17p abnormalities do not always have p53 mutations (reviewed by Gallagher et al., 1997). In MDS mutational inactivation of p53 is rare with an incidence of less than 5% in most cases but found in up to 15% of cases with a more progressed phenotype (Tang et al., 1998). Despite this, the presence of p53 mutations served as a significant prognostic indicator of resistance to chemotherapy and short survival and has also been detected in AML transformed from MDS (Misawa et al., 1998). In a study by Horiike et al., (1999), mutations of p53 were associated with deletions of chromosomes 5 and 7 and coinciding microsatellite instability with replication error phenotype in t-AML/MDS. The authors suggested that some patients may be predisposed to MDS after chemotherapy for their primary malignancy. Similar observations were made by Ben-Yehuda et al., 1996.

The p53 pathway can be triggered by cellular stress, including DNA damage, hypoxia and oncogene activation. A number of cellular proteins including MDM2, ARF, ING1, BRCA1 and various kinases modulate p53 stability. The best known biochemical function of p53 is activation of gene expression, including that of target genes *WAF1, MDM2* and *GADD45*, thus controlling cell cycle, apoptosis, differentiation and genome stability (Figures 5,6). Altered expression of p53 at the protein level together with that of MDM2 (which binds to p53 and renders p53 non-functional) and p21WAF1, has been shown to coincide with an unfavorable prognosis in childhood leukemia and MDS (Gustafsson et al., 2000; Kanavaros et al., 1999). In this study, Kanavaros reported the increased frequency of p53 over-expression in AML secondary to MDS compared with *de novo* AML. Finally, the high incidence of apoptosis in MDS has also triggered studies targeting p53 in these syndromes (discussed in later section).

GROWTH FACTORS AND RECEPTORS

The cytokine receptor superfamily includes genes encoding receptors for IL-3, IL-4, IL-5, IL-6, IL-7, IL-9, GM-CSF, G-CSF, erythropoietin, LIF, oncostatin M, growth hormone and prolactin. No difference in the levels of GM-CSF or IL-3 receptors was observed in MDS patient bone marrow cells as compared with normals, although increased levels of circulating GM-CSF, but not IL-3, were measured in approximately 25% of patients in one study (reviewed by Gallagher et al., 1997). In long-term cultures, IL-1 beta expression, but not IL-3, TPO, or Epo, was reduced in MDS marrows compared with normal, although the MDS cultures were hematopoietically defective (Tennant et al., 2000). Thrombopoietin (TPO), a major cytokine involved in megakaryocystopoiesis / thrombopoiesis, may be effective for the treatment of thrombocytopenia associated with myelodysplastic syndromes (Hofmann et al., 1999). The endogenous TPO level was found to be elevated in MDS patients, especially in those with RA (Ogata et al., 2000). Furthermore, this study revealed that the levels of expression of the TPO-receptor (encoded by *MPL*) were significantly reduced in MDS compared with normal subjects. The lack of correlation between endogenous TPO levels and the platelet and megakaryocyte counts in RAEB and RAEB-t suggests that TPO may induce blast proliferation in some cases (Ogata et al., 2000; Luo et al., 2000; Hashimoto et al., 2000). Previously, expression of *MPL* was found to be increased in 26 of 51 AML and 5 of 16 MDS patients in a study where expression correlated with poor survival. TPO receptor signalling has recently been addressed showing TPO dependant activation of STAT3 and STAT5 proteins as well as MAPkinase (Kalina et al., 2000). Phosphorylation of these STAT proteins, found to be lower in MDS subjects than in normals, was further enhanced by stimulation with recombinant TPO. Diminished STAT5 activation in response to erythropoietin has also been demonstrated in MDS patients (Hoefsloot et al., 1997). The balance of STAT proteins will also influence the biological effects of *RAS* with respect to differentiation versus proliferation. STAT5 promotes proliferation and the finding that it is deregulated in MDS may account for the reduced proliferative capacity of an MDS cell as it progresses (Figure 5).

Other growth factor receptors that have been implicated in MDS include KIT, the receptor for Stem cell factor. The proto-oncogene *KIT* encodes the receptor tyrosine kinase for stem/mast cell growth factor. In MDS and AML *KIT* mutations have not been found at the equivalent postions of codons 301 and 969 of the *FMS* gene. It is possible that elevated levels of *KIT* expression could maintain growth of the abnormal clone in MDS evidenced by increased expression of *KIT*, at both the RNA and protein levels, in bone marrow CD34+ cells from MDS patients. Over-expression of the gene product rather than mutational activation of the gene can activate oncogene-signaling pathways. A role for mast cell growth factor (MGF), ligand for the gene product of *KIT*, in the improvement of colony forming capacity of myelodysplastic cells, has been reported. Synergistic effects of MGF and erythropoietin have been demonstrated using *in vitro* methods (reviewed by Gallagher et al., 1997). The full potential of MGF in the treatment of MDS remains to be established.

MOLECULAR ANALYSIS OF CLONALITY IN MDS

The presence of pancytopenia in MDS suggests that all cell lineages are affected by the myelodysplastic lesion(s). Characterization of an MDS clone exploits the high frequency of activated oncogenes and chromosomal abnormalities. Numerical chromosomal aberrations, commonly trisomy 8, monosomy 7 or deletions in the long arm of chromosome 5 can be used to characterize the MDS clone. The disadvantage of applying these markers to MDS clonality investigations is that these lesions may arise at various stages in the disease. This problem has been overcome by the use of X-chromosome-linked restriction fragment length polymorphism (RFLP) assay, which is based on differences in X-chromosome inactivation, a DNA methylation dependent process. The polymorphic glucose 6 phosphate dehydrogenase (G6PD), hypoxanthine phosphoribosyl- transferase (HPRT) and phosphoglycerate kinase (PGK) genes or a locus recognized by the M27β probe and the human androgen receptor (HUMARA) are used to study clonality in small populations of cells from various bone marrow and peripheral blood cell lineages (reviewed in Gale, 1999). A monoclonal pattern in MDS has been reported whilst polyclonal T-lymphocytes in MDS have also been reported. Because lymphocytes are long-lived cells and it is unclear whether they are derived from unaffected progenitor cells or that their origin could antedate the onset of MDS, subsets of memory and naive T cells were analyzed separately. A polyclonal pattern, however, was observed in both subsets of cells. In addition, polyclonal granulocytes and lymphocytes have been observed in MDS patients with monoclonal erythrocytes (reviewed by Gallagher et al., 1997). X-chromosome inactivation analysis of *in vitro* cultured progenitor cells has shown the existence of non-clonal progenitor cells that produced erythroid and non-erythroid colonies upon growth factor stimulation, suggesting that non-clonal hematopoietic progenitors can persist in substantial numbers in MDS (reviewed by Gallagher et al., 1997). The conclusion that can be drawn from these studies is that in most cases evidence of monoclonal hematopoisis of the granulocytes can be found with polyclonal lymphocytes. Monoclonal erythrocytes in the presence of apparently polyclonal granulocytes and lymphocytes suggest that abnormalities of the erythroid lineage may be the earliest event. This is consistent with the retroviral studies where introducing mutant *RAS* into CD34+ cells derived from cord blood gives rise to erythroid abnormalities characteristic of the MDS cell (Darley et al., 1997). Skewed Lionization patterns, relying on ratios of alleles comparing patterns to control tissues, may well confirm that the abnormality in myeloid leukemia lies in progenitors which give rise to myeloid and erythroid lineages (reviewed in Gale, 1999).

MOLECULAR MECHANISMS OF APOPTOSIS IN MDS AND PROGRESSION TO AML

Pancytopenia has been identified as the hallmark of the myelodysplastic syndromes and has been ascribed to ineffective hemopoiesis. After intramedullary apoptosis in bone marrow biopsies of MDS patients was first described, later reported to be the possible mechanism for premature intramedullary cell death in MDS (Yoshida et al., 1993).

Since these early reports, other investigators have reported apoptosis in up to and greater than 50% of MDS bone marrow cells (Raza et al., 1995; Greenberg et al., 1998; Parcharidou et al., 1999). A debate arose as to whether the degree of apoptosis is indeed as high as had been previously reported. In 1996, Lepelley failed to detect increased apoptosis in bone marrow aspirates as determined by the terminal deoxynucleotidyl transferase (TdT) incorporation of nucleotides on the 3'-ends of DNA (TUNEL technique). Taken together with the data already published on apoptosis in bone marrow, the discrepancy between apoptosis levels in bone marrow biopsies and aspirates was identified (Raza et al., 2000a). The authors suggested that the level of apoptosis in bone marrow aspirates may be underestimated if only that of the low-density fraction of bone marrow mononuclear cells is reported. The same authors have now reported that rather the high-density fraction may have a significant proportion of apoptotic cells (Shetty et al., 2000).

The focus is now on the molecular mechanisms by which apoptosis in myelodysplastic syndromes occur. Several genes have been identified to play a role in myelodysplastic cell death and attempts are also now being made to investigate their prognostic significance. In most 'low risk' MDS cases, RA and RARS, higher levels of apoptosis have been reported to correlate significantly with a poorer prognosis and also with the levels of the marker for proliferating cells, MIB-1 and with CD34+ cells in the bone marrow

(Shimazaki et al., 2000). In addition, measurements of apoptosis together with cytokine expression have been shown to provide important biological information which helps to distinguish RA and RARS patients (with higher apoptosis, lower TNF-alpha exppresion, higher hemoglobin, lower blast counts and higher numbers of macrophages) from RAEB and RAEB-t patients. This was supported by another group reporting that CD34+ cell apoptosis was significantly increased in MDS subtypes RA and RARS (Parker et al., 1998).

The apparent paradox of simultaneous proliferation and apoptosis in the bone marrow cells of MDS patients has been specifically examined (Raza et al., 1997). One recent study used a double-labelling technique to demonstrate that a characteristically high number of S-phase cells were simultaneously apoptotic in MDS, but not in other diseases state including secondary AML and NHL (Mundle et al.,2000). This observation was further linked to an altered expression of the region of E2F1 transcription factor that specifically binds retinoblastoma protein.

BCL-2 and p53

When the expression of genes traditionally related to apoptosis was studied in total and separated mononuclear marrow cells, the absence of expression of c-*MYC* and p53 in total marrow cells correlated with significant degrees of apoptosis. In CD34+ and CD34- marrow cells, the phenomenon was inversely correlated with the level of *BCL*-2 expression (Tsoplou et al., 1999; Parker et al., 2000). Furthermore, apoptosis and BAX/BAD:BCL-2/BCL-X ratios were found to be inversely correlated with the IPSS and cytogenetic risk groups (Parker et al., 2000). Earlier studies have suggested a correlation between p53 overexpression and enhanced apoptosis in MDS (reveiewed by Gallagher, 1997). The apoptotic rate in AML and MDS with p53 overexpression was at least twice that in cases without p53 overexpression. 17p deletion has also been reported to correlate with the presence of a particular type of dysgranulopoiesis and with a high incidence of p53 mutation. P53 was shown to be over-expressed in the majority of RA patients whilst all normal and aplastic anaemia patients showed no over-expression of p53 in the marrow (Elghetany et al., 1998). P53 was suggested to be useful as a tool for the differential diagnosis of aplastic anaemia and RA MDS. Amifostine (AMF), a phosphorylated aminothiol, has been used to treat MDS where it stimulates hemopoiesis in the bone marrow. In MDS cell culture, AMF was found to be cytotoxic with the induction of apoptosis, however, these observations were made independently of alterations of p53 expression (Ribizzi et al., 2000).

FAS and TNF-alpha

Regulatory molecules such as tumour necrosis factor (TNF)-alpha, FAS and FAS-ligand, which negatively affect hemopoiesis by way of apoptosis are upregulated in MDS. FAS antigen (CD95/APO-1) is a cell-surface molecule that can transduce an apoptotic signal into cells. It belongs to the tumour necrosis factor and the nerve growth factor superfamily. FAS cross-linking by the FAS ligand or an agonistic anti-FAS antibody can deliver a cell death signal (Figure 6). While FAS antigen is expressed on various normal tissues (Leithauser et al., 1993) and in the blood on some populations of normal lymphocytes, neutrophils, monocytes and eosinophils, normal human bone marrow CD34+ cells have been reported to express none or little (up to 10% CD34+ cells) FAS antigen (Lepelley et al., 1998; Maciejewski et al., 1995). Up-regulation of FAS antigen in MDS marrow CD34+ cells was, however, observed (Bouscary et al., 1997; Gupta et al., 1999). MDS patients studied by Mundle et al, (1999) showed consistent low expression of a negative regulator of FAS, called FAS associated phosphatase-1 (Fap-1). Furthermore, TNF-alpha treatment of HL60 cells induced the up-regulation of FAS and the down-regulation of Fap-1. This study suggests that down-regulation of Fap-1 by TNF-alpha in MDS BM cells, may underlie the increased apoptosis of hematopoietic cells in MDS patients

Erythropoietin (epo), is the growth factor required for normal erythroid cell proliferation, survival and differentiation, and is dispensable for BFU-E generation and differentiation to CFU-E. CFU-E is, however, dependent on epo and/or epo-R for differentiation and epo deprivation leads to apoptosis. Impairment of erythroid progenitor growth was found to be statistically correlated to an elevated FAS expression (Fontenay-Roupie et al., 1999) but not with the lack of erythropoietin receptor signal transduction to STAT5 DNA binding activity.

Bone marrow samples from 80 patients with MDS with regard to TNF-alpha and FAS-ligand levels were examined and correlated with disease parameters and risk factors (Deeg et al., 2000). TNF-alpha levels were elevated in comparison to samples from normal donors. However, no significant correlation with FAB subtype, cytogenetic subgroup or score by the IPSS was observed. In another study, however, patients with excess of blasts showed high or intermediate TNFalpha expression in their marrow trephine biopsies (Molnar et al., 2000).

Caspases

Different groups have demonstrated a role for caspases, especially caspase 1 (Interleukin 1 beta converting enzyme[ICE]) and caspase 3 (Yama/Apopain/CPP32), in MDS BM cell apoptosis (Ali et al., 1999; Mundle et al., 1996). Caspases have now been identified to be an integral part of a downstream signalling machinery used by TNF-alpha and FAS-ligand in hematopoietic cells. Indeed, Bouscary et al., (2000) also refer to other studies reporting that neutralization of both TNF-alpha and FAS-L suppresses apoptosis and improve *in vitro* growth of MDS BM cells. When cultured *in vitro*, MDS BM mononuclear cells (MNC) demonstrated an increased apoptotic index within 4h as measured by in situ-labelling of fragmented DNA that was significantly correlated with a concomitant increase in caspase-3-like specific activity (Ali et al., 1999). In this study, caspase-1-like specific activity was detected early and transiently at approximately 15min, followed by a gradual increase in caspase-like-3 specific activity that peaked at 2h. Apoptosis was attenuated by inclusion of the broad-spectrum caspase inhibitor, Z-VAD.FMK, which the authors suggest, may be of useful therapeutic value.

The P39/Tsugane cell line is a myelomonocytoid line derived from a patient with AML with a preceding MDS. The cells readily undergo apoptosis in response to various agents and have been suggested as a useful tool in the study of MDS apoptosis. ATRA- and etoposide-induced apoptosis in these cells were both mediated through the caspase pathway and were partially blocked with the general inhibitor ZVAD-FMK (Hassan et al., 1999) whereas the FAS system did not play a part in these apoptotic pathways.

AML Progression

The study of sequential bone marrow biopsies of MDS patients has provided evidence to support the hypothesis that progression from MDS to AML is related to the accumulation of immature myeloid cells with an increase in *BCL*-2 expression and decreased apoptosis (Davies and Greenberg, 1998; Parker et al., 2000). The frequency of apoptotic cells in bone marrow specimens from a range of MDS patients was examined and the relationship of apoptosis to the immunohistochemical expression of *BCL*-2 and p53 was investigated (Kurotaki et al., 2000). The frequency of apoptosis was greater in MDS as compared with MDS-derived AML, de novo AML and controls. RAEB-t exhibited a lower frequency of apoptotic cells and a higher frequency of *BCL*-2 and p53-positive cells than patients with RAEB did. When the RAEB transformed to AML, the level of apoptosis was significantly reduced, while the frequency of *BCL*-2 and p53-positive cells was greater. In contrast to MDS-derived AML, the majority of the de novo AML cases showed few p53-positive cells. Using Ki-67 as a marker for proliferation it was found that low risk groups of RA and RARS had increased apoptosis relative to proliferation (Parker *et al.*, 2000). Cells from patients with RAEB had increased proliferation, which decreased upon progression to RAEB-t and AML. Progression to AML was also associated with a decrease in apoptosis and upregulation of BCL-2. The findings from these studies confirm that apoptosis has a definite role to play in dysplastic and ineffective hemopoiesis. There is much evidence to support the hypothesis whereby the suppression of apoptosis with enhanced p53 and *BCL*-2 expression increase the probability of developing leukemia in MDS (Davies & Greenberg, 1998), and that oncogenic development might be different between MDS-derived AML and *de novo* AML. Increased *BCL-2* expression may, therefore, be viewed as an accelerator of leukemia progression.

In an animal acute promyelocytic leukemia (APL) model, the *PML/RAR*α transgenic mice had an accelerated disease onset and reduced survival when crossed to BCL-2 transgenic mice (Kogan et al., 2001). Inv16 with the CBFβ/MYH11 fusion or mutant N-*RAS* double transgenic mice developed an MDS-like disease when crossed to BCL-2 transgenic mice (Padua, unpublished).

The emergence of novel genes found to be regulated in the process of apoptosis in myelodysplastic syndromes will help to fully elucidate the molecular mechanisms involved and possibly leads to the advancement of genetically-directed therapy in MDS.

NOVEL PREDICTORS OF PROGRESSION OF MDS TO AML: GENETIC MARKERS

In the final section of this chapter, we will discuss some of the more recent genetic predictors of leukaemic cell progression from MDS to AML.

GST

Genetic polymorphisms of detoxification enzymes have been associated with susceptibility to therapy-related leukemia and MDS. Gluathione S-transferase (*GST*) M1 and *GST*T1 are polymorphic genes.

Absence of enzyme activity is due to homozygous inherited deletion of the gene, reducing detoxification of carcinogens. The frequency of *GST*M1 null was found to be significantly increased in AML/MDS cases compared with control whereas the frequency of *GST*T1 null genotype in AML/MDS was not (Davies et al., 2000). This agrees with the original findings in MDS where there was no difference in the *GST*T1 null genotype in MDS and normals (Preudhomme et al., 1997), however, a significantly lower frequency was seen in cases with previous exposure to mineral dusts and exhaust gases. Similar occurrence was noted in a study by Sasai et al., (1999) where no association between the null phenotype and either N-*RAS* or *p53* mutation was found. These results suggest that the *GST* null genotype may play a role in an increased risk of myelodysplasia, which is independent of other established mechanisms such as chromosomal aberrations and oncogene mutations.

NQO1

NAD(P)H-quinone oxidoreductase (NQO1) in an enzyme which converts benzene-derived quinones to hydroquinones. A point mutation at codon 187 results in loss of enzyme activity in homozygous individuals, compared to normal activity in homozygous wild type subjects. Lack of NQO1 activity has been found to be associated with benzene poisoning, leading to hemotoxicity (Rothman et al., 1997). There appears to be variation of this polymorphism in the different ethnic groups with a gene frequency of 0.79 for the wild type allele and 0.29 for the mutated allele amongst Northern European and Caucasian Americans. The frequency of the mutated allele is slightly higher among African Americans and considerably higher among Hispanics and Asians. Although a naturally occurring polymorphism, it has been found that NQO1 mutations were significantly increased in myeloid leukemia, particularly those with chromosomal abnormalities of 5 and 7 and t-AML (Larson et al., 1999). Polymorphisms of NQO1, (but not of CYP3A4, was frequently associated with both MDS and AML, with different allelic frequencies of NQO1 in MDS and de novo AML (Naoe et al., 2000).

Matrix Metalloproteinases

The matrix metalloproteinases (MMP's) and their inhibitors, tissue inhibitors (TIMP's) play key roles in tissue remodeling and tumor invasion by digestion of extracellular matrix barriers (Baker et al., 2000). Recent studies have shown that BM mononuclear cells continuously produce MMP-9 and TIMP-1 while leukaemic blast cells additionally secrete MMP-2 (Ries et al.,

1999). MMP-2 secretion was found to be absent in all healthy donors. MMP-2 secretion may represent a potential marker for monitoring leukemic cell progression in myeloproliferative malignancies.

MLF1

MLF1 is a novel protein identified as the nucleophosmin (NPM-MLF1) chimeric protein produced by a t(3;5)(q25.1;q34) chromosomal translocation (Table 2). This chimera is associated with MDS, often prior to AML, except for M3 (Matsumoto et al., 2000). NPM-MLF1 contributes to the genesis of MDS/AML in part by the overexpression of MLF1 within hematopoietic tissues. High levels of MLF1 were found in patients with relatively immature subtypes of AML (M1, M2, M6 and M7) and high risk MDS (RAEB and RAEB-t). MLF1 normally functions in multi-potent progenitor cells and its dysregulation may take part in leukemogenesis from MDS. NPM contributes to two other fusion proteins found in lympho-hematopoietic malignancies, anaplastic large cell lymphoma (NPM-ALK) and acute promyelocytic leukemia (APL)(NPM-RARα) (Hitzler et al., 1999).

WT1

The Wilms' tumour gene, WT1, is expressed in a limited set of tissues during fetal development, consistent with its role in nephrogenesis and in the development of the gonads. It is also expressed in acute leukemia and in $CD34^+$ hematopoeitic progenitor cells (Takahashi et al., 2000). The expression of this gene is downregulated during the differentiation of hematopoietic progenitor cells and it has been reported that about 10-15% of acute nonlymphoid leukemia has the mutation of the WT1 gene. The WT1 gene is a potential tumour marker for leukaemic blast cells and a recent study has monitored WT1 expression in the peripheral blood of patients with overt AML evolved from MDS. It was shown to be significantly decreased by effective chemotherapy or allogeneic stem cell transplantation and became undetectable in long-term survivors (Tamaki et al., 1999). These results clearly showed that WT1 expression levels are a tumour marker for preleukaemic or leukaemic blast cells of MDS and thus reflect the disease progression of MDS. WT1 mRNA is a new marker of leukaemic blast cells for AML, ALL, and CML. Interestingly, recent studies have used WT1 mRNA detection by reverse transcriptase-polymerase chain reaction as a useful and predictive determinant of minimal residual disease (Ashihara et al.,

1999; Sugiyama, 2000; Pan et al., 2000). Detection of frequencies as low as 1 in 10^3 to 10^4 normal bone marrow cells and 1 in 10^5 normal peripheral blood mononuclear cells were observed. The Wilms' tumour protein, represses transcription from several growth factor genes. WT1 transcription is regulated in erythroid and myeloid lineages by the transcription factor GATA-1 (Patmasiriwat et al., 1999).

EVI1

*EVI*1, located at chromosome band 3q26, encodes a 1051 amino acid zinc finger protein expressed in the leukaemic cells of 2-5% of AML and MDS patients but not in normal marrow or cord blood cells (reviewed in Nucifora, 1997). The activation of *EVI*1 often follows a chromosomal rearrangement involving band 3q26, and the two most frequent rearrangements are the t(3;3)(q21;q26) and the inv(3)(q21q26). Other translocation partners include AML1 and TEL (Table 2). *EVI*1 exists also as a longer protein that includes 188 additional amino acids at the N-terminus, named MDS1/*EVI1*. Both genes are expressed at very low levels in the normal bone marrow. (Soderholm et al., 1997). A recent study suggests *EVI1* blocks cellular differentiation by binding to *GATA*-1 or other specific DNA sequences controlling gene expression which may lead to pathogenesis of some AML (Xi et al., 1997)

GATA-1 / GATA-2

GATA-1 and GATA-2 transcription factors are required for effective hemopoiesis. These regulatory proteins present overlapping yet distinct patterns of expression in hematopoietic cells. Absence of GATA-2 leads to defective hemopoiesis and an embryonic lethal phenotype. Disruption of GATA-1 results in a compensatory increase in GATA-2 in early erythroid cells and incomplete erythropoiesis (Ikonomi et al., 2000). GATA-2 expression analyses in leukaemic cell lines as well as primary patient samples are compatible with the hypothesis that 3q21 aberrations contribute to leukemogenesis through deregulation of the hematopoietic transcription factor GATA-2 (Wieser et al., 2000).

p15(INK4b)

p15(INK4b) gene is an inhibitor of cyclin-dependent kinase (CDK) 4 and CDK6 whose expression is induced by transforming growth factor (TGF)beta. It was recently shown that the promoter of the *p15INK4b* but not the *p16INK4a* gene is frequently and selectively hypermethylated in MDS and *de novo* AML (reviewed in Quesnel & Fenaux, 1999; Uchida et al., 1998). Methylation of the *p15(INK4b)* in MDS is correlated with blastic bone marrow involvement and increases with disease evolution toward AML. These studies would strongly suggest that *p15INK4b* methylation is a mechanism allowing leukemic cells to escape to inhibitory signals from the bone marrow environment, presumably that of TGFbeta. Association of frequent and strong methylation with high-risk MDS suggested that promoter methylation of *p15INK4B* gene plays an important role as a late event during MDS progression (Figure 6).

FLT3

*FLT*3 and its ligand FL is a receptor tyrosine kinase important for the survival and development of hematopoietic stem and progenitor cells (reviewed in Lyman, 1998). FL has been found to be elevated in 48.3% of RA and not in RAEB, RAEB-t or CMML (Zwierzina et al., 1999). Tandem duplication of *FLT3* has been found in MDS, who then rapidly evolved to AML (Horiike et al., 1997), in a single case of RAEB (of 37 MDS cases examined)(Yokota et al., 1997) but not in childhood MDS (Xu et al., 1999). Wild type *FLT*3 is thought to have a proliferative effect by signalling through RAS/RAF/MAPK pathways. *FLT*3 mutations of internal tandem duplications activate STAT5, which is important for proliferation (Mizuki et al., 2000). In MDS, Erythropoietin-induced activation of STAT5 is absent or suppressed (Hoefsloot et al., 1997). This suggests that in early MDS, cells are less proliferative and acquire increased proliferation as suppression of STAT5 is released by activation of progression genes. As *FLT*3 abnormalities are found in 27% of AML patients (of 854) with poor prognostic consequences, this gene may contribute to disease progression (Kottaridis et al., 2000). Mice with targeted disruption of FLT3 develop as adults with normal mature hematopoietic cells, but with abnormalities in primitive progenitors (Mackarehtschian et al.,1995).

Folate Binding Protein

The membrane-associated folate receptor type beta is elevated in the spleen in patients with CML and AML (Ross et al., 1999). The increase of the folate binding protein expression in these conditions, besides ensuring the growth of resistant cells by its contribution to the reduced folate intake, also participates in the methotrexate resistance. The internalization of folate cofactor, which would compete with methotrexate, hinders the effective inhibition of dihydrofolate reductase by the antifolate. A study of the clinical significance of reduced folate carrier present in MDS and its relationship with multi-drug resistance MDR has revealed that the reduced folate carrier, was present only on the leukemic cell and there was a direct correlation with multidrug resistance (MDR) expression (Chen et al., 1998). The reduced folate carrier may thus have a significant predictor role as MDR in MDS patients.

P-glycoprotein

P-glycoprotein (P-gp) is the product of the multi-drug resistance *MDR*1 gene. *MDR*1 expression in MDS is present in cells with an immature phenotype and is frequently observed in patients who have an abnormal karyotype and a high risk of leukemic transformation. In MDS, P-gp expression is clinically associated with drug resistance and evidence suggests that an important role in determining therapy outcome is played by P-gp in MDS (Wattel et al., 1999) and secondary leukemia (Damiani et al., 1998). Using quinine as a reversal agent in high risk MDS, a significantly higher proportion (52%) of P-gp positive patients who received quinine achieved complete remission compared with 18% who received chemotherapy alone. An important therapeutic modality and avenue of great interest will thus be the use of MDR-reversal agents in the attempts to improve on chemotherapeutic efficacy (Boogaerts et al., 1996; Krishna & Mayer, 2000; Tan et al., 2000).

POST GENOME THERAPY

MDS has no effective treatment and most therapies employed are palliative. The hope is that in addition to providing precise tools to facilitate diagnosis and monitoring of minimal residual disease, dissecting the genes involved in the genesis and progression of MDS and secondary AML will lead to the design of improved therapeutic strategies.

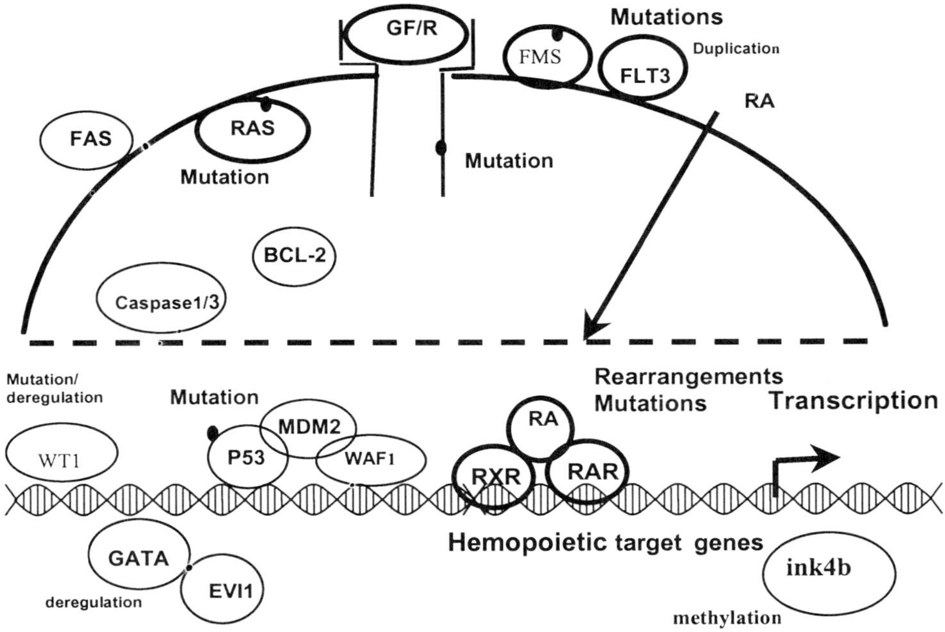

Figure 6. *Preleukaemia: Model of Cellular Transformation. A succession of genetic abnormalities alter signaling proteins result in leukaemogenesis. Deregulation of interactions between transcription factors such as GATA2 and oncogenes such as p53, expediate the progression from MDS to AML*

A gene-targeted approach may prove effective. Small molecules can be designed to inhibit pathways, such as has been found with the tyrosine kinase inhibitors now in clinical trials for BCR/ABL bearing chronic myelogenous leukemia (CML) with encouraging results. As histone deacetylase (HD) is involved in nucleosomal remodelling, inhibitors such as butyrate and its analogue trichostatin, may well prove effective in fusions such as AML1/ETO, CBFβ/MYH11 and AML1/MDS1, which disrupt chromatin modelling (reviewed in Redner et al., 1999). The most successful outcome of cloning a gene fusion, which has translated to direct benefit for patient treatment is the use of the differentiation agent *all*-trans retinoic acid (ATRA) for APL with t(15;17) translocations targeting the PML/RARα fusion. Trichostatin, has also been found to be effective in APLs. This fusion also binds the co-repressor NCOR and HD, as do the 4 other fusions involving RARα associated with APL (reviewed in Parrado et al 2000). Farnesyl transferase inhibitors, which interfere with the post translational modification of RAS (reviewed in Beaupre & Kurzrock, 1999), is now in clinical trials for

AML. Another approach is to use the abnormal gene itself as an immunogen and to develop DNA vaccination. Using this immunological approach is currently in clinical trials for lymphoma (Stevenson et al., 1999). Reagents directed towards the apoptosis pathway, such as amifostine or caspase inhibitors such as Z-VAD.FMK may also have efficacy (Ali et al., 1999; Raza et al., 2000b). Reagents, which inhibit the MDR genes such as quinidine and PSC388, are currently in clinical trials with encouraging results (Advani et al., 1999). Emerging techniques of comparative genomic hybridization (CGH), spectral karyotyping (SKY) or M-FISH (Figure 7) and arrays will enable us to determine which genes are associated and functional assays will help us understand how they interact. The years ahead will be a challenge, having the sequence of the entire human genome to hand.

ACKNOWLEDGEMENTS

We thank Ellie Nacheva, Tony Green, Rina Jaju, Lyndal Kearney, Jim Wainscoat and Christine Harrison for contributing their FISH images, to Christine Chomienne and Scott Kogan for useful discussions, the Leukemia Research Fund for their support over the years and Vysis for their contribution towards publication of the FISH images.

REFERENCES

Adams, J.M. & Corey, S. (1992) Oncogene co-operation in leukaemogenesis. *Cancer Surveys*, **15**, 119-141.

Advani, R., Visani, G., Milligan, D., Saba, H., Tallman, M., Rowe, J.M., Wiernik, P.H., Ramek, J., Dugan, K., Lum, B., Villen, J., Davis, E., Paietta, E., Litchman, M., Covelli, A., Sikic, B. & Greenberg, P. (1999) Treatment of poor prognosis AML patients using PSC833 (valspodar) plus mitoxanthrone, etoposide, and cytarabine (PSC-MEC). *Advances in Experimental Medical Biology*, **457**, 47-56.

Ali, A., Mundle S.D., Ragasa, D., Reza, S., Shetty, V., Mativi, B.Y., Cartlidge, J.D., Azharuddin, M., Qawi, H., Dar, S. & Raza, A. (1999) Sequential activation of caspase-1 and caspase-3-like proteases during apoptosis in myelodysplastic syndromes. *Journal of Hematotherapy Stem Cell Research*, **8**, 343-56.

Ahuja, H.G., Felix, C.A. & Aplan, P.D. (1999) The t(11;20)(p15;q11) chromosomal translocation associated with therapy-related myelodysplastic syndrome results in an NUP98-TOP1 fusion. *Blood*, **94**, 3258-3261.

Arai, Y. Hosoda, F., Kobayashi, H., Arai, K., Hayashi, Y., Kamada, N., Kaneko, Y. & Ohki, M. (1997) The inv(11)(p15q22) chromosome translocation of de novo and therapy-related myeloid malignancies results in fusion of the necleoporin gene, NUP98, with the RNA helicase gene, DDX10. *Blood* **89**, 3936-3944.

Ashihara, E., Shimazaki, C., Okamoto, A., Shimura, K., Takahashi, R., Sumikuma, T., Hirai H., Inaba T., Fujita, N. & Nakagawa, M. (1999) Successful peripheral *Blood* stem cell transplantation for myelodysplastic syndrome. *Bone Marrow Transplant*, **24**, 1343-1345.

Atlas, M., Head, D., Behm, F., Schmidt, E., Zeleznik-Le, N.H., Roe, B.A., Burian, D. & Domer, P.H. (1998) Cloning and sequence analysis of four t(9;11) therapy related leukemia breakpoints. *Leukemia*, **12**, 1895-1902.

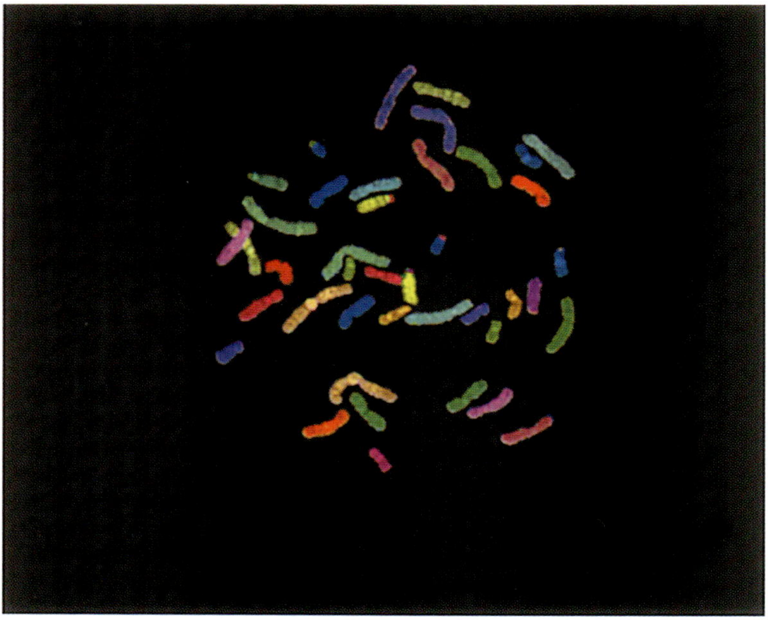

Figure 7A. Multiplex-fluorescence in situ hybridization (M-FISH) showing a normal human karyotype. *Courtesy of Harrison, Royal free Hospital, London)*

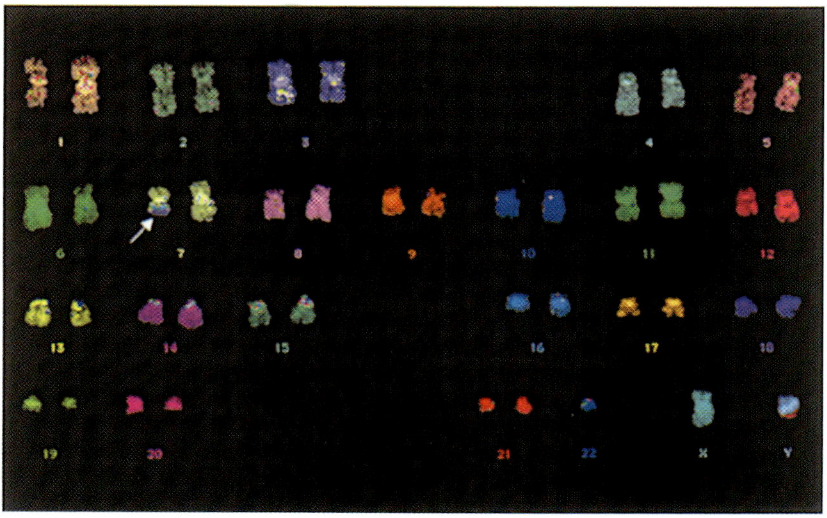

Figure 7B. *M-FISH karyotype of a bone marrow metaphase from a patient with MDS-RAEBt. G-banding reported a del(7)(q22q31). However, M-FISH analysis revealed that this was an unbalanced der(7)t(3;7) (arrow). One chromosome 22 was missing from this cell only, and does not represent a clonal abnormality. Courtesy of Kearney, Oxford*

Aul, C., Bowen, D.T. & Yoshida Y. (1998) Pathogenesis, etiology and epidemiology of myelodysplastic syndromes. *Haematologica,* **83**, 71-86.

Baker, A.H., Ahonen, M. & Kahari, V.M. (2000) Potential applications of tissue inhibitor of metalloproteinase (TIMP) overexpression for cancer gene therapy. *Advances in Experimental Medical Biology*, **465,** 469-483.

Baker, A., Cachia, P., Ridge S., McGlynn, H., Clarke, R., Whittaker, J., Jacobs, A. & Padua R.A. (1995) FMS mutations in patients following cytotoxic therapy for lymphoma. *Leukemia Research*, **19**, 309-318.

Baker, D., Maher, J., Roberts, I. and Dibb, N. (1994) Evidence that ras and myc mediate the synergy between SCF or M-CSF and other haemopoietic growth factors. *Leukemia* **8**, 1970-1981.

Bench, A.J., Nacheva, E.P., Hood, T.L., Holden, J.L., French, L., Swanton, S., Champion, K.M., Li, J., Whittaker, P., Stavrides, G., Hunt, A.R., Huntly, B.J., Campbell, L.J., Bentley, D.R., Deloukas, P. & Green, A.R. (2000) Chromosome 20 deletions in myeloid malignancies: reduction of the common deleted region, generation of a PAC/BAC contig and identification of candidate genes. *Oncogene*, **19**, 3902-13.

Ben-Yehuda, D., Krichevsky, S., Capsi, O., Rund, D., Polliack, A., Abeliovich, D., Yahalom, V., Paltiel, O., Or, R., Peretz, T., Ben-Neriah, S., Yehuda, O., Rachmilwitz, E.A. (1996) Microsatellite instability and p53 mutations in therapy-related leukemia suggest mutator phenotype. *Blood*, **88**, 4296-4303.

Beaupre, D.M. & Kurzrock, R. (1999) RAS and leukemia: from basic mechanisms to gene-directed therapy. *Journal of Clinical Oncology*, **17**, 1071-1079.

Blutters-Sawatski, R., Borkhardt, A., Grathwohl, J., Repp, R., Rheinisch-Becher, I. Bohle, R.M. & Lampert, F. (1995) Secondary acute myeloid leukemia with translocation (4;11) and MLL/AF4 43arrangement in a 15-year-old boy treated for a common acute lymphoblastic leukemia 11 years earlier. *Annals of Hematology*, **70**, 31-35.

Boer, J., Bonten-Surtel, J., Grosveld, G. (1998) Overexpression of the nucleoporin CAN/NUP214 induces growth arrest, nucleocytoplasmic transport defects, and apoptosis. *Molecular and Cellular Biology*, **18**, 1236-1247.

Boogaerts, M.A., Verhoef, G.E. & Demuynck H. (1996) Treatment and prognostic factors in myelodysplastic syndromes. *Baillieres Clinics in Haematology*, **9**, 161-183.

Borkhardt, A., Bojesen, S., Haas, O.A., Fuchs, U., Bartelheimer, D., Loncarevic, I.F., Bohle, R.M., Harbott, J., Repp, R., Jaeger, U., Viehmann, S., Henn, T., Korth, P., Scharr, D. & Lampert, F. (2000) The human GRAF gene is fused to MLL in a unique t(5;11)(q31;q23) and both alleles are disrupted in three cases of myelodysplastic syndrome/acute leukemia with a deletion 5q. Proceedings of the National Academy of Sciences USA, **97**, 9168-9173.

Boultwood, J., Strickson, A.J., Jabs, E.W., Cheng, J.F., Fidler, C. & Wainscoat, J.S. (2000a) Physical mapping of the human ATX1 homologue (HAH1) to the critical region of the 5q- syndrome within 5q32, and immediately adjacent to the SPARC gene. Human Genetics, **106**, 127-129.

Boultwood, J., Fidler, C., Strickson, A.J., Watkins, F., Kostrzewa, M., Jaju, R.J., Muller, U. & Wainscoat, J.S. (2000b) Transcription mapping of the 5q- syndrome critical region: cloning of two novel genes and sequencing, expression, and mapping of a further six novel cDNA. *Genomics*, **66**, 26-34.

Bouscary, D., Chen, Y.L., Guesnu, M., Picard, F., Viguier, F., Lacombe, C., Dreyfus, F. & Fontenay-Roupie M. (2000) Activity of the caspase-3/CPP32 enzyme is increased in "early stage" myelodysplastic syndromes with excessive apoptosis, but caspase inhibition does not enhance colony formation in vitro. *Experimental Hematology*, **28**,784-791.

Bouscary, D., De Vos, J., Guesnu, M., Jondeau, K., Viguier, F., Melle, J., Picard, F., Dreyfus F. & Fontenay-Roupie M. (1997) Fas/Apo-1 (CD95) expression and apoptosis in patients with myelodysplastic syndromes. *Leukemia* , **11**, 839-845.

Buijs, A., van Rompaey, L., Molijn, A.C., Davis, J.N., Vertegaal, A.C., Potter, M.D., Adams, C., van Baal, S., Zwarthoff, E.C., Roussel, M.F. & Grosveld, G.C. (2000) The MN1-TEL fusion protein, encoded by the translocation t(12;22)(p13;q11) in myeloid leukemia, is a transcription factor with transforming activity. *Molecular and Cellular Biology*, **20**, 9281-9293.

Buske, C., Humphries, R.K. (2000) Homeobox genes in leukaemogenesis. *International Journal of Hematology*, **71**, 301-308.

Cachia, P.G., Taylor C., Thompson, P.W., Tennant, G.B., Masters, G., Pettersson, T., Whittaker, J.A., Burnett, A.K., Jacobs, A. & Padua R.A. (1994) Non-dysplastic myelodysplasia. *Leukemia* , **8**, 677-681.

Castilla, L.H., Wijmenga, C., Wang, Q. Stacey, T., Speck, N.A., Echaus, M., Marin-Padilla, M., Collins, F.S., Wynshaw-Boris, A. & Liu, P.P. (1996) Failure of embryonic hematopoiesis and lethal hemorrhages in mouse embryos heterozygous for a knock-in leukemia gene CBFβ-MYH11. *Cell*, **87**, 687-696.

Carter, G., Hughes, D.C., Clark, R.E., McCormick, F., Jacobs, A., Whittaker, J.A. & Padua R.A. (1990) Ras mutations in patients following cytotoxic therapy for lymphoma. *Oncogene*, **5**, 411-416.

Castro, P.D., Liang, J.C., Nagarajan, L. (2000) Deletions of chromosome 5q13.3 and 17p loci cooperate in myeloid neoplasms. *Blood*, **95**, 2138-2143.

Chen, J., Li, R., Yan, S., Li, Q., Bai, T. & Wang S. (1998) Analysis of the characteristics of folate binding proteins and its relationship with expression of multidrug resistance P-glycoprotein in myelodysplastic syndromes. *Chinese Medical Journal*, **111**, 235-238.

Counter, C.M., Gupta, J., Harley, C.B., Leber, B. & Bacchetti, S. (1995) Telomerase activity in normal leukocytes and in haematological malignancies. *Blood*, **85**, 2315-2320.

Crane, M. M., Strom, S.S., Halabi, S., Berman, E.L., Fueger, J.J., Spitz, M.R.& Keating M.J. (1996) Correlation between selected environmental exposures and karyotype in acute myelocytic leukemia. *Cancer Epidemiology Biomarkers & Prevention,* **5**, 639-644.

Cuenco, G.M., Nucifora, G. & Ren, R. (2000) Human AML1/MDS1/EVI1 fusion protein induces an acute myelogenous leukemia (AML) in mice: a model for human AML. *Proceedings of the National Academy of Sciences USA*, **97**, 1769-1765.

Damiani, D., Michieli, M., Ermacora, A., Candoni, A., Raspadori, D., Geromin, A., Stocchi, R., Grimaz, S., Masolini, P., Michelutti, A., Scheper, R.J. & Baccarani, M. (1998) P-glycoprotein (PGP), and not lung resistance-related protein (LRP), is a negative prognostic factor in secondary leukemias. *Haematologica*, **83**, 290-297.

Darley, R.L., Hoy, T.G., Baines, P., Padua, R.A. & Burnett, AK. (1997) Mutant *N-RAS* induced erythroid lineage dysplasia in human CD34+ cells. *Journal of Experimental Medicine* **185**:1337-1347.

Davies, S.M., Robison, L.L., Buckley, J.D., Radloff, G.A., Ross, J.A. & Perentesis, J.P. (2000) Glutathione S-transferase polymorphisms in children with myeloid leukemia: A Children's Cancer Group study. *Cancer Epidemiology Biomarkers and Prevention*, 9, 563-566.

Davis, R.E. & Greenberg P.L. (1998) Bcl-2 expression by myeloid precursors in myelodysplastic syndromes: relation to disease progression. *Leukemia Research*, **22**, 767-777.

Deeg, H.J., Beckham, C., Loken, M.R., Bryant, E., Lesnikova, M., Shulman, H.M. & Gooley T. (2000) Negative regulators of hemopoiesis and stroma function in patients with myelodysplastic syndrome. *Leukemia & Lymphoma*, **37**, 405-414.

De Souza, F.T., Menezes de Souza, J., Macedo Silva, M.L., Tabak, D. & Abdelhay, E. (1998) Correlation of N-ras point mutations with specific chromosomal abnormalities in primary myelodysplastic syndrome. *Leukemia Research*, **22**, 125-134.

Dissing, M., Le beau, M.M. & Pedersen-Bjergaard, J. (1998) Inversion of chromosome 16 and uncommon rearrangements of CBFB and MYH11 genes in the therapy-related acute myeloid leukemia:rare events related to DNA-topoisomerase II inhibitors. *Journal of Clinical Oncology*, **16**, 1890-1896.

Dobson, D.L., Warren, A.J., Pannell, R. Forster, A., Lavenir, I., Corral, J., Smith, A.J. & Rabbitts, T.H. (1999) The MLL-AFP gene fusion in mice controls myeloproliferation and specifies acute myeloid leukemogenesis. *EMBO J*, **18**, 3564-3574.

Dreyling, M.H., Schrader, K., Fonatsch, C., Schlegelberger, B., Haase, D., Schoch, C., Ludwig, W., Loffler, H., Buchner, T., Wormann, B., Hiddemann, W. & Bohlander SK. (1998) MLL and CALM are fused to AF10 in morphologically distinct subsets of acute leukemia with translocation t(10;11): both rearrangements are associated with a poor prognosis. *Blood*, **91**, 4662-4667.

Dunbar, C.E., Crosier, P.S. & Nienhuis, AW. (1991) Induction of an activated ras oncogene into murine BM lymphoid progenitors via retroviral gene transfer results in thymic lymphomas. *Oncogene Research*, **6**, 39-51.

Elghetany, M.T., Vyas, S. & Yuoh, G. (1998) Significance of p53 overexpression in bone marrow biopsies from patients with bone marrow failure: aplastic anemia, hypocellular refractory anemia, and hypercellular refractory anemia. *Annals of Hematology*, **77**, 261-264.

Fagioli, F., Cuneo, A., Piva, N., Carli, M.G., Previati, R., Balboni, M., Tomasi, P., Cariani, D., Scapoli, G. & Castoldi, G. (1992) Distinct cytogenetic and clinicopathologic features in acute myeloid leukemia after occupational exposure to pesticides and organic solvents. *Cancer,* **70**, 77-85.

Felix, C.A. (1998) Secondary leukemias induced by topoisomerase-targeted drugs. *Biochimica Biophysics Acta*, **1400**, 233-155.

Fornerod, M., Boer, J., van Baal, S., Morreau, H. & Grosveld, G. (1996) Interaction of cellular proteins with the leukemia specific fusion proteins DEK-CAN and SET-CAN and their normal counterpart, the nucleoporin CAN. *Oncogene*, **13**, 1801-1908.

Fontenay-Roupie, M., Bouscary, D., Guesnu, M., Picard, F., Melle, J., Lacombe, C., Gisselbrecht, S., Mayeux, P. & Dreyfus, F. (1999) Ineffective erythropoiesis in myelodysplastic syndromes: correlation with Fas expression but not with lack of erythropoietin receptor signal transduction. *British Journal of Haematology*, **106**, 464-473.

Friedman, A.D. (1999) Leukaemogenesis by CBF proteins. *Leukemia*, **13**, 1932-1942.

Fujisawa, S. Togawa, J., Tanaka, M., Koharazawa, H., Aoba, M. Fijita, H., Murata, T., Kanamori, H., Matsuzaki, M., Mohri, H., Ishigatsubo, Y. (1999) De novo acute myelogenous leukemia with trilineage myelodysplasia associated with t(8;21)(q22;q22). *Internal Medicine*, **38**, 607-611.

Gale, R.E. (1999) Evaluation of clonality in myeloid stem-cell disorders. *Seminars in Hematology*, **36**, 361-372.

Gallagher, A.P., Burnett, A.K., Bowen, D.T., Darley, R.L. (1998) Mutant RAS selectivity promotes sensitivity of myeloid leukemia cells to apoptosis by a protein kinase C-dependent process. Cancer research, **58**, 2029-2035

Gallagher, A.P., Darley, R.L., Padua, R.A. (1997) The molecular basis of myelodysplastic syndromes. Haematologica, 82, 191-204.

Gamou, T., Kitamura, E., Hosoda, F., Shimizu, K., Shinohara, K., Hayashi, Y, Nagase, T., Yokoyama, Y. & Ohki, M. (1998) The partner gene of AML1 in t(16;21) myeloid malignancies is a novel member of the MTG8(ETO) family. *Blood*, **91**, 4028-4037.

Golomb, H.M., Alimena, G., Rowley, J.D., Vardiman, J.W., Testa, J.R. & Sovik, C. (1982) Correlation of occupation and karyotype in adults with acute nonlymphocytic leukemia. *Blood,* **60**, 404-411.

Golub, T.R., Barker, G.F., Lovett, M. & Gilliland, D.G. (1994) Fusion of PDGF receptor beta to a novel ets-like gene, tel, in chronic myelomonocytic leukemia with t(5;12) chromosomal translocation. *Cell* **77**, 307-316.

Golub, T.R. (1997) TEL gene rearrangements in myeloid malignancy. *Hematological Oncology Clinics of North America*, **11**, 1207-1220.

Greenberg P.L. (1998) Apoptosis and its role in the myelodysplastic syndromes: implications for disease natural history and treatment. *Leukemia Research*, **22**, 1123-1136.

Greenberg, P., Cox, C., Le Beau, M.M., Fenaux, P., Morel, P., Sanz, G., Sanz, M., Vallespi, T., Hamblin, T.,Oscier, D., Ohyashiki, K., Toyama, K., Aul, C., Mufti, G. & Bennett J.(1997) International scoring system for evaluating prognosis in myelodysplastic syndromes. *Blood*, **15,** 2079-2088.

Gupta, P., Niehans, G.A., LeRoy, S.C., Gupta, K., Morrison, V.A., Schultz, C., Knapp, D.J. & Kratzke R.A. (1999) Fas ligand expression in the bone marrow in myelodysplastic syndromes correlates with FAB subtype and anemia, and predicts survival. *Leukemia* , **3**, 44-53.

Gustafsson, B., Christenson, B., Hjalmar, V. & Winiarski J. (2000) Cellular expression of MDM2 and p53 in childhood Leukemia s with poor prognosis. *Medical Pediatric Oncology*, **34**, 117-124.

Hashimoto, S., Toba, K., Watanabe, K., Takahashi, H., Abe, T., Yano, T., Kioke, T., Takahashi M. & Aizawa Y. (2000) Thrombopoietin activates the growth of megakaryoblasts in patients with chronic myeloproliferative disorders and myelodyplastic syndrome. *European Journal of Haematology*, **64**, 225-230.

Hassan, Z., Fadeel, B., Zhivotovsky, B. & Hellstrom-Lindberg, E. (1999) Two pathways of apoptosis induced with *all*-trans retinoic acid and etoposide in the myeloid cell line P39. *Experimental Hematology*, **27**, 1322-1329.

Hatake, K., Tomizuka, H., Ikeda, M., Terui, Y. & Miura Y. (1998) Apoptosis-gene expression in hematopoietic system: normal and pathological conditions (Review). *International Journal of Molecular Medicine*, **1**, 121-129.

Hatano, Y., Miura, I., Nakamura, T., Yamazaki, Y., Takahashi, N. & Miura, A.B. (1999) Molecular heterogeneity of the NUP98/HOXa9 fusion transcript in myelodysplastic syndromes associated with t(7;11)(p15;p15). *British Journal of Haematology*, **107**, 600-604.

Haupt, Y., Harris, A.W. & Adams, J.M. (1992) Retroviral infection accelerates T lymphomagenesis in E mu-N-ras transgenic mice by activating c-myc or N-myc. *Oncogene*, **7**, 981-986.

Hawley, R.G., Fong, A.Z., Ngan, B.Y., Hawley, T.S. (1995) Hematopoietic transforming potential of activated ras in chimeric mice. *Oncogene*, **11**, 1113-1123.

Hitzler, J.K., Witte, D.P., Jenkins, N.A., Copeland, N.G., Gilbert, D.J., Naeve, C.W., Look, A.T. & Morris, S.W.(1999) cDNA cloning, expression pattern, and chromosomal localization of Mlf1, murine homologue of a gene involved in myelodysplasia and acute myeloid leukemia . *American Journal of Pathology*, **155**, 53-59.

Hoefsloot, L.H., van Amelsvoort, M.P., Broeders, L.C., van der Plas, D.C., van Lom, K., Hoogerbrugge, H., Touw, I.P. & Lowenberg B. (1997) Erythropoietin-induced activation of STAT5 is impaired in myelodyplastic syndrome. *Blood*, **89**, 1690-1700.

Hofmann, W.K., Kalina, U., Wagner, S., Seipelt, G., Ries, C., Hoelzer, D. & Ottmann, O.G. (1999) Characterization of defective megakaryocytic development in patients with myelodysplastic syndromes. *Experimental Hematology*, **27**, 395-400.

Horrigan, S.K., Arbieva, Z.H., Xie, H.Y., Kravarusic, J., Fulton, N.C., Naik, H., Le, T.T. & Westbrook C.A. (2000) Delineation of a minimal interval and identification of 9 candidates for a tumour suppressor gene in malignant myeloid disorders on 5q31. *Blood*, **95**, 2372-2377.

Horiike, S., Misawa, S., Nakai, H., Kaneko, H., Yokota, S., Taniwaki, M., Yamane, Y, Inazawa, J., Abe, T. & Kashima, K. (1994) N-ras mutation and karyotypic evolution are closely associated with leukemic transformation in myelodysplastic syndrome. *Leukemia* **8**, 1331-1336.

Horiike, S., Misawa, S., Kaneko, H., Sasi, Y., Kobayashi, M., Fujii, H., Tanaka, S., Yagita, M., Abe, T., Kashima, K. & Taniwaki M. (1999) Distinct genetic involvement of the TP53 gene in therapy-related leukemia and myelodysplasia with chromosomal losses of Nos 5 and/or 7 and its possible relationship to replication error phenotype. *Leukemia*, **13**, 1235-1242.

Horiike, S., Yokota, S., Nakao, M., Iwai, T., Sasai, Y., Kaneko, H., Taniwaki, M., Kashima, K., Fujii, H. Abe, T. & Misawa, S. (1997) Tandem duplication of the FLT3 receptor gene are associated with leukemic transformation of myelodysplasia. *Leukemia*, **11**, 1442-1446.

Ikeda, T., Ikeda, K., Sasaki, K., Kawakami, K. & Takahara, J. (1999) The inv(11)(p15;q22) chromosome translocation of therapy-related myelodysplasia with NUP98-DDX10 and DDX10-NUP98 fusion transcripts. *International Journal of Hematology*, **69**, 160-164.

Ikonomi, P., Rivera, C.E., Riordan, M., Washington, G., Schechter, A.N. & Noguchi, C.T. (2000) Overexpression of GATA-2 inhibits erythroid and promotes megakaryocyte differentiation. *Experimental Hematology*, **28**, 1423-143

Jacobs, A. (1991) Genetic abnormalities in myelodysplastic syndrome. [Review]. *Cancer Genetics & Cytogenetics* **56**, 1-6.

Jaju, R., Boultwood, J., Olover, F.J., Kostrzewa, M., Fidler, C., Parker, N., McPherson, J.D., Morris, S.W., Muller, U. Wainscoat, J.S. Kearney, L. (1998) Molecular cytogenetic delineation of the critical deleted region in the 5q- syndrome. *Genes Chromosomes Cancer* **22**, 251-251.

Jaju, R.J., Haas, O.A., Neat, M., Harbott, J., Saha, V., Boultwood, J., Brown, J.M., Pirc-Danoewinata H., Krings, B.W., Muller, U., Morris, S.W., Wainscoat, J.S. & Kearney L. (1999) A new recurrent translocation, t(5;11)(q35;p15.5), associated with del(5q) in childhood acute myeloid leukemia. The UK Cancer Cytogenetics Group. *Blood*, **94**, 773-780.

Jaju, R.J., Jones M., Boultwood, J., Kelly ,S., Mason D.Y., Wainscoat, J.S., Kearney L (2000) Combined immunophenotyping and FISH identifies the involvement of B-cells in 5q-syndrome. *Genes Chromosomes & Cancer,* **29**, 276-280.

Jaquet, K., Kreipe, H., Felgner, J., Boultwood, J. & Parwaresch, M.R. (1993) Myelodysplastic disorders with hemizygous M-CSF receptor gene loss do not show point mutations of codon 969 within the remaining allele. *Leukemia* **7**, 650-652.

Jiang, Y., Liang H., Guo, W., Kottickal, L.V. & Nagarajan, L. (2000) Differential expression of a novel C-terminally truncated splice form of SMAD5 in hematopietic stem cells and leukemia. *Blood*, **95**, 3945-3950.

Kalina, U., Hofmann, W., Koschmieder, S., Wagner, S., Kauschat, D., Hoelzer, D. & Ottmann, O.G. (2000) Alteration of c-mpl-mediated signal transduction in CD34(+) cells from patients with myelodyplastic syndromes. *Experimental Hematology*, **28**,1158-1163.

Kanavaros, P., Stefanaki, K., Rontogianna, D., Darivianaki, K., Vlychou, M., Papadaki, E., Eliopoulos, G., Bakiri, M., Matsouka, C., Kakolyris, S. & Georgoulias, V. (1999) Immunohistochemical detection of p53, mdm2, wafl/p21, and Ki67 proteins in bone marrow biopsies in myelodysplastic syndromes, acute myelogenous leukemias and chronic myeloproliferative disorders. *Clinics of Experimental Pathology*, **47**, 231-238.

Kogan, S.C., Brown, D., Shultz, D.B., Truong, B.T., Lallemand-Breitenbach, V., Guillemin, M., Lagasse, E.,Weissman, I. & Bishop, J.M. (2001) BCL-2 cooperates with PMLRARα to block neutrophil differentiation and initiate acute leukemia. *Journal of Experimental Medicine*, **193**, 531-544..

Kogan, S.C., Lagasse, E., Atwater, S. Bae, S.C., Weissman, I, Ito, Y., & Bishop, J.M. (1998) The PEBP2betaMYH11 fusion created by Inv(16)(p13;q22) in myeloid leukemia impairs neutrophil maturation and contributes to granulocytic dysplasia. *Proceedings of the National Academy of Sciences USA*, **95**,11863-11868.

Kottaridis, P.D., Gale, R.E., Frew, M.E., Harrison, G., Langabeer, S.E., Belton, A.A., Walker, H., Wheatley, K., Bowen, D.T., Burnett, A.K. (2000) The presence of a FLT3 mutation in AML adds important prognostic information to cytogenetic risk group and response to the first cycle of chemotherapy: analysis of 854 patients from the MRC AML 10 and 12 trials. *Blood*, **96**: 825a.

Krishna, R. & Mayer, L.D. (2000) Multidrug resistance (MDR) in cancer. Mechanisms, reversal using modulators of MDR and the role of MDR modulators in influencing the pharmacokinetics of anticancer drugs. *European Journal of Pharmacological Science*, **11**, 265-283.

Kurotaki, H., Tsushima, Y., Nagai, K. & Yagihashi, S.(2000) Apoptosis, bcl-2 expression and p53 accumulation in myelodysplastic syndrome, myelodysplastic-syndrome-derived acute myelogenous leukemia and de novo acute myelogenous leukemia . *Acta Haematology*, **102**, 115-123.

Larson, R.A., Le Beau, M.M., Vardiman, J.W. & Rowley J.D. (1996) Myeloid leukemia after hematotoxins. *Environmental Health Perspectives*,**104**, 1303-1307.

Larson R.A., Wang Y., Banerjee M, Wiemels J., Hartford C., Le Beau M.M. & Smith, M.T. (1999) Prevalence of the inactivating $^{609}C \rightarrow T$ polymorphism in the NAD(P)H:quinone oxidoreductase (NQO1) gene in patients with primary and therapy-related myeloid leukaemia. *Blood* **94**:803-807.

Lavau, C., Du, C., Thirman, M. & Zeleznik-Le, N. (2000) Chromatin-related properties of CBP fused to MLL generate a myelodysplastic-like syndrome that evolves into myeloid Leukemia . *EMBO Journal*, **19**, 4655-4664.

Leithauser, F., Dhein, J., Mechtersheimer, G., Koretz, K., Bruderlein, S., Henne, C., Schmidt, A., Debatin, K.M., Krammer, P.H. & Moller, P. (1993) Constitutive and induced expression of APO-1, a new member of the nerve growth factor/tumor necrosis factor receptor superfamily, in normal and neoplastic cells. *Laboratory Investigations*, **69**, 415-29

Lepelley, P., Campergue, L., Grardel, N., Preudhomme, C., Cosson, A. & Fenaux P. (1996) Is apoptosis a massive process in myelodysplastic syndromes? *British Journal of Haematology*, **95**, 368-371.

Lepelley, P., Grardel, N., Erny, O., Iaru, T., Obein, V., Cosson, A. & Fenaux, P. (1998) FAS/APO-1 (CD95) expression in myelodysplastic syndromes. *Leukemia & Lymphoma*, **30**, 307-312.

Li, B., Yang, J. Andrews, C., Chen, T.X., Toofanfard, P. Huang, R.W. Horvathe, E., Chopra H., Raza, A. & Priesler, H.D. (2000) Telomerase activity in preleukemia and acute myelogenous leukemia. *Leukemia & Lymphoma*, **36**, 579-587.

Lubbert, M., Mirro, J., Jr., Kitchingman, G., McCormick, F., Mertelsmann, R., Herrmann, F. & Koeffler, H.P. (1992) Prevalence of N-ras mutations in children with myelodysplastic syndromes and acute myeloid leukemia. *Oncogene* **7**, 263-268.

Luo, S.S., Ogata, K., Yokose, N., Kato, T. & Dan, K. (2000) Effects of thrombopoietin on proliferation of blasts from patients with myelodyplastic syndromes. *Stem Cells*, **18**, 112-119.

Lyman, S.D. (1998) Biologic effects and potential clinical applications of FLT3 ligand. *Current Opinion in Hematology*, **5**, 192-196.

Lyons, J., Janssen, J.W., Bartram, C., Layton, M. & Mufti, G.J. (1988) Mutation of Ki-ras and N-ras oncogenes in myelodysplastic syndromes. *Blood* **71**, 1707-1712.

Mackarehtschian, K., Hardin, J.D., Moore, K.A., Boast, S., Goff, S.P. & Lemischka, I.R. (1995) Targeted disruption of the flk2/flt3 gene leads to deficiencies in primitive hematopoietic progenitors. *Immunity*, **3**, 147-161.

MacKenzie, K.L., Doinikov, A., Millington, M., Shounan, Y., Symonds, G. (1999) Mutant N-ras induces myeloproliferative disorders and apoptosis in bone marrow repopulated mice. *Blood*, **93**,2043-2056.

Maher, J., Baker, D., Dibb, N. & Roberts, I. (1996) Mutant ras promotes haemopoietic cell proliferation or differentiation in a cell-specific manner. *Leukemia* **10**, 83-90.

Maher, J., Baker, D.A., Manning, M., Dibbs, N.J., Roberts, I.A. (1995) Evidence for cell-specific differences in transformation by N-, H- and k-ras. *Oncogene*, **11**, 1639-1647.

Maher, J., Colona, F., Baker, D., Luzzatto, L. & Roberts, I. (1994) Retroviral-mediated gene transfer of a mutant H-ras gene into normal human bone marrow alters myeloid cell proliferation and differentiation. *Experimental Hematology,* **22**, 8-12.

Maciejewski, J.P., Selleri, C., Sato, T., Anderson, S. & Young, N.S. (1995) Increased expression of Fas antigen on bone marrow CD34+ cells of patients with aplastic anaemia. *British Journal of Haematology*, **91**, 245-252.

Matsumoto, N., Yoneda-Kato, N., Iguchi, T., Kishimoto, Y., Kyo,T., Sawada, H., Tatsumi, E. & Fukuhara S. (2000) Elevated MLF1 expression correlates with malignant progression from myelodysplastic syndrome. *Leukemia*, 14, 1757-1765.

McGlynn, A.P., Padua, R.A., Burnett, A.K. & Darley, R.L. (2000) Alternative effects of RAS and RAF oncogenes on the proliferation and apoptosis of factor dependent FDC-P1 cells. *Leukemia Research*, **24,**47-54.

McGlynn, H., Baker, A.H. & Padua R.A. (1998) Biological consequences of a point mutation at codon 969 of the FMS gene. *Leukemia Research*, **22**, 365-372.

McGlynn, H., Kapelko, K., Baker, A.H. & Padua R.A. (1997) Allelic loss of the FMS gene in acute myeloid leukemia . *Leukemia Research*, **21**, 919-923.

Melnick, A. Carlile, G.W., McConnell, M.J., Polinger, A., Hiebert, S.W. & Licht, J.D. A(2000) ML-1/ETO fusion protein is a dominant negative inhibitor of transcriptional repression by the promyelocytic leukemia zinc finger protein. *Blood*, **96**, 3939-3947.

Merlat, A., Lai, J.L., Sterkers, Y., Demory, J.L., Bauters, F., Preudhomme, C. & Fenaux, P. (1999) Therapy-related myelodysplastic syndrome and acute myeloid leukemia with 17p deletion: A report on 25 cases. *Leukemia*, 13, 250-257.

Michaux, L., Wlodarska, I., Dierlamm, J., Mugneret, F., Herens, C., Beverloo, B., Verhest, A., Verellen-Dumoulin, C., Verhoef, G., Selleslag, D., Madoe, V., Lecomte, M., Deprijck, B., Ferrant, A., Delannoy, A., Marichal, S., Duhem, C., Dicato, M. & Hagemeijer A. (2000) MLL amplification in myeloid Leukemia s: A study of 14 cases with multiple copies of 11q23. *Genes Chromosomes & Cancer*, **29**, 40-47.

Misawa, S., Horiike, S., Kaneko, H., Sasi, Y., Ueda, Y., Nakao, M., Yokot, S., Tanaka, S., Taniwaki, M., Fujii, H., Nakagawa, H., Tsuda, S. & Kashima, K. (1998) Significance of chromosomal alterations and mutations of the N-RAS and TP53 genes in relation to leukemogenesis of acute myeloid leukemia. *Leukemia Research*, **22**, 631-637.

Mitelman, M.F., Brand, L. & Nilsson, P.G. (1978). Relation array occupational exposure to potential mutagenic carcinogenic agents, clinical findings and bone marrow chromosomes in acute lymphocytic leukemia. *Blood*, **52,** 1229-1237.

Mizuki, M. Fenski, R., Halfter, H., Matsumara, I., Schmidt, R., Muller, C., Gruning, W., Kratz-Albers, K., Serve, S., Steur, C., Buchner, T., Kienast, J., Kanakura, Y. Berdel, W.E.,Serve, H. (2000) FLT3 mutations from patients with acute myeloid leukemia induce transformation of 32D cells mediated by the RAS and STAT5 pathways. *Blood,* **96**, 3907-3914.

Molnar, L., Berki, T., Hussain, A., Nemeth, P. & Losonczy, H. (2000) Detection of TNFalpha exon in the bone marrow and determination of TNFalpha production of peripheral blood mononuclear cells in myelodysplastic syndrome. *Pathology & Oncology Research*, **6**, 18-23.

Mundle, S.D., Mativi, B.Y., Bagai, K., Feldman, G., Cheema, P., Gautam, U., Reza, S., Cartlidge, J.D., Venugopal, P., Shetty, V., Gregory, S.A., Robin, E., Rifkin, S., Shah, R. & Raza, A. (1999) Spontaneous down-regulation of Fas-associated phosphatase-1 may contribute to excessive apoptosis in myelodysplastic marrows. *International Journal of Hematology*, **70**, 83-90.

Mundle, S.D., Mativi, B.Y., Cartlidge, J.D., Dangerfield, B., Broady-Robinson, L., Li, B., Shetty, V., Venugopal, P., Gregory, S.A., Preisler, H.D. & Raza A. (2000) Signal antonymy unique to myelodysplastic marrows correlates with altered expression of E2F1. *British Journal of Haematology*, **109**, 376-81.

Mundle, S.D., Reza, S., Ali, A., Mativi, Y., Shetty, V., Venugopal, P., Gregory, S.A. & Raza A. (1996) Correlation of tumor necrosis factor alpha (TNF alpha) with high Caspase 3-like activity in myelodysplastic syndromes. *Cancer Letters*, **40**, 201-207.

Nakao, K., Nishino, M., Takeuchi, K., Iwata, M., Kawano, A., Arai, Y. & Ohki, M. (2000) Fusion of the nucleoporin gene NUP98 and the putative RNA helicase gene, DDX10, by inversion 11 (p15q22) chromosome translocation in a patient with etoposide-related myelodysplastic syndrome. *Internal Medicine* **39**, 412-415.

Naoe, T., Takeyama, K., Yokozawa, T., Kiyoi, H., Seto, M., Uike, N., Ino, T., Utsunomiya, A., Maruta, A., Jin-nai, I., Kamada, N., Kubota, Y., Nakamura, H., Shimazaki, C., Horiike, S., Kodera, Y., Saito, H., Ueda, R., Wiemels, J. & Ohno, R. (2000) Analysis of genetic polymorphism in NQO1, GST-M1, GST-T1, and CYP3A4 in 469 Japanese patients with therapy-related leukemia / myelodysplastic syndrome and de novo acute myeloid leukemia. *Clinical Cancer Research*, **6**, 4091-4095.

Narod S.A. & Dube I.D. (1989) Occupational history and involvement of chromosomes 5 and 7 in acute nonlymphocytic leukemia. *Cancer Genetics & Cytogenetics,*. **38**, 261-269.

Nishiyama, M., Arai, Y., Tsunematsu, Y., Kobayashi, H., Asami, K., Yabe, M., Kato, S., Oda, M., Eguchi, H., Ohki, M. & Kaneko, Y. (1999) 11p15 translocations involving the NUP98 gene in childhood therapy-related acute myeloid leukemia/myelodysplastic syndrome. *Genes Chromosomes & Cancer*, **26**, 215-220.

Nisse, C., Lorthois, C., Dorp, V., Eloy, E., Haguenoer, J.M. & Fenaux P. (1995) Exposure to occupational and environmental-factors in myelodysplastic syndromes - preliminary-results of a case-control study. *Leukemia,* **9**, 693-699.

Nucifora, G. (1997) The EVI1 gene in myeloid leukemia. *Leukemia*, **11**, 2022-2031.

Nucifora, G., Begy, C.R., Kobayashi, H., Roulston, D., Claxton, D. Pedersen-Bjergaard, J., Parganas, E., Ihle, J.N. & Rowley, J.D. (1994) Consistent intergenic splicing and production of multiple transcripts between AML1 at 21q22 and unrelated genes at (3;21)(q26;q22) translocations. *Proceedings of the National Academy of Sciences USA*, **91**, 4004-4008.

Ogata, K. & Tamura, H. (2000) Thrombopoietin and myelodyplastic syndromes. *International Journal of Hematology*, **72**, 173-177.

Ohyashi, J.H., Iwama, H., Yahata, N., Ando, K., Hayashi, S. Shay, J.W. Ohyashiki, K. (1999) Telomere stabiltiy is frequently impaired in high-risk groups of patients with myelodysplastic syndromes. *Clinical Cancer Research*, **5**, 1155-1160.

Padua, R.A, Guinn, B., Al-Sabah, A., Smith, M., Taylor, C., Pettersson, T., Ridge, S., Carter, G., White, D., Oscier, D., Chevret, S., & West, R. (1998) *RAS*, *FMS* and *p53,* mutations and poor clinical outcome in myelodysplasia: a 10-year follow-up. *Leukemia,* **12,** 887-892.

Padua, R.A. & West, R.R. (2000) Oncogene mutation and prognosis in the myelodysplastic syndromes (MDS). *British Journal of Haematology*, **111,** 873-874, 2000.

Pan, L., Ohnishi, K., Zhang, W.J., Yoshida, H., Maksumova, L., Muratkhodjaev, F., Shigeno, K., Nakamura, S., Luo, J.M., Hao, H.L., Fujisawa, S., Naito, K., Shinjo, K., Takeshita, A. & Ohno, R.(2000) *In vitro* IL-12 treatment of peripheral blood mononuclear cells from patients with leukemia or myelodysplastic syndromes: increase in cytotoxicity and reduction in WT1 gene expression. *Leukemia*, **14**, 1634-1641.

Paquette, R.L., Landaw, E.M., Pierre, R.V., Kahan, J., Lubbert, M., Lazcano, O., Isaac, G., McCormick, F. & Koeffler, H.P. (1993) N-ras mutations are associated with poor prognosis and increased risk of leukemia in myelodysplastic syndrome. *Blood* **82**, 590-599.

Parcharidou, A., Raza, A., Economopoulos, T., Papageorgiou, E., Anagnostou, D., Papadaki, T. & Raptis, S. (1999) Extensive apoptosis of bone marrow cells as evaluated by the in situ end-labeling (ISEL) technique may be the basis for ineffective haematopoiesis in patients with myelodysplastic syndromes. *European Journal of Haematology*, **62**, 19-26.

Parker, J.E., Fishlock, K.L., Mijovic, A., Czepulkowski, B., Pagliuca, A. & Mufti G.J. (1998) 'Low-risk' myelodysplastic syndrome is associated with excessive apoptosis and an increased ratio of pro- versus anti-apoptotic bcl-2-related proteins. *British Journal of Haematology*, **103**, 1075-1082.

Parker, J.E., Mufti, G.J., Rasool, F., Mijovic, A., Devereux, S., & Pagliuca, A. (2000) The role of apoptosis, proliferation, and the bcl-2-related proteins in the myelodysplastic syndromes and acute myeloid leukemia secondary to MDS. *Blood*, **96**, 3932-3938.

Parrado, A., Chomienne, C., & Padua, R.A. (2000) Retinoic acid receptor alpha (*RARα)* mutations in human leukemia. *Leukemia & Lymphoma*, **39**, 271-282.

Patmasiriwat, P., Fraizer, G., Kantarjian, H. & Saunders, G.F. (1999) WT1 and GATA1 expression in myelodysplastic syndrome and acute leukemia . *Leukemia*, **13**, 891-900.

Peeters, P., Wlodarska, I., Baens, M., Criel, A., Selleslag, D., Hagemeijer, A., van den Berghe, H., & Marynen, P. (1997) Fusion of ETV6 to MDS/EVI1 as a result of t(3;12)(q26;p13) in myeloproliferative disorders. *Cancer Research*, **57**, 564-569.

Preudhomme, C. Nisse, C., Hebbar, M., Vanrumbeke, M., Brizard, A., Lai, J.L., Fenaux, P. (1997) Glutatione S transferase theta 1 gene defects in myelodysplastic syndromes: correlation with karyotype and exposure to potential carcinogens. *Leukemia,* **11,** 1580-1582.

Quesnel, B. & Fenaux, P. (1999 P15INK4b gene methylation and myelodysplastic syndromes. *Leukemia & Lymphoma*, **35**, 437-443.

Raza, A., Alvi, S., Borok, R.Z., Span, L., Parcharidou, A., Alston, D., Rifkin, S., Robin, E., Shah, R. & Gregory, S.A. (1997) Excessive proliferation matched by excessive apoptosis in myelodysplastic syndromes: the cause-effect relationship. *Leukemia & Lymphoma*, **27**, 111-118.

Raza, A., Mundle, S., Iftikhar, A., Gregory, S., Marcus, B., Khan, Z., Alvi, S., Shetty, V., Dameron, S. & Wright, V. (1995) Simultaneous assessment of cell kinetics and programmed cell death in bone marrow biopsies of myelodysplastics reveals extensive apoptosis as the probable basis for ineffective hematopoiesis. *American Journal of Hematology*, **48**, 143-154.

Raza, A., Mundle, S., Shetty, V., Alvi, S., Chopra, H., Span, L., Parcharidou, A., Dar, S., Venugopal, P., Borok, R., Gezer, S., Showel, J., Loew, J., Robin, E., Rifkin, S., Alston, D., Hernandez, B., Shah, R., Kaizer, H., Gregory, S. & Preisler, H. (2000a) A paradigm shift in myelodysplastic syndromes. *Leukemia*, 10, 1648-1652.

Raza, A., Qawi, H., Lisak, L., Andric, T., Dar, S., Andrews, C., Venugopal, P., Gezer, S., Gregory, S., Loew, J., Robin, E., Rifkin, S., Hsu, W.T. & Huang, R.W. (2000b) Patients with myelodysplastic syndromes benefit from palliative therapy with amifostine, pentoxifylline, and ciprofloxacin with or without dexamethasone. *Blood*, **1**:1580-7.

Redner, R., Wang, J., & Liu, J.M. (1999) Chromatin remodelling and leukemia: new therapeutic paradigms. *Blood*, **94**, 417-428.

Ribizzi, I., Darnowski, J.W., Goulette, F.A., Sertoli, M.R.& Calabresi, P. (2000) Amifostine cytotoxicity and induction of apoptosis in a human myelodysplastic cell line. *Leukemia Research*, **24**, 519-525.

Ries, C., Loher, F., Zang, C., Ismair, M.G. & Petrides, P.E . (1999) Matrix metalloproteinase production by bone marrow mononuclear cells from normal individuals and patients with acute and chronic myeloid leukemia or myelodysplastic syndromes. *Clinical Cancer Research*, **5**, 1115-1124.

Rigolin, G.M., Cuneo, A., Roberti, M.G., Bardi, A., Bigoni, R., Piva, N., Minotto, C., Agostini, P., Del Senno, L., Spanedda, R. & Castoldi, G. (1998) Exposure to myelotoxic agents and myelodysplasia: case-control study and correlation with clinicobiological findings. *British Journal of Haematology,* **103,**189-197.

Ross, J.F., Wang, H., Behm, F.G., Mathew, P., Wu, M., Booth, R. & Ratnam, M. (1999) Folate receptor type beta is a neutrophilic lineage marker and is differentially expressed in myeloid leukemia. *Cancer*, **85**, 348-357.

Rothman, N., Smith, M.T., Hayes, R.B., Traver, R.D., Hoener, B., Campleman, S., Li, G.L., Dosemeci, M., Linet, M., Zhang, L., Xi, L., Wacholder, S., Lu, W., Meyer, K.B., Titenko-Holland, N., Stewart, J.T., Yin, S. & Ross, D. (1997) Benzene poisoning, a risk factor for hematological malignancy, is associated with the NQO1 609C-->T mutation and rapid fractional excretion of chlorzoxazone. *Cancer Research*, **15**, 2839-42.

Roulston, D. Espinosa, R., Nucifora, G., Larson, R.A., Le Beau, M.M & Rowley, J.D. (1998) CBA2(AML1) translocation with novel partner chromosomes in myeloid leukemias: association with prior therapy. *Blood*, **92**, 2879-2885.

Rowley, J.D. & Golomb, H.M. (1984) The 4th international workshop on chromosomes in leukemia - a prospective-study of acute nonlymphocytic leukemia Chicago, Illinois, USA, September 2-7, 1982. *Cancer Genetics & Cytogenetics,* **11**, 249-360.

Rowley, J.D., Reshmi, S., Sobulo, O., Musvee, T., Anastasi, J., Raimondi, S.,Schneider, N.R., Barredo, J.C., Cantu, E.S., Schlegelberger, B., Behm, F., Doggett, N.A., Borrow, J. & Zeleznik-Le, N. (1997) All patients with the t(11;16)(q23;p13.1) that involves MLL and CBP have treatment-related haematologic disorders. *Blood*, **90**, 535-541.

Sasai, Y., Horiike, S., Misawa, S., Kaneko, H., Kobayashi, M., Fujii, H., Kashima, K. & Taniwaki, M. (1999) Genotype of glutathione S-transferase and other genetic configurations in myelodysplasia. *Leukemia Research*, **23**, 975-81.

Schnittger, S., Kinkelin, U., Schoch, C., Heinecke, A., Haase, D., Haferlach, T., Buchner, T., Wormann, B., Hiddemann, W. & Griesinger, F. (2000) Screening for MLL tandem duplication in 387 unselected patients with AML identify a prognostically unfavorable subset of AML. *Leukemia*, **14**, 796-804.

Sheng, X.M., Kawamura, M., Ohnishi, H., Hanada, R., Kojima, S., Kobayashi, M., Bessho, F., Yanagisawa, M. & Hayashi, Y. (1997) Mutations of the *RAS* genes in childhood acute myeloid leukemia, myelodysplastic syndrome and juvenile chronic myelocytic leukemia. *Leukemia Research,* **21**, 697-701.

Shetty, V., Hussaini, S., Broady-Robinson, L., Allampallam, K., Mundle, S., Borok, R., Cartlidge, J., Broderick, E., Mazzoran, L., Zorat, F., & Raza, A. (2000) Intramedullary apoptosis of hematopietic cells in myelodysplastic syndrome patients can be massive: apoptotic cells recovered from high density fraction of bone marrow aspirates. *Blood*, **96**, 1388-1392.

Shimada, H., Arai, Y., Sekiguchi, S., Ishii, T., Tanitsu, S. & Sasaki, M. (2000) Generation of the NUP98-HOXD13 fusion transcript by a rare translocation, t(2;11)(q31;p15), in a case of infant leukemia. *British Journal of Haematology*, **10**, 210-213.

Shimazaki, K., Ohshima, K., Suzumiya, J., Kawasaki, C.& Kikuchi, M. (2000) Evaluation of apoptosis as a prognostic factor in myelodysplastic syndromes. *British Journal of Haematology*, **110**, 584-590.

Smith, M.A., McCaffrey, R.P. & Karp, J.E. (1996) The secondary leukemias: challenges and research directions. *Journal of the National Cancer Institute*, **88**, 407-418.

Soderholm, J., Kobayashi, H., Mathieu, C., Rowley, J.D. & Nucifora, G. (1997) The *Leukemia* -associated gene MDS1/EVI1 is a new type of GATA-binding transactivator. *Leukemia*, **11**, 352-358.

Soekarman, D., von Lindern, M., Daenen, S., de Jong, B., Fonatsch, C., Heinze, B.,Bartram, C., Hagemeijer A. & Grosveld, G. (1992) The translocation (6;9)(p23;q34) shows consistent rearrangement of two genes and defines a myeloproliferative disorder with clinical features. *Blood*, **79**, 2990-2007.

Stevenson, F.K., King, C.A., Spellerberg, M.B., Zhu, D., Rice, J., Sabota, S., Thompsett, A., Radl, J. & Hamblin, T.J. (1999) DNA vaccines against haematological malignacies. *Haematologica*, **84**, 11-13.

Stillman, W.S., Varella-Garcia, M. & Irons, R.D. (2000) The benzene metabolite, hydroquinone, selectively induces 5q- and -7 in human CD34+CD19- bone marrow cell. *Experimental hematology*, **28,** 169-76.

Suciu, S., Kuse, R., Weh, H.J. & Hossfeld, D.K. (1990) Results of chromosome-studies and their relation to morphology, course, and prognosis in 120 patients with *de novo* myelodysplastic syndrome. *Cancer Genetics & Cytogenetics*, **44**, 15-26.

Sugiyama, H. (2000) Genetic diagnosis of leukemia: diagnosis of relapse and complete remission, and prediction of leukemia onset. *Rinsho Byori*, **48**, 155-161.

Takahashi, T., Yamamoto, R., Tanaka, K., Kamada, N. & Miyagawa, K. (2000) Mutation analysis of the WT1 gene in secondary leukemia . *Leukemia*, **14**, 1316-1317.

Tamaki, H., Ogawa, H., Ohyashiki, K., Ohyashiki, J.H., Iwama, H., Inoue, K., Soma, T., Oka, Y., Tatekawa, T., Oji, Y., Tsuboi, A., Kim, E.H., Kawakami, M., Fuchigami, K., Tomonaga, M., Toyama, K., Aozasa, K., Kishimoto, T. & Sugiyama, H. (1999) The Wilms' tumor gene WT1 is a good marker for diagnosis of disease progression of myelodysplastic syndromes. *Leukemia* , **13**, 393-399.

Tan, B., Piwnica-Worms, D., & Ratner, L. (2000) Multidrug resistance transporters and modulation. *Current Opinion in Oncology*, **12**, 450-458.

Tang, J.L., Tien, H.F., Lin, M.T., Chen, P.J. & Chen, Y.C. (1998) P53 mutation in advanced stage of primary myelodysplastic syndrome. *Anticancer Research*, **18**, 3757-3761.

Taylor, C., Hughes, D.C., Zappone, E., Cazzola, M., Carter, G., Jacobs, A., & Padua, R.A. (1995a) A screen for RAS mutations in individuals at risk of secondary leukemia due to occupational exposure to petrochemicals. *Leukemia Research*, **19**, 299-301.

Taylor, C., McGlynn, H., Carter, G. Baker, A., Warren, N., Ridge, S.A., Owen, G., Thompson, E., Thompson, P.W., Jacobs, A., Padua, R.A. (1995b) RAS and FMS mutations following therapy of childhood acute lymphoblastic leukaemia. *Leukemia*, **9**, 466-470.

Taylor, C., Larghero, J., Thomas, K., Warren, N., Carter, G., Hughes, D., Culligan, D., Al-Sabah, A., Whittaker, J., Chomienne, C. & Padua, R.A. (2000) *HRAS* mutations in haematologically normal individuals. *Hematology Journal*, **1**, 399-402, 2000.

Tennant, G.B., Walsh, V., Truran, L.N., Edwards, P., Mills, K.I. & Burnett, A.K. (2000) Abnormalities of adherent layers grown from bone marrow of patients with myelodysplasia. *British Journal of Haematology*, **111**, 853-862.

Tosi, S., Harbott, J., Teigler-Schlegel, A., Haas, O.A., Pirc-Danoewinata, H., Harrison, C.J., Biondo, A., Cazzaniga, G., Kempsi, H., Scherer, S.W. & Kearney, L. (2000) t(7;12)(q36;p13), a new recurrent translocation involving ETV6 in infant leukemia. *Genes Chromosomes & Cancer*, **29**, 325-332.

Tsoplou, P., Kouraklis-Symeonidis, A., Thanopoulou, E., Zikos, P., Orphanos, V. & Zoumbos, N.C. (1999) Apoptosis in patients with myelodysplastic syndromes: differential involvement of marrow cells in 'good' versus 'poor' prognosis patients and correlation with apoptosis-related genes. *Leukemia*, **13**, 1554-1563.

Uchida, T., Kinoshita, T., Hotta, T., & Murate, T. (1998) High-risk myelodysplastic syndromes and hypermethylation of the p15Ink4B gene. *Leukemia & Lymphoma*, **32**, 9-18.

van Kamp, H., de Pijper, C., Verlaan-de Vries, M., Bos, J.L., Leeksma, C.H., Kerkhofs, H., Willemze, R., Fibbe, W.E. & Landegent, J.E. (1992) Longitudinal analysis of point mutations of the N-ras proto-oncogene in patients with myelodysplasia using archived blood smears. *Blood* **79**, 1266-1270.

Vanleeuwen F.E. (1996) Risk of acute myelogenous leukemia and myelodysplasia following cancer-treatment. *Baillieres Clinical Haematology*, **9**, 57-85.

Vieira, L., Marques, B., Ambrosio, A.P., Chumbo, M., Reis, A.B., Junior, E.C. & Boavida, M.G. (2000) TEL and MN1 fusion in myelodysplastic syndrome:new evidence for therapy-related event. *British Journal of Haematology*, **10**, 238-239.

Wattel, E., Solary, E., Hecquet, B. Caillot, D., Ifrah, N., Brion, A., Milipied, N., Janvier, M., Guerci, A., Rochant, H., Cordonnier, C., Dreyfus, F., Veil, A., Hoang-Ngoc, L., Stoppa, A.M., Gratecos, N., Sadoun, A., Tilly, H., Brice, P. Lioure, B., Desablens, B., Pignon, B., Abgrall, J.P., Leporrier, M., Fenaux, P. et al. (1999) Quinine improves results of intensive chemotherapy (IC) in myelodysplastic syndromes (MDS) expressing P-glycoprotein (PGP). Updated results of a randomized study. Groupe Francaise des Myelodysplasies (GFM) and Groupe GOELAMS. *Avances in Experimental Medicine and Biology*, **457**, 35-46.

West, R.R., Stafford, D.A., Farrow, A., & Jacobs, A. (1995) Occupational and environmental exposures and myelodysplasia - a case- control study. *Leukemia Research,* **19**, 127-139.

West, R.R., Stafford, D., White, A.D., Bowen, D.T., Padua, R.A. (2000) Cytogenetic abnormalities in the myelodysplastic syndromes and occupational or environmental exposure. *Blood,* **95**, 2093-2097.

Westbrook, C.A., Hsu, W., Chyna, B., Litvak, D., Raza, A. & Horrigan, S.K. (2000a) Cytogenetic and molecular diagnosis of chromosome 5 deletions in myelodysplasia. *British Journal of Haematology*, **110**, 847-855.

Westbrook, C.A., Hu, Z., Arbieva, Z., Kravarusic, J., Chyna, B., Edassery, S. & Horrigan, S.K. (2000b) Novel nuclear receptor coactivator is a candidate for the del(5q) leukemia tumor suppressor gene. *Experimental Hematology*, **28**, 1492.

White, A.D., Hoy, T.G. & Jacobs, A. (1994) Extended cytogenetic follow-up and clinical progression in patients with myelodysplastic syndromes (MDS). *Leukemia & Lymphoma*, **12**, 401-412.

White, A.D., Jones, B.M., Clark, R.E. & Jacobs A. (1992) Chromosome aberrations following cytotoxic therapy in patients in complete remission from lymphoma. *Carcinogenesis*, **13,** 1095-1099.

Wieser, R., Volz, A., Vinatzer, U., Gardiner, K., Jager, U., Mitterbauer, M., Ziegler, A. & Fonatsch, C. (2000) Transcription factor GATA-2 gene is located near 3q21 breakpoints in myeloid leukemia. *Biochemical Biophysical Research Communications*, **273**, 239-245.

Wilbanks, A.M., Mahajan, S., Frank, D.A., Druker, B.J., Gilliland, D.G. & Carroll, M. (2000) TEL/PDGFbetaR fusion protein activates STAT1 and STAT5 a common mechanism for transformation by tyrosine kinase fusion proteins. *Experimental Hematology*, **28**, 584-593.

Xi, Z.F., Russell, M., Woodward, S., Thompson, F., Wagner, L. & Taetle, R. (1997) Expression of the Zn finger gene, EVI-1, in acute promyelocytic leukemia. *Leukemia*, **11**, 212-220.

Xu, F. Taki, T., Yang, H.W., Hanada, R., Hongo, T., Ohnishi, H., Kobayashi, M, Bessho, F., Yanagisawa, M. & Hayashi, Y. (1999) Tandem duplication of the FLT3 gene is found in acute lymphoblastic leukemia as well as acute myeloid leukemia, not in myelodysplastic syndrome or juvenile chronic myelogenous leukemia in children. *British Journal of Haematology*, **105**, 155-162.

Yagasaki, F., Jinnai, I., Yoshida, S., Yokoyama, Y., Matsuda, A., Kusumoto, S., Yobayashi, H., Terasaki, H., Ohyashiki, I., Bessho, M., & Hirashima, K. (1999) Fusion of TEL/ETV6 to a novel ACS2 in myelodysplastic syndrome and acute myelogenous leukemia with t(5;12)(q31;p13). *Genes Chromosomes & Cancer*, **26**, 192-202.

Yergeau, D.A., Hetherington, C., Wang, Q., Zhang, P., Sharpe, A.H., Binder, M., Marin-Padilla, M., Tenen, D.G., Speck, N.A. & Zhang, D.E. (1997) Embryonic lethality and impairment of hematopoiesis in mice heterozygous for an AML-ETO fusion gene. *Nature Genetics*, **15**, 303-306.

Yin, S.N., Hayes, R.B., Linet, M.S., Li, G.L., Dosemeci, M., Travis, L.B., Li, C.Y., Zhang, Z.N., Li, D.G., Chow, W.H., Wacholder, S., Wang, Y.Z., Jiang, Z.L., Dai, T.R., Zhang, W.Y., Chao, X.J., Ye, P.Z., Kou, Q.R., Zhang, X.C., Lin, X.F., Meng, J.F., Ding, C.Y., Zho, J.S. & Blot, W.J. (1996) A cohort study of cancer among benzene-exposed workers in China - overall results. *American Journal Of Industrial Medicine,* **29**, 227-235.

Yokota, S., Kiyoi, H. Nakao, M., Iwai, T. Misawa, S., Okuda, T. Sonoda, Y., Abe, T., Kahsima, K. Matsuo, Y. & Naoe, T. (1997) Internal Tandem duplication of the FLT3 gene is preferentially seen in acute myleoid leukemia and myelodysplastic syndrome among various haematological malignancies. A study on a large series of patients and cell lines. *Leukemia*, **11**, 1605-1609.

Yoshida, Y. (1993) Hypothesis: apoptosis may be the mechanism reponsible for the premature intramedullary cell death in the myelodysplastic syndrome. *Leukemia*, **7**,144-146.

Yu, B.D., Hanson, R.D., Hess, J.L., Horning, S.E.& Korsemeyer, S.J. (1998) MLL, a mammalian trithorax-group gene functions as a transcriptional maintenance factor in morphogenesis. Proceedings of the Nartional Academy of Sciences USA, 95, 10632-10636.

Yunis, J.J., Boot, A.J., Mayer, M.G. & Bos, J.L. (1989) Mechanisms of ras mutation in myelodysplastic syndrome. *Oncogene* **4**, 609-614.

Zhang, L.P., Wang, Y.X., Shang, N., Smith, M.T. (1998) Benzene metabolites induce the loss and long arm deletion of chromosomes 5 and 7 in human lymphocytes. *Leukemia Research,* **22**:105-113.

Zwierzina, H., Anderson, J.E., Rollinger-Holzinger, I., Torok-Storb, B., Nuessler, V. & Lyman, S.D. (1999) Endogenous FLT-3 ligand serum levels are associated with desease stage in patients with myelodysplastic syndromes. *Leukemia*, **13**, 553-557.

9

STEM CELL TRANSPLANTATION FOR MYELODYSPLASIA

Hans – G. Klingemann* and H. Joachim Deeg+
**Section of Bone Marrow Transplant and Cell Therapy at RUSH Cancer Institute, Chicago, IL, and the +Fred Hutchinson Cancer Research Center, Seattle, WA*

The natural course of MDS varies considerably depending upon patient age and findings at the time of diagnosis. Life expectancy ranges from years in early stages to only a few months in advanced stages. The disease can rapidly progress to acute leukemia, and the prognosis for patients with advanced MDS (RAEB, RAEBT) and therapy-related (secondary) MDS is generally less than 12 months. CMML generally referred to as MDS has recently been reclassified as a myeloproliferative disorder (MPD), although myelodysplastic features are usually present. The median survival is 8 - 30 months. Since most transplant studies for MDS include CMML, this review will consider CMML as well. While patients with RA or RARS may fair well with conventional treatment, they frequently require transfusion support with red blood cells and platelets which results in iron overload and allo-sensitization. Prolonged neutropenia may facilitate infections which can significantly increase the risk of post-transplant complications.

With respect to the best timing of transplantation, the international prognostic scoring system (IPSS) appears to be useful. For example, a patient with high-risk cytogenetic abnormalities, a high number of blasts in the marrow, and peripheral cytopenia has a median life expectancy of only a few months and clearly should consider an allogeneic transplant without delay. Investigators at the Fred Hutchinson Cancer Research Center analyzed results in 251 patients transplanted (allogeneic) for MDS over a period of 15 years, and found the IPSS score to be the most powerful predictor for outcome (Appelbaum & Anderson, 1998). The five year relapse-free survival (RFS) was 60 % for patients with low, 35% for intermediate-1 and 28 % for intermediate -2 and high risk patients. Older age, longer disease duration, a mismatched donor, male gender and therapy-related MDS significantly increased non-relapse mortality. The Vancouver group studied 84 patients, and found cytogenetic abnormalities prior to transplant to be significant predictors of outcome after allogeneic BMT.

Stem cells transplantation is currently the only curative approach for MDS and is primarily offered to younger patients as the perception prevails from several earlier clinical studies that transplant-related complications are unacceptably high in recipients who are older than 40 years. However, it is time to revisit this issue since allogeneic transplantation using less toxic regimens as well as autografting present transplant options that are now available even for older patients.

ALLOGENEIC STEM CELL TRANSPLANTATION

An incidence of transplant-related mortality in the range of 30-50 % even in younger patients with MDS has discouraged many physicians from considering transplantation for newly diagnosed patients. Prolonged pre-transplant transfusion support and iron deposition is thought to contribute to post-transplant organ failure such as veno-occlusive disease (VOD) of the liver. Further, prolonged neutropenia pre-transplant increases the risk of opportunistic infections. Prolonged pre-transplant antibiotic use may also leave patients colonized with resistant pathogenic flora, especially fungi. Considering these factors, outcome would be expected to be more favorable if the transplant was performed early after diagnosis.

The Seattle group reported their experience in 70 patients with RA who received allogeneic transplants (Anderson et al., 1996a). Between 1981 and 1990 patients were conditioned with a standard CY/TBI regimen. Non-relapse mortality was relatively high (37%), while the relapse rate was low (only 1/40 patients relapsed). In an attempt to reduce regimen-related toxicity a non-TBI regimen consisting of busulfan/cyclophosphamide (BU/CY) was designed, and 38 patients were transplanted between 1990 and 1993. Disease free survival at three years post-transplant was 60 % for the CY/TBI and 63% for the BU/CY regimen. No differences in relapse probability (only one patient relapsed) and non-relapse mortality (37 % in both groups) were reported. The study confirmed that advanced patient age and longer disease duration were adverse prognostic factors. Actuarial survival was 78% for patients < 20 years, 58% for 20-29 years of age, 47% for 30 - 39 years of age and 46 % for patients 40 years and older. At five years, 58% of patients whose disease duration was less than 1 year at the time of transplant were disease free, compared to only 30 % of patients who had been diagnosed with their disease for more than five years. As non-relapse mortality was high with both regimens, but relapse was infrequent, the data suggested that a less intensive regimen might yield better results. The same group of investigators, therefore used a reqimen of CY plus TBI with lung and liver shielding. This trial however, was closed after only sixteen patients since the relapse rate was projected to be 36%. Presumably clonal precursors were protected during shielding, suggesting that "systemic" therapy with a stem cell-toxic agent is required.

A meta analysis of those studies raises the following issues: (i) since post-transplant relapse of RA was a rare occurrence, less intensive preparative regimens should be considered for this form of MDS. (ii) patients with adverse prognostic features (high number of marrow blasts, complex cytogenetics, multiple cytopenias) ought to be considered for BMT early after diagnosis ; (iii) conversely, patients who have an indolent course should be transplanted when cytopenia develops and transfusion requirements increase .

***Table 1**. Allogeneic stem cell transplantation for RA (Ia) and advanced MDS (Ib). Comparison of two different preparative regimen (Anderson et al,1996a)*

Ia:

	Bu/Cy2	Cy/TBI
Patients	28	38
DFS at 3 years	60 %	63 %
Relapse	4 %	0 %
TRM	37 %	37 %

Ib:

	Bu/Cy/TBI	Cy/TBI
Patients	31	44
DFS at 3 yrs	23 %	30 %
Relapse	28 %	54 % (n.s.)
TRM	68 %	36 %

Patients with *advanced MDS* (RAEB, RAEB-T and CMML) have a poorer outcome, largely due to a high relapse rate. In an effort to reduce disease recurrence post-transplant, the Seattle group tested a conditioning regimen consisting of busulfan 7mg/kg, cyclophosphamide (50 mg/kg) and 6 x 200 cGy of TBI (Anderson et al., 1996b). Compared to a historical group of patients who had been given standard CY/TBI conditioning, actuarial disease free survival was similar (23% versus 30%). However, the non-relapse mortality was unacceptably high in the BU/CY/TBI group (68% versus 36%). The conclusion form this and similar studies from other centers was that either novel, less toxic conditioning regimen should be applied or transplantation at an earlier disease stage needed to be considered.

Favorable single center results were recently reported by Okamoto et al. (1999), who treated 13 patients with advanced MDS (RAEB: n =4, RAEB-T: n=1 and secondary MDS: n=8) with a combination of radiation (6 x 200 cGy) followed by cytosine arabinoside (Ara-C) at a dose of 3 g/m^2 every 12 hours for 4 consecutive days. In addition, G-CSF was administered by continuous infusion, which was commenced 12 hours before the first dose of Ara-C and discontinued at the completion of the last dose of Ara-C. G-CSF was administered with the rationale of driving MDS cells into cell cycle and render them more susceptible to the cytotoxic effect of Ara-C. Projected RFS and overall survival rates at 5 years were 67.7% and 75.5%, respectively. Projected relapse and non-relapse mortality rates at 5 years were 8.3% and 26.7%, respectively.

MDS is primarily a disease of older patients with a median age of 65-70 years at the time of diagnosis. With proper patient selection and earlier transplantation would it be safe to offer allogeneic transplantation even to older patients? The Seattle team has reviewed their experience in 50 patients who were between 55 and 66 years old at the time of transplant (Deeg et al., 2000). Relapse rate was low in patients with RA (1/13), whereas 19% of patients with RAEB and 37% with RAEB-T/AML relapsed. The actuarial 3 year survival for patients with de novo RA, RAEB and RAEB-T/AML was 57%, 52% and 45% respectively. In all groups results were best among patients prepared with a regimen of "targeted" BU in combination with CY. Using IPSS scores , survival for the 4 risks groups was 100%, 54%, 44% and 30% respectively. These data show that transplantation can be carried out successfully in older patients, and confirm that the pre-transplant IPSS score also affects the outcome after stem cell transplantation.

Table 2. *Outcome of allogeneic stem cell transplantation in patients age 55-65 years. Actuarial survival at 3 years according to diagnosis or IPSS score.*

Diagnosis	**RFS**
RA:	57 %
RAEB:	52 %
RAEB-T/AML:	45 %
IPSS Score	
IPSS 1:	100 %
IPSS 2:	54 %
IPSS 3:	44 %
IPSS 4:	30 %

ALLOGENEIC TRANSPLANTATION USING REDUCED DOSE INTENSITY REGIMENS

Over the past few years so called "mini-transplants" have emerged as a treatment modality. These transplants rely on conditioning regimens that are predominantly immunosuppressive (fludarabin, anti-T-cell antibodies, low dose total body radiation) in combination with post-transplant immunotherapy, and usually peripheral blood derived progenitors rather than marrow as a source of stem cells. Chemotherapy is given usually at non-myeloablative doses. The primary objective of such an approach is to allow donor cell engraftment and to achieve a donor derived anti-cancer response (graft-versus-leukemia, GVL) effect. Because of the reduced toxicity of these regimens, these transplants can even be performed in the outpatient setting. These transplants also allow to extend the age range for transplantation, and some centers will now accept patients up to 70 or 75 years of age.

Such an approach seems to be most appropriate for early stage MDS with low tumor cell burden. Preliminary results are encouraging. Compared to transplantation using high doses of chemotherapy, the duration of aplasia was significantly shorter, and transplant related mortality was generally lower (e.g. day 100 mortality 10% vs 15 – 20 %) than with high dose conditioning. However, despite the enthusiasm for reduced intensity conditioning regimens (mini-transplants), one has to keep in mind that follow-up so far is short. There is also some concern that especially older patients may experience significant acute and chronic GVHD.

RESPONSE TO DONOR LYMPHOCYTE INFUSIONS (DLI)

Patients with relapsed AML and MDS do not respond as well to DLI as patients with recurrent CML, low grade lymphoma or myeloma. Still, MDS appears to be responsive to manipulations of the recipient's immune system. One case report describes a patient with progressive secondary MDS who responded to IL-2 injections with a cytogenetic remission of limited duration. There are also some, albeit limited, data from patients with MDS who were treated with DLI. In the study by Porter et al. (1996) 3 patients (RAEB: n=1, CMML: n=1, RA: n=1) were given DLI. Only the patient with RA entered a CR: the patient with RAEB had only transient hematologic improvement. As of August 98 the European Bone Marrow Transplant EBMT group had reported 9 evaluable patients with MDS, 4 of whom achieved a complete remission (44%). Similar results (unpublished) have been observed by the Seattle group. This response rate is similar to that in patients with AML, but significantly inferior to the response rate seen after DLI for relapsed CML. Patients who receive chemotherapy (e.g. high dose cytosine arabinoside) prior to DLI seem to have a better response, possibly due to cytoreduction and immune suppression to avoid donor cell rejection.

Autologous stem cell transplantation

The rationale for autologous transplantation in MDS is based on the observation that clonogenic cells co-exist with a residual population of normal hematopoietic progenitor cells in the marrow. Not unexpectedly, transplant related mortality is generally lower after autologous (14 %) than after allogeneic BMT (38%). Of note, however, is the delayed neutrophil (median: 48) and platelet (median: 95days) recovery seen after autologous transplant.

There is indirect evidence for the notion that autologous transplant, if considered, should be performed early in the course of the disease. Studies in patients with CML have shown that the pool of normal stem cells is larger at an early stage of the disease. Although similar data are not yet available for MDS, there is concern about the depletion of the normal hematopoietic stem cell compartment which develops over the course of the disease. Furthermore, progressive defects in the bone marrow stroma and the development of myelofibrosis can also occur as the disease evolves. Finally, data suggest that the multidrug-resistant (MDR) gene is over-expressed on myeloblasts evolving from MDS.

Obtaining a stem cell inoculum (either bone marrow or PBSC) which is free of malignant precursors is essential for the prevention of relapse. There is strong evidence that all patients who continue to have clonal precusors in the harvest product, relapse after autologous transplantation. But even some patients who received a perfectly 'clean' graft (as determined by the best available techniques) experienced disease recurrence after autologous transplantation. As with other malignancies, malignant cells surviving in the patient may cause relapse if not contained by a graft-versus-leukemia effect.

The EBMT Group retrospectively compared outcome in 130 patients who received an autologous transplant with 177 patients who received an HLA matched unrelated donor transplant (Gassmann et al., 1996). Cohorts were well matched for diagnosis, age, stage of disease and interval from diagnosis to transplant. Not unexpectedly, transplant related mortality was significantly higher in unrelated recipients (55%) than in autologous BMT patients (22%). The RFS at three years was the same in both groups. The conclusion of this study was that patients with more advanced MDS should receive induction chemotherapy and if they enter a complete remission, could be considered for an autologous BMT.

Table 3. *Autologous stem cell transplantation for MDS. Data from a review presented by Witte et al. at the American Society of Hematology Meeting in 1999*

	Number	RFS	TRM	Relapse
Overall	266	27	29	62
CR-1	185	32	22	59
no CR1	81	14	50	72
p=		<0.001	0.001	0.02

TRANSPLANTATION FOR SECONDARY MDS

Secondary MDS (therapy-related) has a particularly poor prognosis with an estimated one year survival of 10% - 15% with supportive care alone. Ballen et al. (1997) reported 18 patients with therapy-related MDS who received an allogeneic BMT at a median age of 32 years. At three years the actuarial disease free survival was 24 %. In the Seattle study by Anderson et al., (1996a) in patients older than 55 years, eight patients were included who were transplanted for secondary MDS with similar outcome as reported by Ballen et al. The French Society of BMT reported outcome of 77 patients with secondary AML/MDS following cytotoxic exposure. Similar to the other studies, the 5 years disease free survival was 24%. However there was a statistically significant difference between patients who achieved a CR with chemotherapy before BMT (55 %) versus those who did not (10 %).

Results from 20 allogeneic stem cell transplants in children with secondary MDS have recently been reported. FAB classification was RA/RARS in 6, RAEB in 7, RAEB-T in 6 and unclassified in1. Five patients received transplants from matched siblings, 14 from either an unrelated donor (marrow: n=8; placental blood n=3), a partially matched related donor (n=3) or an autologous BMT [n= 1]. With a median follow-up of 16 months, disease free and overall survival for the group were 50% and 60% respectively.

If secondary MDS develops following autologous BMT, the outcome is generally very poor. The Boston group (Friedberg et al., 1999) reported 11 patients (4 with RA or RARS, 7 with advanced MDS) who received transplants from HLA identical siblings (n=6) or unrelated donors (n=5). All patients died (sepsis: n=6, VOD: n=2, alveolar hemorrhage n=1) with a median survival of 1.6 months after BMT.

Table 4. *Outcome of patients receiving an allogeneic transplant for secondary MDS*

Study	N	Age (median)	TRM	RFS
Ballen et al.	18	32		24% at 3 yrs
Seattle	8	59		24% at 3 yrs
City of Hope	8			25% at 2 yrs
French BMT Soc	77	38	47%	24% at 5 yrs
			(55% vs. 10% when CR at BMT)	
Boston*	11	n/a	91%	0% at 1 yr
Children	20	n/a	n/a	50% at 2 yrs

**secondary MDS after autologous BMT*

Conclusions

Allogeneic stem cell transplantation from a matched related donor for the treatment of MDS is indicated if the patient has high risk features or clinically relevant cytopenias are developing. If non-myeloablative transplants prove to provide long term disease free survival, the age range for allogeneic transplants may well go beyond 60 years. In patients younger than 50 years without a matched related donor, an unrelated donor transplant should be considered. Although transplants in patients with MDS who lack high risk features may be difficult to justify, it is important to emphasize that transplants at an early stage have a very favorable outcome. Autologous BMT at this point has to be considered investigational.

ACKNOWLEDGEMENTS

Dr. Klingemann acknowledges the Coleman Foundation and Dr. Deeg acknowledges grants CA87948 and HL 36444 and, the Gabrielle Rich Leukemia Fund for their support.

REFERENCES

Anderson, J.E., Appelbaum, F.R., Schoch, G. Gooley, T., Anasetti, C., Bensinger, W.I., Bryant, E., Dean Buckner, C, Chauncey, T, Clift, R.A., Doney, K., Flowers, M., Hansen, J.A., Martin, P.J., Matthews, D.C., Sanders, J.E., Shulman, H., Sullivan, K.M., Witherspoon, R.P., & Storb, R. (1996a) Allogeneic Marrow Transplant for Refractory Anemia: A comparison of two preparative regimens and analysis of prognostic factors. *Blood*, **87,** 51-58.

Anderson, J.E., Appelbaum, F.R., Schoch, G. Gooley, T., Anasetti, C., Bensinger, W.I., Bryant, E., Dean Buckner, C, Chauncey, T, Clift, R.A., Joachim Deeg, H., Doney, K., Flowers, M., Hansen, J.A., Martin, P.J., Matthews, D.C., Nash, R.A., Sanders, J.E., Shulman, H., Sullivan, K.M., Witherspoon, R.P., & Storb, R. (1996b) Allogeneic marrow transplantation for myelodysplastic syndrome with advanced disease morphology: A phase II study of Busulfan, Cyclophosphamide, and total-body irradiation and analysis of prognostic factors. *Journal of Clinical Oncology*, **14,** 220-226.

AppeLbaum, F., & Anderson, J. (1998) Allogeneic bone marrow transplantation for myelodysplastic syndrome: outcomes analysis according to IPSS score. *Leukemia*, **12, Supplement 1**, S25-S29.

Ballen, K.K., Gilliland, D.G., Guinan, E.C., Hsieh, C-C., Parsons, S.K., Rimm, I.J., Ferrara, J.L.M., Bierer, B.E., Weinstein, H.J., & Antin, J.H. (1997) Bone marrow transplantation for therapy-related myelodysplasia: comparison with primary myelodysplasia. *Bone Marrow Transplantation*, **20**, 737-743.

Deeg, H.J., Shulman, H.M., Anderson, J.E., Bryant, E.M., Gooley, T.A., Slattery, J.T., Anasetti, C., Fefer, A., Storb, R., & Appelbaum, F.R. (2000) Allogeneic and syngeneic marrow transplantation for myelodysplastic syndrome in patients 55 to 66 years of age. *Blood*, **95,** 1188-1194.

Friedberg, J.W., Neuberg, D., Stone, R.M., Alyea, E., Jallow, H., LaCasce, A., Mauch, P.M., Gribben, J.G., Ritz, J., Nadler, L.M., Soiffer, R.J., & Freedman, A.S. (1999) Outcome in patients with myelodysplastic syndrome after autologous bone marrow transplantation for non-Hodgkin's lymphoma. *Journal of Clinical Oncology*, **17,** 3128-3135.

Gassmann, W., Schmitz, N., Loffler, H., & DeWitte, T. (1996) Intensive chemotherapy and bone marrow transplantation for myelodysplastic syndromes. *Seminars in Hematology*, **33,** 196-205.

Okamoto, S., Takahashi, S., Wakui, M., Ishida, A., Tanosaki, R., Ikeda, Y., & Asano, S. (1999) Treatment of advanced myelodysplastic syndromes with a regimen including recombinant human granulocyte colony-stimulating factor preceding allogeneic bone marrow transplantation. *British Journal of Haematology,* **104**: 569-573.

Porter, D.L., Roth, M.S., Lee, S.J., McGarigle, C., Ferrara, J.L.M., & Antin, J.H. (1996) Adoptive immunotherapy with donor mononuclear cell infusions to treat relapse of acute leukemia or myelodysplasia after allogeneic bone marrow transplantation. *Bone Marrow Transplantation*, **18**, 975-980.

10

MYELODYSPLASTIC SYNDROMES COMPLICATING HEMATOPOIETIC STEM CELL TRANSPLANTATION

Athanasios B.-T. Fassas and Guido Tricot
Myeloma and Transplantation Research Center,
University of Arkansas for Medical Sciences, Little Rock, AR

INTRODUCTION

The development of therapy-related myelodysplasia (t-MDS) and acute myelogenous leukemia (t-AML) has been increasingly recognized as an important problem following high-dose chemotherapy and autologous hematopoietic stem cell transplantation (AHSCT) (Stone et al., 1994; Deeg et al. 1998; Pedersen-Bjergaard et al., 2000). The significance of this issue is better appreciated in light of the expanding indications for AHSCT early in the treatment course along with its limited related mortality. Any discussion of t-MDS/AML complicating AHSCT should take into account the contribution of chemotherapy, especially with alkylating agents, administered prior to transplantation and the difficulty of establishing the diagnosis solely on morphologic grounds. Several reports over the last 10 years, have extensively discussed many aspects of t-MDS/AML, such as origin of the disease, risk factors, cytogenetic abnormalities and available therapeutic options. However, important questions especially regarding the relative contribution of prior chemotherapy, the extent to which total body irradiation (TBI) increases the risk of t-MDS/AML, and the significance of MDS-related chromosomal changes in the absence of bone marrow dysplasia still remain.

CAUSE OF DISEASE

Despite the considerable debate concerning the cause of t-MDS/AML, it is safe to conclude that most cases should be attributed to relatively low-dose conventional chemotherapy administered prior to the AHSCT. These relatively low doses of cytotoxic agents are sufficient to induce genetic damage into the hematopoietic stem cells (HSC), but are not lethal. Several studies delineate, albeit in different ways, the significant impact of the primary chemotherapeutic regimen with alkylating agents (Stone et al., 1994; Wheeler et al., 1997; Pedersen-Bjergaard et al., 2000; Harrison et al., 1998; Milligan et al., 1999; Govindarajan et al., 1996). The very short latent period between the AHSCT and the development of t-MDS/AML (while the interval between original diagnosis and t-MDS/AML is comparable otherwise to that observed in conventionally treated patients who developed t-MDS/AML) and the finding that the actual risk of t-MDS/AML following AHSCT is similar to that seen in patients treated with intensive chemotherapy (without, however, stem cell rescue) (Pedersen-Bjergaard et al., 1987) support this conclusion. More importantly, the same chromosomal abnormalities seen in t-MDS/AML were retrospectively identified by fluorescence in situ hybridization (FISH) in the stem cell grafts of 9 out of 12 examined patients, lending further support to the notion that the HSC were abnormal prior to the transplantation (Abruzzese et al., 1999).

Some other findings, however, point to the transplant event as, at least, a contributing factor. Some patients treated only with six courses of CHOP (a regimen not known to be leukemogenic) have developed t-MDS/AML after AHSCT (Stone et al., 1994). Normal bone marrow karyotype at the time of harvesting (in patients who subsequently developed t-MDS/AML) suggests that the reinfused cells at the time of AHSCT were normal(Miller et al., 1994; Micallef et al., 2000; Krishnan et al., 2000). It needs to be pointed out, however, that the use of conventional cytogenetic analysis may not detect preleukemic clones in the asymptomatic phase because these clones have not yet acquired a growth advantage over the normal HSC or, alternatively, because they have not yet accumulated major DNA damage, resulting in cytogenetic abnormalities. Approximately 70% of *de novo* MDS patients with refractory anemia and refractory anemia with ringed sideroblasts have normal karyotypes (Weh et al., 1987). The reports of increased risk of t-MDS/AML following TBI conditioning (Stone et al., 1994; Wheeler et al., 1997; Milligan et al., 1999; Darrington et al., 1994; Friedberg et al., 1999; Ketterer et al., 1998; Berglund et al., 2000; Park et al., 2000; Micallef et al., 2000) suggest a leukemogenic role of the transplant procedure. However, the expected complete marrow ablation by TBI has not resulted in an increased incidence of treatment-related MDS/AML in the allogeneic transplant setting. In this setting mixed chimerism has been observed in many patients conditioned with TBI and cyclophosphamide (Roy et al., 1990). Therefore, surviving but genetically damaged HSC could give rise to t-MDS/AML. An effect of the high-dose chemotherapy is also suggested by the finding that the risk is increasing with the number of the transplants performed (Milligan et al., 1999). Finally, the higher risk seen, at least in some studies, with peripheral blood stem cell transplants (compared to bone marrow harvests) indicates a potential contribution of the mobilization chemotherapy (Miller et al., 1994; Krishnan et al., 2000; Bhatia et al., 1996). From this perspective, it would be interesting to follow the course of patients who received stem cell transplants mobilized only with growth factors as well as the course of patients transplanted for autoimmune diseases (multiple sclerosis, systemic lupus) with a limited or no exposure to previous chemotherapy.

In a recent study, Harrison et al. reported on a comparative retrospective analysis of 4576 patients with Hodgkin's disease, 595 of whom received autologous transplant. The risk of developing t-MDS/AML was dominated by the quantity of prior treatment and exposure to MOPP regimen or lomustine. After adjustment for these factors in the multivariate model, the relative risk associated with high-dose chemotherapy and transplantation itself was only 1.83 (95% CI: 0.66-5.11, p: 0.25).

RISK FACTORS

Several studies have evaluated the actuarial risk of t-MDS/AML following AHSCT (Stone et al., 1994; Wheeler et al., 1997; Pedersen-Bjergaard et al., 2000; Harrison et al., 1998; Milligan et al., 1999; Govindarajan et al., 1996; Miller et al., 1994; Darrington et al., 1994; Friedberg et al., 1999; Park et al., 2000; Micallef et al., 2000; Krishnan et al., 2000; Bhatia et al., 1996; Traweek et al., 1994; Taylor et al., 1997; André et al., 1998; Laughlin et al.; 1998; Kollmannsberger et al., 1998; Del Cañizo et al, 2000). Most reports included patients with lymphoma, while multiple myeloma (Govindarajan et al., 1996), breast cancer (Laughlin et al., 1998) and germ cell tumor (Kollmannsberger et al., 1998) patients were analyzed each in one study (Table I). The cumulative risk has varied widely between 1.1% at 20 months to 24.3% at 43 months post-transplant (Table 1). The differences observed can be attributed to different patient follow-up periods, small number of events (MDS/AML), different patient populations as well as pre-transplant conditioning used.

Table 1. *Risk of t-MDS/AML following autologous hematopoietic stem cell transplantation: review of the literature*

Authors	Primary tumor	No. patients t- MDS/ No patients t-AML/ *No patients treated*	Actuarial risk
Miller et al.	HD	3/0/68	14.5% at 4 y
	NHL	3/1/138	
Bhatia et al.	HD	9/1/258	13.5% at 6 y
	NHL		
Traweek et al.$	HD	2/2/108	9% at 3 y
	NHL	5/1/167	
Krishnan et al.*	HD	11/218	8.6% at 6 y
	NHL	11/394	
Darrington et al.	HD	4/2/249	4% at 5 y
	NHL	6/0/262	
Stone et al.	NHL	18/2/262	18% at 6 y
Friedberg et al.	NHL	41/0/552	19.8% at 10 y
Wheeler et al.*	HD	6/300	4.2% at 5 y
	NHL		
Taylor et al.#	HD	0/1/52	1.1 % at 1.6 y
	NHL	0/0/62	
Pedersen-Bjergaard et al.	HD	1/1/27	24.3% at 3.5 y
	NHL	3/1/49	
André et al.	HD	5/3/467	4.3% at 5 y
Harrison et al.*	HD	8/595	3.1% at 5 y
Milligan et al.	HD	51/15/4998	4.6% at 5 y
	NHL		3.0 % at 5 y
Govindarajan et al.	MM	0/0/71†	0%
		7/0/117‡	12% at 4 y
Laughlin et al.	Breast carcinoma	3/2/864§	1.6% at 4 y
Kollmannsberger et al.	Germ cell tumors	2/4/302	1.3% at 4.3 y
Del Cañizo et al.•	HD	4/2/225	Not reported
	NHL	4/1/308	
Park et al. @	HD	1/2/69	6.3% at 10 y
	NHL	2/4/299	
Micallef et al. +	NHL	25/2/230	Not reported

*Abbreviations: HD: Hodgkin's disease, NHL: non-Hodgkin lymphoma, MM: multiple myeloma; *No distinction between t-MDS and t-AML; •2 more cases of t-MDS were observed in patients with multiple myeloma and acute myelogenous leukemia; # 1 patient with chronic myelogenous leukemia;§ 1 patient with acute lymphoblastic leukemia;† Previously treated only with one course of cytotoxic chemotherapy; ‡ Previously treated with more than one course of cytotoxic chemotherapy; @ 2 patients with acute lymphoblastic leukemia; + 1 patient with chronic myelomonocytic leukemia; $ patients were included in the study on the basis of clonal chromosomal abnormalities*

The risk of t-MDS/AML was found to increase with patient **age** and **prior treatment** with alkylating agents (Table II). Age over 35 and 40 years at the time of transplant was a risk factor in the lymphoma studies from

Minnesota (Miller et al., 1994) and Nebraska (Darrington et al., 1994), respectively. The EBMT cooperative study (Milligan et al., 1999) also confirmed this finding. The amount and duration of prior chemotherapy and exposure to alkylating agents were significant risk factors in the study from the Dana Farber Institute (Stone et al., 1994; Wheeler et al., 1997). The myeloma study from Arkansas (Govindarajan et al., 1996) identified all 7 patients with t-MDS in a group of 117 transplanted patients who had received more than one cycle of chemotherapy prior to enrollment in the transplant study. No t-MDS/AML was seen in a group of 71 patients who were transplanted after no or only one cycle of conventional chemotherapy. Other studies indirectly confirmed the significance of prior treatment by showing the importance of the time interval between the original diagnosis and AHSCT and the number of previous lymphoma relapses (Stone et al., 1994; Wheeler et al., 1997; Milligan et al., 1999).

Table 2. *Risk Factors for t-MDS/AML following autologous stem cell transplantation*

Older age	Milligan et al., 1999; Miller et al., 1994; Darrington et al., 1994; Micallef et al., 2000
Previous chemotherapy (cumulative dose/duration) (alkylating agents)	Stone et al., 1994; Wheeler et al., 1997; Pedersen-Bjergaard et al., 1997; Harrison *et al*, 1998; Milligan et al., 1999; Govindarajan et al.; 1996; Park et al., 2000; Del Cañizo et al., 2000
(topoisomerase II inhibitors)	Krishnan et al., 2000; Kollmansberger et al., 1998
Total body irradiation (TBI)	Stone et al., 1994; Wheeler et al., 1997; Milligan et al., 1999; Darrington et al., 1994; Ketterer et al., 1998
Previous radiotherapy	Stone et al., 1994; Wheeler et al., 1997; Park et al., 2000
Fludarabine	Ketterer et al., 1998; Micallef et al., 2000
Splenectomy	André et al., 1998

Conditioning with **TBI** might also contribute to an increased risk of t-MDS/AML (Table 2). Ketterer et al. (1998) in an abstract form reported a statistically significant association between the use of TBI and development of MDS, especially when used in patients previously exposed to **fludarabine,** which effectively depletes the HSC pool. The EBMT study confirmed that radiotherapy used in the conditioning regimen was an independent and significant risk factor (Milligan et al., 1999). A marked decrease in the incidence of t-MDS/AML was appreciated in two parallel studies from the Dana Farber Institute, after the use of TBI was abandoned from the conditioning regimen (Stone et al., 1994; Wheeler et al., 1997). Total body irradiation reached statistical significance as a risk factor for t-MDS in the report of lymphoma patients from Nebraska (Darrington et al., 1994). In a recent, small study of 22 patients with follicular lymphoma who received AHSCT, 3 cases of t-MDS were diagnosed, all in TBI-treated patients (Berglund et al., 2000). TBI in the conditioning regimen was also associated with t-MDS/AML in another study of 395 lymphoma patients from France (Park et al., 2000). The St Bartholomew's transplant group observed no further cases of t-MDS (although with a limited follow-up) after discontinuation of the TBI use (Micallef et al., 2000). The same group recently confirmed that exposure to fludarabine was associated with an increased risk of t-MDS/AML.

Prior splenectomy as a risk factor for subsequent myelodysplasia in patients with Hodgkin's disease was reported by André et al.. The finding was not confirmed in the British cooperative study (Harrison et al., 1998). Use of **etoposide** (Table II) as part of the stem cell mobilization chemotherapy was associated with the development of t-AML with the typical 11q23/21q22 chromosomal abnormalities, characteristic for the edipodophyllotoxins. Such "priming" treatment conferred a 12.3-fold higher risk of developing t-AML in a study of lymphoma patients from the City of Hope Medical Center (Krishnan et al, 2000). A cumulative dose of etoposide greater than 2 gr/m^2 was found to correlate with t-AML in patients with advanced germ cell tumors who underwent AHSCT (Kollmannsberger et al., 1998). Of note, the incidence of t-MDS/AML in the two studies of AHSCT for solid tumors (breast cancer, germ cell tumors) was much lower than that reported for the patients with hematologic malignancies, probably reflecting the lower intensity of prior chemotherapy and the younger age of the treated patients. Finally, **radiotherapy** treatment prior to preparation for autologous transplantation was found to be a significant risk factor for t-MDS/AML in three studies (Stone et al., 1994; Wheeler et al., 1997; Park et al., 2000). Although no convincing data exist regarding a potential association between the number of stem cells infused and the development of t-MDS/AML, it is tempting to speculate that patients who are transplanted with minimal numbers of stem cells are more likely to develop t-MDS. A small population of stem cells will result in constant stress on the bone marrow and continuous proliferation, additionally driven by the administration of hematopoietic growth factors, thus enhancing the possibility of genetic damage. Conversely, however, the inability to collect adequate stem cells may reflect bone marrow damage inflicted by the previously administered chemoradiotherapy.

SOURCE OF STEM CELLS

Over the last 10 years, the collection of hematopoietic progenitors from the peripheral blood, either after "priming" chemotherapy and/or with hematopoietic growth factors, has almost completely replaced the harvest of bone marrow cells. As no prospective comparison of peripheral blood and bone marrow grafts on the outcome of the primary malignancy and the risk of post-transplant t-MDS/AML has been conducted (and it would be extremely difficult to design now), we have to rely on the results of retrospective studies. Three independent studies (Miller et al., 1994; Bhatia et al., 1996; André et al., 1998) have shown an increased risk of t-MDS/AML after transplantation with peripheral blood stem cells, when compared to bone marrow harvests. A recent analysis of more than 1400 patients from Spain (Del Cañizo et al., 2000) found no difference in the crude incidence of t-MDS/AML according to the source of progenitor cells. However, the median time between AHSCT and t-MDS/AML was significantly longer for patients who received bone marrow than for those who received peripheral blood. Although the issue is by no means resolved, it is challenging to consider the biologic differences between HSC from the peripheral blood and the bone marrow. It is possible that the peripheral stem cell grafts contain hematopoietic progenitors, which were damaged by the priming chemotherapy and were unable to subsequently completely repair their DNA damage. These cells are reinfused after a myeloablative preparative regimen and then forced to proliferate, further stimulated by hematopoietic growth factors. Therefore, they may be more prone to subsequent development of t-MDS/AML compared to "steady state" bone marrow progenitors collected without chemotherapy "priming". Alternatively, peripheral blood grafts may contain more preleukemic clones than the bone marrow harvests because of differences in adhesive properties between normal and preleukemic stem cells. Of course, the early diagnosis of t-MDS/AML in the recent years by routinely performing cytogenetic analyses coincided with the switch from bone marrow to peripheral blood as a source of stem cells.

PRESENTATION, CYTOGENETICS ANALYSIS OF OUTCOME OF T-MDS/AML

The diagnosis, classification and prognosis of *de novo* MDS is based on the French-American-British (FAB) cooperative group criteria (Bennett et al., 1976; Bennett et al., 1982; Greenberg et al., 1997). Peripheral blood cytopenias in the presence of dysplastic features and/or excess blasts in the bone marrow usually establish the diagnosis, which is further supported by the detection of characteristic cytogenetic abnormalities. The diagnosis of MDS in the post-AHSCT is much more problematic. The marrow is frequently fibrotic and hypocellular with dysplastic changes; peripheral cytopenias are frequently present for months or even years post-transplant, caused by infusion of inadequate numbers of stem cells, without showing clear evidence of MDS. Therefore, neither the diagnosis nor the prognosis can be solely based upon morphologic examination of bone marrow except in the presence of excess of bone marrow blasts, unequivocal Auer rods or more than an occasional blast in the peripheral blood (Amigo et al., 1999). The diagnosis relies heavily on the detection of clonal chromosomal abnormalities in the presence of cytopenias of at least 6-12 months duration post-transplant. Two forms of the syndrome have been characterized; an indolent form manifested by persistent cytopenias years after transplant with or without clonal cytogenetic changes and an aggressive form with multiple line dysplasia and rather “malignant”clinical behaviour with rapid evolution to acute leukemia (Wilson et al., 1997).

The disease presents much more frequently as t-MDS than as t-AML (approximate ratio: 4:1). This excess of MDS has also been observed following treatment with alkylating agents (Le Beau et al., 1986; Johansson et al., 1991; Pedersen-Bjergaard et al., *1995)*. Details about the interval between AHSCT and t-MDS/AML have been reported for 151 patients (Table 3).

Table 3. *Latent period between autologous stem cell transplantation and development of t-MDS/AML: review of the literature*

Latent Period (months)	t-MDS Number of patients	t-AML* Number of patients
1-6	5	4
7-12	16	6
13-24	27	6
25-36	20	6
37-48	22	6
49-60	10	4
>60	16	3

Data from references: (Stone et al., 1994; Pedersen-Bjergaard et al., 1997; Govindarajan et al., 1996; Miller et al., 1994; Darrington et al., 1994; Park et al., 2000; Micallef et al., 2000; Traweek et al., 1994; Taylor et al., 1997; Laughlin et al., 1998; Kollmansberger et al., 1998; Del Cañizo et al., 2000; Gale et al., 1996; Sobecks et al., 1999; Marolleau et al., 1993; Rege et al., 1998; Roman-Unfer et al., 1995)

**Includes 4 patients with acute lymphoblastic leukemia and 1 patient each with chronic myelogenous leukemia and chronic myelomonocytic leykemia.*

Only four patients were diagnosed with acute lymphoblastic and one with chronic myelogenous leukemia following AHSCT. Approximately one fourth of the patients were diagnosed with t-MDS/AML during the first year following AHSCT while it was only rarely observed more than 5 years post-transplant. In five additional studies the median intervals between AHSCT and t-MDS/AML were 1.9 years (y) for a group of 22 patients, 2.4 y for a group of 6 patients, 4.4 y for a group of 27 patients, 3.8 y for a group of 70 patients and 3.9 y for a group of 41 patients, respectively (Table 4). Therefore, although the general risk decreases 5 years after AHSCT, t-MDS/AML may develop late after transplantation, emphasizing the need for prolonged surveillance.

Table 4. *Latent period between autologous stem cell transplantation and development of t-MDS/AML : review of the literature*

Reference	Number of patients	Median (years)	Range (years)
Friedberg et al.	41	3.9	1-10.8
Krishnan et al.	22	1.9	N/A
Wheeler et al.	6	2.4	0.5-4.6
Micallef et al.	27	4.4	0.9-8.8
Yakoub-Agha et al.	70	3.8	0.9-15.3

Detailed cytogenetic analysis has been reported for at least 249 patients with t-MDS/AML. Only 24 patients had a normal karyotype probably reflecting the difficulty of diagnosing t-MDS/AML in the absence of cytogenetic abnormalities. Not unexpectedly, the most common abnormalities were the loss or deletion of the long arms or the loss of the whole chromosomes 5 and/or 7, observed after exposure to alkylating agents in at least 142 patients. Balanced translocations involving chromosome bands 11q23 or 21q22 were detected in 18 patients, who had been exposed to DNA topoisomerase II inhibitors. Trisomy 8 was seen in 14 patients.

The prognosis of t-MDS/AML is poor. A compilation of data from the published series is presented in Table 5. The median survival after the establishment of diagnosis is 6 months. Conventional antileukemic therapy appears to be only of minimal benefit. Differentiating agents, retinoids, vitamin D, interferons and hematopoietic growth factors have no significant impact on survival despite occasional success in the correction of cytopenias.

Table 5. *Survival of patients after the diagnosis of t-MDS/AML following autologous stem cell transplantation*

Survival(months)	Died of t-MDS	Died of t-AML	Died of t-ALL	Still alive
0-6	28	11	3	7
7-12	23	6*		4
13-18	3	4		1
>18	5	2	1	14
Total	59	23	4	26

*Data from references : (Stone et al., 1994; Pedersen-Bjergaard et al., 1997; Miller et al., 1994; Darrington et al., 1994; Park et al., 2000; Micallef et al., 2000; Traweek et al., 1994; Laughlin et al., 1998; Kollmannsberger et al., 1998; Gale et al., 1996; Sobecks et al., 1999);*Includes 1 patient with chronic myelomonocytic leukemia*

The only potentially curative approach (a statement that applies to *de novo* MDS, too) is allogeneic bone marrow/stem cell transplantation (allo-BMT). Initial results with this approach have not been particularly encouraging. Friedberg et al. treated 13 t-MDS/AML patients with allo-BMT. All died, including 10 within the first 100 days after transplant. The median survival time from the allo-BMT was only 1.8 months. Ballen et al. reported an actuarial disease-free survival of 24% at 3 years for a group of 18 rather young patients with therapy-related MDS. None had undergone AHSCT as part of previous treatment. The cytogenetic "profile" of the patients in this series was favorable, as only 2 patients had a complex karyotype and only 4 had abnormalities of chromosomes 5 and 7. In the Seattle experience (Anderson et al., 1997), the results of allo-BMT in therapy-related AML in general were extremely poor with a dismal 5-year survival of only 7.8%. Yakoub-Agha et al. reported a 2-year overall survival, event-free survival, relapse and transplant-related mortality of 30%, 28%, 42% and 49%, respectively. The study included 70 patients. No information was given about prior AHSCT. Approximately one third of the patients had poor-risk cytogenetic abnormalities. Age greater than 37 years, male sex, positive serology for cytomegalovirus, absence of complete remission (CR) status at the time of allo-BMT, presence of poor-risk chromosomal abnormalities and intensive conditioning were associated with poor outcome. The effect of disease status at the time of allo-BMT on the outcome (i.e.CR versus active disease) has not been completely resolved. Confounding issues are lack of referral for allo-BMT in case of refractory disease or complications after induction therapy, different biologic behavior of responsive disease and possibly use of more intensive (and invariably more toxic) conditioning regimens for refractory disease. It is conceivable that nonmyeloablative preparative regimens (so called "mini-transplants") may attenuate the early transplant-related mortality. Only very few "mini-transplants" for MDS have been performed. Although a graft-versus-leukemia effect has been observed in *de novo* MDS, no such response has been seen so far for therapy-related MDS (Barrett et al., 2000).

An alternative to allo-BMT could be autologous stem cell transplantation. It has been shown that normal stem cells coexist with the malignant clone in *de novo* and therapy-related MDS (Delforge et al., 1995; Carella et al., 1996). These normal progenitors can be harvested following intensive antileukemic chemotherapy and, at least theoretically, could support one or more cycles of high-dose chemotherapy given with curative intent. A recent report from EBMT (de Witte et al., 2000) which compiled data from 1378 transplants (for *de novo* MDS and secondary AML) confirmed the benefit of autologous transplantation (versus unrelated donor transplants) in patients older than 40 years of age and suggested a possible role of the procedure even in much younger patients who lack a suitable sibling donor. In this study, the estimated 3-year disease-free survival was 25% for the 198 patients transplanted from unrelated donors, 28% for the 91 patients transplanted from alternative family donors and 33% for the 126 patients autografted in first complete remission. For comparison, the estimated disease-free survival and relapse rate at 3 years were 36% for both parameters in 885 patients transplanted from matched siblings.

The generally poor results with available therapeutic options dictate major efforts to prevent the development of the disease. One approach could be to perform AHSCT early in the course of the primary malignancy (i.e. transplantation in first CR at least in patients with poor prognostic disease features), limiting thereby the exposure to conventional chemotherapy. Restricting the use of conditioning regimens which include TBI and possibly substituting the alkylating agents and the edipodophyllotoxins by drugs lacking leukemogenic potential in the "priming" chemotherapy phase should also be considered. In addition, every possible effort should be made towards the detection of typical cytogenetic abnormalities prior to AHSCT and exclusion of patients with these abnormalities from autologous transplants. Given the above mentioned limitations of the conventional technique, fluorescence in situ hybridization using probes directed at the well characterized chromosomal targets of MDS should be more widely used (Abruzzese et al., 1999).

Evaluation of clonality has been examined in several studies in an attempt to identify clonal populations in informative females after high-dose chemotherapy or marrow regeneration from a limited stem cell pool. Gale et al. reported on three patients in whom serial examinations of X-chromosome inactivation patterns (XCIPs) were used to predict development of t-MDS/AML. The method may be very difficult to interpret in patients with imbalanced or skewed constitutive patterns (i.e. >75% expression of one allele) unless the emerging (abnormal) clone comes from a cell expressing the minor allele. Mach-Pascual et al. investigated the predictive value of clonal bone marrow hematopoiesis for t-MDS/AML development, as defined by an X-inactivation based clonality assay at the human androgen receptor locus, in a group of patients who received AHSCT for NHL. T-MDS/AML developed in 2 of 53 patients with polyclonal hematopoiesis and in 4 of 10 with clonal hematopoiesis. The applicability of this technique to the clinical practice is currently unknown. Telomere length in stem cells has been shown to be abnormal in *de novo* MDS and following AHSCT (Boultwood et al., 1997; Engelhardt et al., 1998). Telomeres which are critically shortened are subject to increased incidence of cytogenetic abnormalities and may contribute to leukemic transformation (Ball et al., 1998). Evaluation of the telomere length in a prospective fashion might reveal patients at high risk for t-MDS/AML development.

The significance of clonal chromosomal abnormalities in the bone marrow after AHSCT, especially when uncharacteristic for myelodysplasia, is unknown. Imrie et al. reported the detection of cytogenetic abnormalities in 7 of 62 AML patients after AHSCT. Four had a complex karyotype while three had a single structural abnormality. Deletions of chromosomes 5 and 7 and of the long arm of chromosome 20 were detected among other abnormalities. No patient developed cytopenia or franc MDS/AML up to 70 months after detection of the abnormal clone. In a group of 60 breast cancer patients who received AHSCT, clonal chromosomal abnormalities were detected in 3 (Martínez-Climent et al., 2000). These were trisomy X in 2 cases and t(1;6) in one case. Cytopenias were observed in 2 of the three patients. MDS/AML could not be diagnosed with a median follow-up of 36 months post-transplant. It appears that occasional patients develop cytogenetic changes, either characteristic or uncharacteristic for t-MDS/AML, which may persist or fluctuate over time and may or may not be accompanied by bone marrow morphologic changes, peripheral blood cytopenias or evolution to clinical MDS/AML.

REFERENCES

Abruzzese, E., Radford, J.E., Miller, J.S., Vredenburgh, J.J., Rao, P.N., Pettenati, M.J., Cruz, J.M., Perry, J.J., Amadori, S. & Hurd, D.D. (1999) Detection of abnormal pretransplant clones in progenitor cells of patients who developed myelodysplasia after autologous transplantation. *Blood*, **94**, 1814-1819.

Amigo, M.L., Del Cañizo, M.C., Rios, A., Garcia, M.A., Caballero, M.D., Martin, A., Bermejo, N., Vilches, P. & San Miguel, J.F. (1999) Diagnosis of secondary myelodysplastic syndromes (MDS) following autologous transplantation should not be based only on morphological criteria used for diagnosis of de novo MDS. *Bone Marrow Transplant*, **23**, 997-1002.

Anderson,J.E., Gooley, T.A., Schoch, G., Anasetti, C., Bensinger, W.I., Clift, R.A., Hansen, J.A., Sanders, J.E., Storb, R. & Appelbaum, F.R. (1997) Stem cell transplantation for secondary acute myeloid leukemia: evaluation of transplantation as initial therapy or following induction chemotherapy. *Blood*, **89**, 2578-285.

André, M., Henry-Amar, M., Blaise, D., Colombat, P., Fleury, J., Milpied, N., Cahn, J.Y., Pico, J.L., Bastion, Y., Kuentz, M., Nedellec, G., Attal, M., Ferme, C. & Gisselbrecht, C. (1998) Treatment-related deaths and second cancer risk after autologous stem-cell transplantation for Hodgkin's disease. *Blood*, **92**, 1933-1940.

Ball, S.E., Gibson, F.M., Rizzo, S., Tooze, J.A., Marsh, J.C. & Gordon-Smith, E.C. (1998) Progressive telomere shortening in aplastic anemia. *Blood*, **91**, 3582-3592.

Ballen, K.K., Gilliland, D.G., Guinan, E.C., Hsieh, C.C., Parsons, S.K., Rimm, I.J., Ferrara, J.L., Bierer, B.E., Weinstein, H.J., Antin, J.H. (1997) Bone marrow transplantation for therapy-related myelodysplasia: comparison with primary myelodysplasia. *Bone Marrow Transplant*, **20**,737-743.

Barrett, J. & Childs, R. (2000) Non-myeloablative stem cell transplants. *British Journal of Haematology*, **111**, 6-17.

Bennett, J.M., Catovsky, D., Daniel, M.T., Flandrin, G., Galton, D.A, Gralnick, H.R. & Sultan, C. (1976) Proposals for the classification of the acute leukaemias. French-American-British (FAB) co-operative group. *British Journal of Haematology*, **33**, 451-458.

Bennett, J.M., Catovsky, D., Daniel, M.T., Flandrin, G., Galton, D.A., Gralnick, H.R. & Sultan, C. (1982) Proposals for the classification of the myelodysplastic syndromes. *British Journal of Haematology*, **51**, 189-199.

Berglund, A., Enblad, G., Carlson, K., Glimelius, B. & Hagberg, H. (2000) Long-term follow-up of autologous stem-cell transplantation for follicular and transformed follicular lymphoma. *European Journal of Haematology*, **65**, 17-22.

Bhatia, S., Ramsay,N.K., Steinbuch, M., Dusenbery, K.E., Shapiro, R.S., Weisdorf, D.J., Robison, L.L., Miller, J.S. & Neglia, J.P. (1996) Malignant neoplasms following bone marrow transplantation. *Blood*, **87**, 3633-3639.

Boultwood, J., Fidler, C., Kusec, R., Rack, K., Elliott, P.J., Atoyebi, O., Chapman, R., Oscier, D.G. & Wainscoat, J.S. (1997) Telomere length in myelodysplastic syndromes. *American Journal of Hematology*, **56**, 266-271.

Carella, A.M., Dejana, A., Lerma, E., Podesta, M., Benvenuto, F., Chimirri, F., Parodi, C., Sessarego, M., Prencipe, E. & Frassoni, F. (1996) In vivo mobilization of karyotypically normal peripheral blood progenitor cells in high-risk MDS, secondary or therapy-related acute myelogenous leukaemia. *British Journal of Haematology*, **95**, 127-130.

Darrington, D.L., Vose, J.M., Anderson, J.R., Bierman, P.J., Bishop, M.R., Chan, W.C., Morris, M.E., Reed, E.C., Sanger, W.G., Tarantolo, S.R., Weisenburger, D.D., Kessinger, A. & Armitage, O. (1994) Incidence and characterization of secondary myelodysplastic syndrome and acute myelogenous leukemia following high-dose chemoradiotherapy and autologous stem-cell transplantation for lymphoid malignancies. *Journal of Clinical Oncology*, **12,** 2527-2534.

Deeg, J.H. & Socié, G. (1998) Malignancies after hematopoietic stem cell transplantation: many questions, some answers. *Blood*, **91**, 1833-1844.

Del Cañizo, M.F., Amigo, M.F., Hernandez, J.M., Sanz, G., Nunez, R., Carreras, E., Alegre, A., Cuesta, B. & Mataix, R. (2000) Incidence and characterization of secondary myelodysplastic syndromes following autologous transplantation. *Haematologica*, **85**, 403-409.

Delforge, M., Demuynck, H., Vandenberghe, P., Verhoef, G., Zachee, P., Van Duppen, V., Marijnen, P., Van den Berghe, H. & Boogaerts, M.A. (1995) Polyclonal primitive hematopoietic progenitors can be detected in mobilized peripheral blood from patients with high-risk myelodysplastic syndromes. *Blood*, **86**, 3660-3667.

De Witte, T., Hermans, J., Vossen, J., Bacigalupo, A., Meloni, G., Jacobsen, N., Buutu,T., Ljungman, P., Gratwohl, A., Runde, V., Niederwieser, D., Van Bieaen, A., Devergie, A., Cornelissen, J., Jouet, J.P., Arnold, R. & Apperley, J. (2000) Haematopoietic stem cell transplantation for patients with myelodysplastic syndromes and secondary acute myeloid leukaemias: a report on behalf of the chronic leukaemia working party of the European group for blood and marrow transplantation (EBMT). *British Journal of Haematology*, **110**, 620.

Engelhardt, M., Ozkaynak, M.F., Drullinsky, P., Sandoval, C., Tugal, O., Jayabose, S. & Moore, M.A. (1998) Telomerase activity and telomere length in pediatric patients with malignancies undergoing chemotherapy. *Leukemia*, **12**, 13-24.

Friedberg, J.W., Neuberg, D., Stone, R.M., Alyea, E., Jallow, H., LaCasce, A., Mauch, P.M., Gribben, J.G., Ritz, J., Nadler, L.M., Soiffer, R.J. & Freedman, A.S. (1999) Outcome in patients with myelodysplastic syndrome after autologous bone marrow transplantation for non-Hodgkin's lymphoma. *Journal of Clinical Oncology*, **17,** 3128-3135.

Gale, R.E., Bunch, C., Moir, D.J., Patterson, K.G., Goldstone, A.H. & Linch, D.C. (1996) Demonstration of developing myelodysplasia/acute myeloid leukaemia in haematologically normal patients after high-dose chemotherapy and autologous bone marrow transplantation using X-chromosome inactivation patterns. *British Journal of Haematology*, **93**, 53-58.

Govindarajan, R., Jagannath, S., Flick, J.T., Vesole, D.H., Sawyer, J., Barlogie, B. &Tricot, G. (1996) Preceding standard therapy is the likely cause of MDS after autotransplants for multiple myeloma. *British Journal of Haematology*, **95**, 349-353.

Greenberg, P., Cox, C., LeBeau, M.M., Fenaux, P., Morel, P., Sanz,.G., Sanz, M., Vallespi, T., Hamblin, T., Oscier, D., Ohyashiki, K., Toyama, K., Aul, C., Mufti, G. & Bennett, J. (1997) International scoring system for evaluating prognosis in myelodysplastic syndromes. *Blood*, **89**, 2079-2088.

Harrison, C.N., Gregory, W., Hudson, G.V., Devereux, S., Goldstone, A.H., Hancock, B., Winfield, D., MacMillan, A.K., Hoskin, P., Newland, A.C., Milligan, D. & Linch, D.C. (1999) High-dose BEAM chemotherapy with autologous haemopoietic stem cell transplantation for Hodgkin's disease is unlikely to be associated with a major increased risk of secondary MDS/AML. *British Journal of Cancer*, **81**, 476-483.

Imrie, K.R., Dubé, I., Prince, H.M., Girouard, C., Crump, M. & Keating, A. (1998) New clonal karyotypic abnormalities acquired following autologous bone marrow transplantation for acute myeloid leukemia do not appear to confer an adverse prognosis. *Bone Marrow Transplant*, **21**, 395-399.

Johansson, B., Mertens, F., Heim, S., Kristoffersson, U. & Mitelman, F. (1991) Cytogenetics of secondary myelodysplasia (sMDS) and acute nonlymphocytic leukemia (sANLL). *European Journal of Haematology*, **47**, 17-27.

Ketterer, N., Salles, G. Raba, M., Eljaafari-Corbin, A., Espinouse, D., Tremisi, P., Dumontet, C., Moullet, I., Neidhardt-Berard, E.M., Bouafia, F., Coiffier, B. (1998) High CD34$^+$ cell counts decrease hematological toxicity of peripheral blood progenitor cell (PBPC) transplantations. [abstract] *British Journal of Haematology*, **102,** 204.

Kollmannsberger, C., Beyer, J., Droz, J.P., Harstrick, A., Hartmann, J.T., Biron, P., Flechon, A., Schoffski, P., Kuczyk, M., Schmoll, H.J., Kanz, L. & Bokemeyer, C. (1998) Secondary leukemia following high cumulative doses of etoposide in patients treated for advanced germ cell tumors. *Journal of Clinical Oncology*, **16**, 3386-3391.

Krishnan, A., Bhatia, S., Slovak, M.L., Arber, D.A., Niland, J.C., Nademanee, A., Fung, H., Bhatia, R., Kashyap, A., Molina, A., O'Donnell, M.R., Parker, P.A., Sniecinski, I., Snyder, D.S., Spielberger, R., Stein, A. & Forman, S.J. (2000) Predictors of therapy-related leukemia and myelodysplasia following autologous transplantation for lymphoma: an assessment of risk factors. *Blood*, **95**, 1588-1593.

Laughlin, M.J., McGaughey, D.S., Crews, J.R., Chao, N.J., Rizzieri, D., Ross, M., Gockerman, J., Cirrincione, C., Berry, D., Mills, L., Defusco, P., LeGrand, S., Peters, W.P. & Vredenburgh, J.J. (1998) Secondary myelodysplasia and acute leukemia in breast cancer patients after autologous bone marrow transplant. *Journal of Clinical Oncology*, **16**, 1008-1012.

Le Beau, M.M., Albain, K.S., Larson, R.A., Vardiman, J.W., Davis, E.M., Blough, R.R., Golomb, H.M. & Rowley, J.D. (1986) Clinical and cytogenetic correlations in 63 patients with therapy-related myelodysplastic syndromes and acute nonlymphocytic leukemia: further evidence for characteristic abnormalities of chromosomes no. 5 and 7.*Journal of Clinical Oncology*, **4**, 325-345.

Mach-Pascual, S., Legare, R.D., Lu, D., Kroon, M., Neuberg, D., Tantravahi, R., Stone, R.M., Freedman, A.S., Nadler, L.M., Gribben, J.G. & Gilliland, D.G. (1998) Predictive value of clonality assays in patients with non-Hodgkin's lymphoma undergoing autologous bone marrow transplant: a single institution study. *Blood*, **91**, 4496-4503.

Marolleau, J.P., Brice, P., Morel, P. & Gisselbrecht, C. (1993) Secondary acute myeloid leukemia after autologous bone marrow transplantation for malignant lymphomas. *Journal of Clinical Oncology*, **11**, 590-591.

Martínez-Climent, J.A., Comes, A.M., Vizcarra, E., Benet, I., Arbona, C., Prósper, F., Solano, C., García Clavel, B., Marugán Lluch, A. & García-Conde, J. (2000) Chromosomal abnormalities in women with breast cancer after autologous stem cell transplantation are infrequent and may not predict development of therapy-related leukemia or myelodysplastic syndrome. *Bone Marrow Transplant*, **25**, 1203-1208.

Micallef, I.N., Lillington, D.M., Apostolidis, J., Amess, J.A., Neat, M., Matthews, J., Clark, T., Foran, J.M., Salam, A., Lister, T.A. & Rohatiner, A.Z. (2000) Therapy-related myelodysplasia and secondary acute myelogenous leukemia after high-dose therapy with autologous hematopoietic progenitor-cell support for lymphoid malignancies. *Journal of Clinical Oncology*, **18**, 947-955.

Miller, J.S., Arthur, D.C., Litz, C.E., Neglia, J.P., Miller, W.J. & Weisdorf, D.J. (1994) Myelodysplastic syndrome after autologous bone marrow transplantation: an additional late complication of curative cancer therapy. *Blood*, **8**, 3780-3786.

Milligan, D.W., Ruiz, De Elvira, M.C., Kolb, H.J., Goldstone, A.H., Meloni, G., Rohatiner, A.Z., Colombat, P. & Schmitz N. (1999) Secondary leukaemia and myelodysplasia after autografting for lymphoma: results from the EBMT. EBMT Lymphoma and Late Effects Working Parties. European Group for Blood and Marrow Transplantation. *British Journal of Haematology*, **106**, 1020-1026.

Park, S., Brice, P., Noguerra, M.E., Simon, D., Rousselot, P., Kerneis, Y., Morel, P., Marolleau, J.P. & Gisselbrecht, C. (2000) Myelodysplasias and leukemias after autologous stem cell transplantation for lymphoid malignancies. *Bone Marrow Transplant*, **26**, 321-326.

Pedersen-Bjergaard, J., Anderson, M..K. & Christiansen, D.H. (2000) Therapy-related acute myeloid leukemia and myelodysplasia after high-dose chemotherapy and autologous stem cell transplantation. *Blood*, 95, 3273-3279.

Pedersen-Bjergaard, J., Pedersen, M., Myhre, J. & Geisler, C. (1997) High risk of therapy-related leukemia after BEAM chemotherapy and autologous stem cell transplantation for previously treated lymphomas is mainly related to primary chemotherapy and not to the BEAM-transplantation procedure. *Leukemia*, **11**, 1654-1660.

Pedersen-Bjergaard, J., Pedersen, M., Roulston, D. & Philip, P. (1995) Different genetic pathways in leukemogenesis for patients presenting with therapy-related myelodysplasia and therapy-related acute myeloid leukemia. *Blood*, **86**, 3542-3552.

Pedersen-Bjergaard, J., Specht, L., Larsen, S.O., Ersboll, J., Struck, J., Hansen, M.M., Hansen, H.H. & Nissen, N.I. (1987) Risk of therapy-related leukaemia and preleukaemia after Hodgkin's disease. Relation to age, cumulative dose of alkylating agents, and time from chemotherapy. *Lancet*, **2**, 83-88.

Rege, K.P., Janes, S.L., Saso, R., Min, T., Swansbury, J., Powles, R.L. & Treleaven, J.G. (1998) Secondary leukaemia characterised by monosomy 7 occurring post-autologous stem cell transplantation for AML. *Bone Marrow Transplant*, **21**, 853-855.

Roman-Unfer, S., Bitran, J.D., Hanauer, S., Johnson, L., Rita, D., Booth, C. & Chen, K. (1995) Acute myeloid leukemia and myelodysplasia following intensive chemotherapy for breast cancer. *Bone Marrow Transplant*, **16**, 163-168.

Roy, D.C., Tantravahi, R., Murray, C., Dear, K., Gorgone, B., Anderson, K.C., Freedman, A.S., Nadler, L.M. & Ritz, J. (1990) Natural history of mixed chimerism after bone marrow transplantation with CD6-depleted allogeneic marrow: a stable equilibrium. *Blood*, **75**, 296-304.

Sobecks, R.M., LeBeau, M.M., Anastasi, J. & Williams, S.F. (1999) Myelodysplasia and acute leukemia following high-dose chemotherapy and autologous bone marrow or peripheral blood stem cell transplantation. *Bone Marrow Transplant,* **23**, 1161-1165.

Stone, R.M. (1994) Myelodysplastic syndrome after autologous transplantation for lymphoma: the price of progress. *Blood,* **83**, 3437-3440.

Stone, R.M., Neuberg, D., Soiffer, R., Takvorian, T., Whelan, M., Rabinowe, S.N., Aster, J.C., Leavitt, P., Mauch, P., Freedman, A.S., et al (1994) Myelodysplastic syndrome as a late complication following autologous bone marrow transplantation for non-Hodgkin's lymphoma. *Journal of Clinical Oncology*, **12**, 2535-2542.

Taylor, P.R.A., Jackson, G.H., Lennard, A.L., Hamilton, P.J. & Proctor, S.J. (1997) Low incidence of myelodysplastic syndrome following transplantation using autologous non-cryopreserved bone marrow. *Leukemia*, **11**, 1650-1653.

Traweek, S.T., Slovak, M.L., Nademanee, A.P., Brynes, R.K., Niland, J.C. & Forman, S.J. (1994) Clonal karyotypic hematopoietic cell abnormalities occurring after autologous bone marrow transplantation for Hodgkin's disease and non-Hodgkin's lymphoma. *Blood*, **84**, 957-963.

Weh, H.J., Calavrezos, A., Seeger, D., Kuse, R. & Hossfeld, D.K. (1987) Cytogenetics studies in 69 patients with myelodysplastic syndromes (MDS). *European Journal of Haematology*, **38**, 166-172.

Wheeler, C., Khurshid, A., Ibrahim, J., Elias, A., Mauch, P. & Antin, J. (1997) Low incidence of post-transplant myelodysplasia/acute leukemia (MDS/AML) in NHL patients autotransplanted after cyclophosphamide, carmustine and etoposide (CBV). *Blood*, **90,** 385b.

Wilson, C.S., Traweek, T., Slovak, M.L., Niland, J.C., Forman, S.J. & Brynes, R.K. (1997) Myelodysplastic syndrome occurring after autologous bone marrow transplantation for lymphoma. Morphologic features. *American Journal of Clinical Pathology*, **108**, 369-377.

Yakoub-Agha, I., De La Salmoniere, P., Ribaud, P., Sutton, L., Wattel, E., Kuentz, M., Jouet, J.P., Marit, G., Milpied, N., Deconinck, E., Gratecos, N., Leporrier, M., Chabbert, I., Caillot, D., Damaj, G., Dauriac, C., Dreyfus, F., Francois, S., Molina, L., Tanguy, M.L., Chevret, S. & Gluckman, E. (2000) Allogeneic bone marrow transplantation for therapy-related myelodysplastic syndrome and acute myeloid leukemia: a long-term study of 70 patients-report of the French society of bone marrow transplantation. *Journal of Clinical Oncology*, **18**, 963-971.

11

EVOLUTION OF SECONDARY HEMATOLOGIC DISORDERS: PREMDS→MDS→sAML

Harvey D. Preisler
Rush Cancer Institute, Rush-Presbyterian-St.Luke's Medical Center, Rush University, Chicago, IL

THE MYELODYSPLASTIC SYNDROMES (MDS)

Introduction

The myelodysplastic syndromes [MDS] and acute myelogenous leukemia [AML] occurring subsequent to toxic exposure constitute the clinically apparent secondary hematologic disorders [sHD]. The incidence of these disorders has significantly increased during the past 40 years. This increase is most likely to be due to at least two phenomena: 1) increased exposure of individuals to hemopoietic toxins as part of treatment for malignant or autoimmune diseases; and 2) the increasing age of our population. It is generally assumed that "spontaneous" myelodysplastic syndromes (no history of toxic exposure) in the elderly are actually the result of a lifetime accumulation of genetic damage resulting from repeated low level toxic exposures in the environment. Despite there being some differences in the frequency of specific chromosomal abnormalities between secondary MDS [sMDS] and spontaneous MDS, these two entities are similar in terms of stem cell involvement, the characteristics of the marrow and peripheral blood, and the clinical courses of these two syndromes. In this chapter these two "types" of MDS, will be considered as one.

The clinical characteristics of the secondary hematologic disorders are most consistent with the proposition that the disorders are the clinical manifestation of the sequential appearance of a series of clones each of which is more aggressive than its predecessors. While at the clinical level it may appear that AML evolves from refractory anemia [RA] via a gradual change through two intermediate states, refractory anemia with excess blasts followed by refractory anemia with excess blasts in transformation, in reality these two intermediate states are likely to be different stages in the progressive replacement of an RA cell population by a newly appearing AML cell population.

Table 1.

The new population may differ from its predecessor[s] by:
1. dividing at a more rapid rate
2. having more cells remain in the proliferative pool after cell division
3. having a longer reproductive life span
4. having a significantly lower death rate
5. being less dependent upon environmental conditions for growth stimulation
    a- by producing its own cytokines
    b- by becoming cytokine independent
6. being less sensitive to feedback inhibitors which have a negative regulatory effect on the predecessor populations
7. being better adapted to new environmental conditions than the previous cell population
8. requiring less sustenance from the environment as the population increases producing food shortage (Malthusian concept)

Given that normal hemopoiesis is polyclonal while MDS and AML are monoclonal, these disorders must result from the appearance of a single abnormal stem cell which together with its progeny have a sufficient proliferative advantage to replace their predecessors. Table 1 lists some differences between a predecessor cell population and a newly emerging population which will lead to the latter replacing the former. Figure 1 presents disease evolution from two perspectives: as a succession of cell populations and in a fitness landscape. The latter is an excellent graphic tool for visualizing competition between cell populations. Also presented in figure 1 is a representation of the effects of a new cell population on the marrow microenvironment, effects which alter the microenvironment to be more favorable to the new population and less favorable to the old.

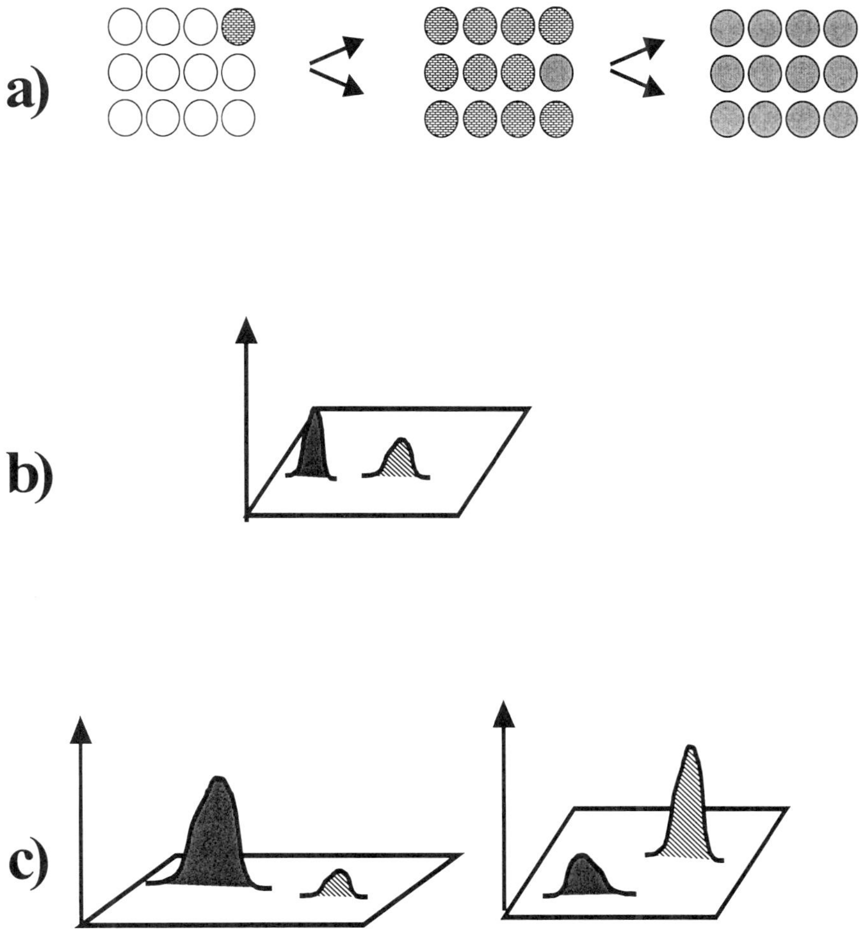

Figure 1. Evaluation of the Secondary Hematologic Disorders (a) Appearance of a new mutation in a single cell leads to the clone replacing the other cells which are present. (b) Fitness landscape showing two different cell populations. Z axis = relative fitness of the population, X axis = characteristic, Y axis is another characteristic (c) Note that when the configuration of the fitness landscape change the relative fitness of the 2 clones also change

Even small changes at the level of the stem cell can have very large effects on competing cell populations. For example, consider the situation in figure 2. Under normal conditions, on average when a hemopoietic stem cell divides one of the daughter cells remains in the stem cell pool and the other differentiates [p=0.5 for probability of remaining a stem cell, in one model of hemopoiesis, Borok and Preisler, unpublished]. If a mutation causes the "p" value to increase to 0.55, the new stem cell and its progeny will replace the old population. Since in this case differentiation of almost one half of the progeny continues there will be little or no effect on the morphology of the marrow. On the other hand, a further increase in the p value to p= ≥0.6 would lead to a preferential increase in primitive marrow cells to 20%. In the discussion of monoclonal hemopoiesis in the elderly, presented later on in this chapter, a reduction in the p value for some stem cells as a normal person ages is postulated to cause a fall in stem cell numbers leading to clonal dominance (Gale et al.,1997).

In summary, differences in the competitive ability between two cell populations can result from differences in the characteristics of the populations as a whole, from differences in the characteristics of stem cells, and from a significant change in the environment which favors one population over the other.

Abnormal states which precede the appearance of the clinically apparent secondary hematologic disorders

The preleukemic syndromes are named such because a significant proportion of patients with preleukemia will eventually develop acute leukemia. These syndromes can be divided into 2 categories: 1) the myelodysplastic disorders, and 2) the myeloproliferative disorders. The recognition that patients who have been cured of lymphoma by chemo/radiotherapy, especially when treatment includes an autologous stem cell transplant, are at especially high risk to develop a secondary hematologic disorder [estimated incidences as high as 15x normal] led to the study of cured lymphoma patients in an attempt to identify the molecular abnormalities which precede the appearance of MDS (Darrington et al., 1994; Mach-Pascual et al., 1998; Traweek et al.,1994; and Stone 1994). The pioneering studies, carried out by the Cardiff group, found monoclonal hemopoiesis to be present in 26% of cured lymphoma patients and N-ras and c-fms mutations to be present in 13 % and 6 % respectively (Carter et al.,1990; Cachia et al.,1993). One limitation of these studies arises from the fact that peripheral blood cells rather than bone marrow cells were studied. The failure to study bone marrow cells in all likelihood led these investigators to be unaware of the marrow abnormalities which were undoubtedly present in a significant number of their patients.

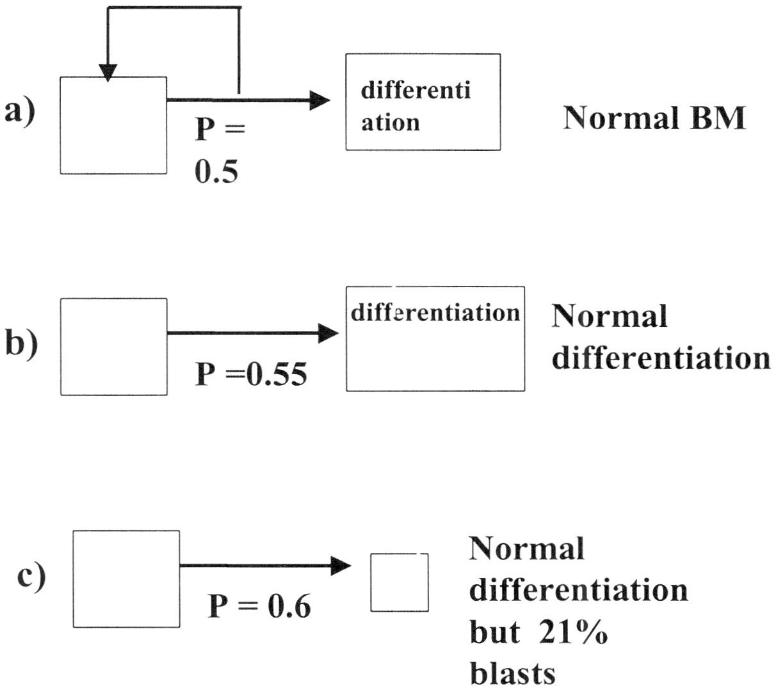

Figure 2. *Self Renewal and Stem Cells :A probability .55% that the stem cell progeny will remain stem cells results in a monoclonal marrow with normal differentiation. An increase in the probablity to 0.6% results in an increase in the % blast cells in the marrow*

Our studies have confirmed and extended those of the Cardif group, in a similar population of cured lymphoma patients detecting N-ras mutations in19.5% and c-fms mutations in 9.8% of the bone marrow aspirates which were studied. Further monoclonal hemopoiesis was detected in 20% of women (Bi et al., 1997).

To our surprise we found significant morphologic abnormalities in the marrows of one half of the cured lymphoma patients who were studied. These abnormalities ranged from minor hyper or hypoplasias to morphologic changes which were indistinguishable from those present in the marrows of patients with MDS.

Consistent with our observations are the recently reported studies of auto transplanted patients in which long lasting hemopoietic abnormalities were demonstrated in patients in whom hemopoiesis was thought to be normal

(Darrington et al., 1994; Mach-Pascual et al., 1998; Stone 1994;Traweek et al.,1994). These abnormalities, including trilineage dysplasia together with cytogenetic abnormalities, were found to be present more than 1+ years after transplantation. Clonal hemopoiesis was common being detected in 10 of 78 marrows at a median time of 14.5 months after transplantation in one study and in 10/83 patients in another study.

***Table 2**. P15 Methylation in 10 Pre-MDS*

Patient #	Diagnosis	Specimen	Date	Methylation%
1	Pre-MDS	BM	04/21/97	50.28
2	Pre-MDS	BM	04/28/97	70.64
3	Pre-MDS	BM	05/29/97	60.58
4	Pre-MDS	BM	05/02/97	44.08
5a	Pre-MDS	BM	01/20/97	68.44
5b	Pre-MDS	BM	07/21/97	19.56
6	Pre-MDS	BM	03/25/98	5.3
7	Pre-MDS	BM	05/28/97	88.8
8	Pre-MDS	BM	01/22/97	11.69
9	Pre-MDS	BM	04/11/97	22.44

Additionally, studies of the tumor suppressor gene p15 have demonstrated levels of methylation which are substantially greater than that present in normal marrow (Table 2 and Figure 3) (Preisler et al., 2001). At the present time it is not known if a level of methylation of 15% or 70% indicates that the gene is methylated to 15% or 70% in all the cells in the population or if the p15 gene is methylated to 100% in 15% -70% of the cells in the population. It is of special interest that the level of methylation in the marrow of one patient fell with time suggesting that these abnormalities are reversible.

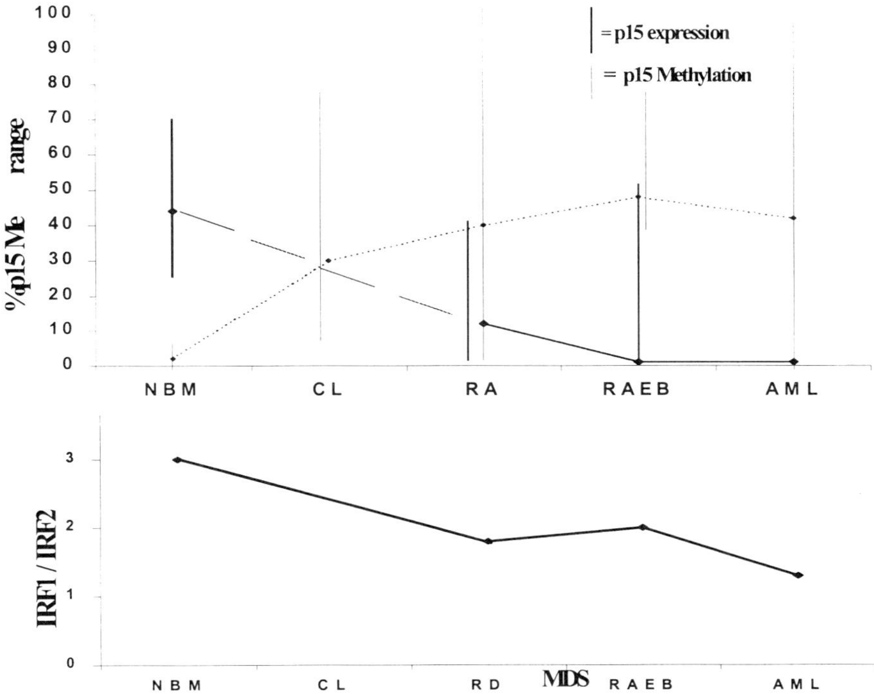

Figure 3. Comparison of molecular biologic characteristics of BM cells obtained from normal individuals, cured lymphoma patients, and from patients with refractory anemia, refractory anemia with excess blasts, or AML. Top ½ of panel - solid line = % methylation of the p15 gene. Dashed line = p15 expression. Bottom ½ of panel - ratio of IRF1/IRF2 expression in the various marrow types. Note that when the "p" for self renewal increases more of the progeny of replication remain as stems cells than differentiate.

These studies clearly demonstrate that the bone marrows of patients who have received extensive cytotoxic therapy are usually abnormal with changes ranging from the morphologic to the molecular biological. The question arises then regarding the likelihood of a patient developing a secondary hematologic disorder if these abnormalities are detected in their marrow at a time that hemopoiesis appears to be normal. This issue will be discussed farther on in the chapter.

The Myelodysplastic Syndromes

The "myelodysplastic syndromes" are a complex of 4 interrelated syndromes and one myeloproliferative disease. Approximately 30% of patients with these syndromes eventually develop AML with the remainder usually expiring from one of the complications of cytopenia. The RA and RARS syndromes are characterized by abnormalities of marrow morphology and peripheral blood cytopenias. RAEB and RAEBt are probably not really discrete syndromes and likely to be intermediate stages in the replacement of RA or RARS marrow or normal marrow by AML cells which developed from the original marrow. In patients with known toxic exposure, and especially those in whom abnormalities of chromosomes 5 and/or 7 are present in the marrow, the course of the sHD to AML can be so rapid that a period of RA/RARS may not have been apparent or perhaps may not have occurred. In fact, the progression of some of these secondary disorders is so rapid that they are often referred to secondary MDS/AML (Pedersen-Bjergaard J et al., 1993; LeBeau et al., 1986).

Despite the fact that marrow cellularity is normal or increased in most MDS patients, the cardinal signs of the disease are various cytopenias which are of special interest since they appear to have at least two causes: 1) the intramedullary death of large numbers of relatively mature hemopoietic cells (Raza et al.,1996a; Raza et al.,1996b) and 2) a state of abnormal differentiation. The fact that stromal cells are also apoptotic, despite not originating from the MDS clone, led to the appreciation that there are toxins in the marrow environment which poison the residents of the marrow. Recognition that TNF-α and possibly IL1β play a role in the induction of apoptosis led to the current innovative anti-TNFα therapies (Raza et al., 1995; Raza et al., 1996c). Despite the clinical importance of extracellular cytokines, it should not be forgotten that the basis of these disorders is the emergence of an abnormal clone of cells. MDS is an excellent example in which there are abnormalities at both the cellular and microenvironment levels, abnormalities which together produce the proliferative advantage which MDS cells enjoy over their more normal competitors [normal cells, pre MDS cells if relevant].

The incidences of N-ras and c-fms mutations in MDS are similar to that in the marrows of cured lymphoma patients with N-ras mutations being detected in 23.5% and c-fms mutations in 5.9% of MDS marrows (Figure 3) (Paquette et al., 1993; Parker and Mufti,1996). The distribution of N-ras mutations among the different MDS classes reveals little difference in most studies although in some studies mutations were more common in CMMoL.

Methylation of the p15 gene has been detected in 25% of MDS marrows reaching 47% in patients with RAEB/RAEBt (Preisler et al., 2001). The IRF1:2 ratio is reduced somewhat in MDS having a median value of 1.82 in RA and 2.01 in RAEBt in contrast to normal marrow cells in which the ratio ranges from 1.9 to 3.7 with a median of 2.97 (Neubauer et al., 1994). p53 mutations are only occasionally detected in MDS marrow cells (Jonveaux et al., 1991; Sugimoto et al., 1993).

Despite the fact that MDS marrows are usually normo or hyperceullar, MDS cells grow poorly in vitro under the same conditions in which normal marrow cells grow quite well (Mayani et al., 1989; Ohmori et al., 1991). This difference must indicate that MDS and normal progenitor cell differ substantially in the optimal conditions for growth.

Acute Myelogenous Leukemia

In AML the in vitro growth defect noted in MDS marrows cells is also present and abnormalities of chromosomes 5 and/or 7 present during the MDS phase persist into the AML phase often accompanied by additional chromosomal abnormalities (Tanaka et al., 1996).

N-ras mutations are detected in approximately 28% of AML marrows and c-fms mutations in 16% Figure 4A) (Bos et al., 1987; Lubbert et al., 1993; Paquette et al., 1993; Radich et al., 1990). Note that except for perhaps a slight increase in the incidence of c-fms mutations when MDS evolves into AML, the incidence of N-ras and c-fms mutations is not significantly different between the marrows of cured lymphoma patients, MDS patients, and patients with AML. As illustrated in Figure 4b the % of marrow cells carrying N-ras and c-fms mutations appears to rise slightly with disease progression but in no case are either mutation present in all of the leukemia cells (Bashey et al., 1992;Toksoz et al., 1987) (Figure 4A). p53 mutations, which are rarely encountered in MDS, are present in the marrow cells of as many as 1/3 of the cases of AML (Figure 4A). Unfortunately, at the present time the proportion of cells carrying this mutation in AML marrows is not known.

The level of methylation of the p15 gene in AML is 42% with expression of the gene absent or abnormally low in 37/44 AML marrows studied. The level of expression of the c-myc gene appears to be elevated in AML (Preisler and Raza, 1987a) and in some leukemias expression of the gene is constitutive (Venugopal et al., 1992a). These characteristics are associated with the failure of marrow cells to differentiate during remission induction therapy (Preisler et al., 1994a) and with poor responsiveness to treatment (Preisler et al., 1989). The level of expression of the c-myb gene is also elevated in many AMLs (Venugopal,1992b) as is the level of expression of the c-fms gene (Preisler et al., 1989). The former is associated with a poor response to treatment while the reverse is the case for the latter (Preisler, 1995a). The IRF1:IRF2 expression ratio is less in AML than in normal or MDS marrow cells [med =1.32 vs 2.97 and 1.9, respectively] (Figure 3).

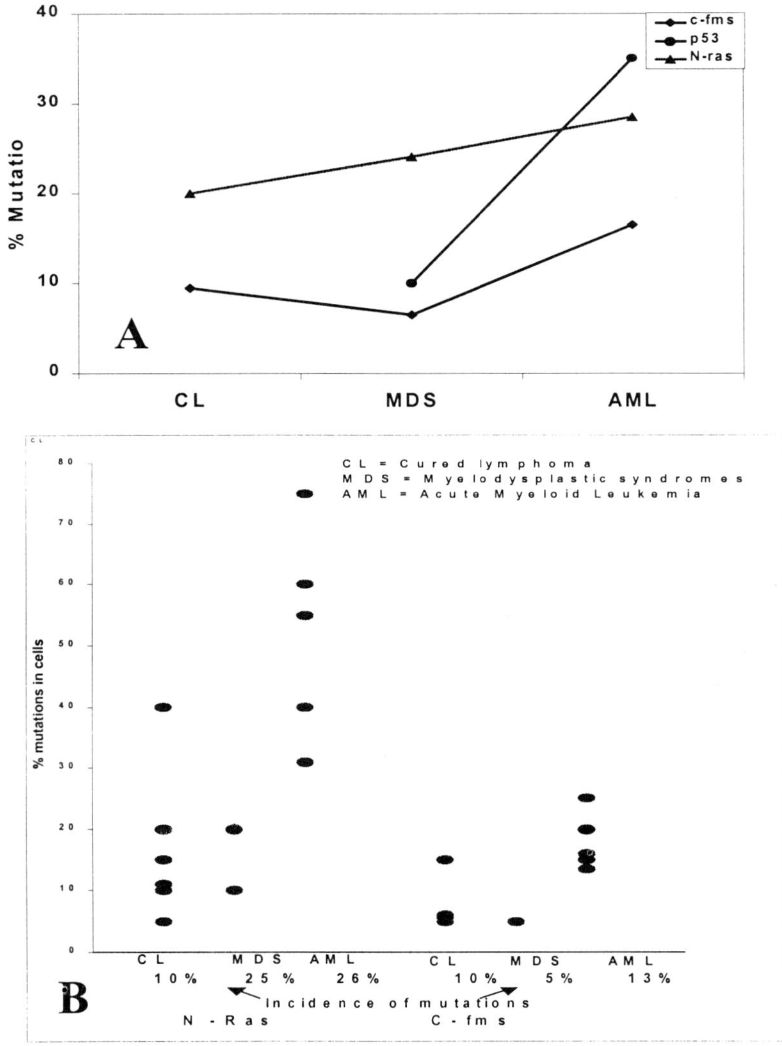

Figure 4. (A) Ras and FMS mutations and the secondary hematologic disorders.Incidence of N-ras, cFMS and p53 mutations in the marrows of cured lymphoma patients, MDS patients, and AML patients.(B) % of cells within a cell population which carry the N-ras or fms mutations.

While the above data represent the situation in AML as a whole, secondary AML (sAML) and "spontaneous" AML do differ in some respects. Expression of the MDR1 gene is higher in secondary AML, as are the presence of abnormalities of chromosomes 5 and/or 7 and the presence of complex karyotypes. At the clinical level, regrowth resistance is also more common and more severe (Preisler and Venugopal, 1994b; Preisler, 1995b) in sAML. Finally, the induction of leukemia cell differentiation during remission induction therapy is more frequent in standard prognosis disease than in poor prognosis AML (Raza et al., 1993).

The level of telomerase activity progressively increases as one goes from normal bone marrow to the marrows of cured lymphoma patients to the marrows of patients with MDS and to AML marrows (Li et al., 2000). This change in telomerase activity is not surprising given the relationship between telomerase activity and the self renewal capacity of cells (Kataoka et al., 1997; Vaziri and Benchimo, 1998) and given that the self renewal capacity of marrow cells progressively increase as evolution to and through the secondary hematologic disorders progress. It seems likely that at least the initial increase in telomerase activity is a reflection of an increase in the proportion of marrow cells which manifest this activity.

While the level of expression of both the myc and myb genes are elevated in acute myelogenous leukemia, no data are available regarding the level of activity of these genes in earlier stages of the secondary hematologic disorders. A detailed discussion of the expression of these genes is presented later on in this chapter.

MODELS FOR THE ORIGIN AND EVOLUTION OF THE SECONDARY HEMATOLOGIC DISORDERS

In vitro models

It has long been recognized that the development of malignant disease is a multi-step process during which genetic damage accumulates, damage which impairs the regulation of proliferation and differentiation. Continued accumulation of genetic abnormalities is responsible for malignant progression as well. This process was modeled by introducing oncogenes into primary cell cultures and observing the biological consequences (Land et al., 1983; Hunter, 1991). It was discovered that while the introduction of a single oncogene into a cell often resulted in an increase in proliferation, cytokine independent proliferation, increased proliferative potential and/or differentiation abnormalities, malignant transformation did not occur (Land et al., 1983, Hunter 1991). "Transformation" was found to require the introduction of more than a single oncogene. Further study demonstrated that oncogenes could be divided into two complimentary groups or classes (those located in the nucleus and those located outside the nucleus) with the simultaneous introduction of one member of each class into a cell resulting in transformation. Careful biological studies of the "transformed" cells demonstrated that even the recipients of double transfections were themselves not fully malignant suggesting that additional changes were necessary for full transformation to occur (Hunter, 1991; Preisler, 1988). Recently, however, it was demonstrated that under the correct conditions the introduction of even a single mutant oncogene can be transforming [see below].

Abnormal oncogene behavior can predispose the affected cells to undergo malignant transformation. The level of predisposition will depend upon the biological effects of the oncogene on the cell into which it has been inserted. For example, an oncogene which doubles the proliferative rate of a cell will not create the same level of predisposition as one which increases cell proliferation 10 fold. Oncogenes can predispose a cell to malignant change by producing one or more of the following effects: genetic instability, an increase in the proliferation rate, an increase in the life span of the cell, interruption of tumor suppressor gene function and so on.

Recently it has been shown that the p53 and IRF1 tumor suppressor genes play a significant role in preventing malignant transformation. Insight into the important contribution of mutation of tumor suppressor genes to neoplastic development was obtained when it was demonstrated that a single mutant gene, which by itself is not transforming, was transforming when introduced into p53 null or IRF1 null mice (Tanaka et al., 1994a). One of the mechanisms by which normal tumor suppressor genes prevent malignant transformation is by triggering apoptosis in cells with damaged DNA and/or in cells whose proliferative characteristics are abnormal (Loew et al.,1993). These functions reduce the likelihood that additional mutations would be acquired. The effects of abnormal p53 expression on malignant transformation in some cases appears to be more than the simple loss of the ability to induce apoptosis since missense mutations can have a greater effect on tumor susceptibility than nonsense mutations. The p53 and IRF1 genes are also tumor suppressors by virtue of the fact that the genes can "sense" the presence of DNA damage and trigger apoptosis (Levin, 1997). Both the p53 genes and the IRF1 genes also play a positive role in cell differentiation (Soddu et al.,1996, Abdollahi et al.,1991), another effect which would be "antimalignant." Additionally, loss of p53 function and presumably a loss in the ability to induce apoptosis can also result in an increase in the growth rate of malignant cells whose proliferation had formerly been restrained by p53 function.

The p15 and p16 tumor suppressor gene families function by inhibiting cell proliferation so that the effects of abnormalities which increases the proliferation rate of cells are dampened (see below).

In vivo models of the genesis of malignant disease

In vivo models of tumor initiation and progression have been developed in transgenic mice. In these studies the introduction of a single oncogene into the genome of a mouse increased the likelihood that the mouse will develop a malignant disease (Adams et al., 1985; Amundadottir et al., 1996). The nature of the promoter which regulates expression of the introduced oncogene determines the tissue or organs in which the oncogene is expressed and thus the organs in which tumors will develop. With rare exceptions these tumors, whether carcinoma of the breast or lymphoma, appear after a latent period which can be fairly long. When tumors do appear they do so in a stochastic manner with the individual tumors being monoclonal. The insertion of 2 complimentary oncogenes [myc and ras for example] results in a shorter latent period. While predisposing to tumor development, the insertion of some oncogenes produce different biological effects which could be limited to a "predisposition" to develop a specific malignant disease or could be associated with an observable abnormality in cell behavior such as hyperplasia or dysplasia. When malignancies appear after the latent period they are often multifocal though each tumor is always monoclonal.

Taken together, these data clearly demonstrate that while abnormalities in cell behavior and an increase in the predisposition to undergo malignant change can occur when an oncogene is introduced into a cell, the development of malignant disease will almost invariably be contingent upon the random acquisition of additional genetic changes. This process does indeed appear to be the case with the development of the secondary hematologic disorders and in fact with the development of most malignant diseases (Vogelstein and Kinzler, 1993). It should be understood that mutated genes or oncogenes produce different effects on cells. This is the case even for oncogenes of the same class. The result is that some combinations will produce very dramatic changes in cell behavior while others will produce only small changes with the latter type of "transformation" requiring additional genetic changes for malignant disease to arise. Additionally, the likelihood that complimentary mutations will occur undoubtedly varies with the specific genes in question. The variability of the effects of different oncogenes, alone and in combination, and the susceptibility of an oncogene to mutation all play a role in determining the length of time between acquiring the first genetic abnormality and malignant transformation. Consideration of the secondary hematologic disorder in this context makes it appear likely that a variety of initial lesions could be responsible for the appearance of RA or RARS and that whether or not evolution of these syndromes to more aggressive forms of MDS and to AML will depend on the probability that a sufficient number of additional mutations will be acquired during the lifetime of the individual.

Of particular note with respect to human leukemia is that the leukemias associated with the avian leukosis virus also occur in a step wise fashion after a long latency period and begin with the appearance of monoclonality. Also of interest is the fact that the avian leukosis virus is not a directly transforming virus but rather transformation is the result of insertional mutagenesis (Benchimo and Minden, 1987).

BIOLOGICAL CHANGES ASSOCIATED WITH THE SECONDARY HEMATOLOGIC DISORDERS

Table 3.

---

a. biological abnormalities
    - monoclonality
    - genetic instability
    - cytogenetic
    - morphologic
    - MDS/AML

a. functional abnormalities
    - ineffective hemopoiesis
    - abnormal cytokine production
    - in vitro proliferation
    - self renewal capacity/telomerase activity

b. molecular
    - N-ras and c-fms mutations
    - p53 mutations
    - IRF1:IRF2 expression
    - p15 expression
    - myc expression

Monoclonal Hemopoiesis

As in transgenic mice the appearance of monoclonal hemopoiesis in the marrow of cured lymphoma patients is likely to be an early event in the development of MDS or AML. In one study of 3 patients who had received a stem cell autograft, clonal dominance was detected among the hemopoietic cells in the marrow (Gale et al., 1996). The extent of dominance increased over time with AML appearing in 2 patients after 4 and 68 months respectively. The marrow of the third patient has shown increasing clonal dominance over time with neutropenia and thrombocytopenia appearing at 14 months. However there has been no further change in hemopoiesis 60 months later.

In a second study 78 patients who had received a stem cell autograft were followed for at least 15 months after transplantation (Mach-Pascual et al., 1998). Monoclonality appeared in the marrows of 10 patients at a median of 14.5 months after transplant. MDS has appeared in 4 of these 10 patients. Cytogenetic studies of the marrows of 7 of the 10 patients with monoclonal hemopoiesis demonstrated the presence of abnormalities of chromosome 5 and/or 7 in 5 patients. In one patient monoclonality and a deletion 7 was present while an abnormal chromosome 7 was present in 16 of 28 metaphases. Within several years all metaphases contained the abnormality. The marrow cells of a second patient with monoclonal hemopoiesis is without morphologic evidence of dysplasia 3 years after transplantation, yet del 13q and del 7 have been detected in some marrow metaphases. It is of interest that MDS has developed in two patients whose marrows seemed to be polyclonal until the clinical onset of MDS. To the present time the lesion[s] which are responsible for monoclonal hemopoesis have yet to be identified.

Taken together, the appearance of monoclonal hemopoiesis in the marrow and blood of cured lymphoma patients in all likelihood indicates that at least one step towards the development of a secondary hematologic disorder has occurred. Further, it is clear that if progression does occur, clonal evolution to secondary acute myelogenous leukemia can take a very long time or may not occur during the lifetime of the individual. Additionally, the appearance of monoclonal hemopoiesis "by itself" is not necessarily an indication that malignant transformation will occur in the near future or will occur at all. Six years ago we detected monoclonal hemoporesis in 3 cured lymphoma patients and to this day a clinically apparent hematological disorder has not appeared.

Monoclonality in the hemopoietic system has been reported to increase in frequency as normal women age (Busque et al., 1996; Champion et al., 1997; and Kassar et al., 1998). In one study monoclonal hemopoiesis was detected in 3-4% of specimens of cord blood and of blood obtained from young women. In contrast clonal hemopoiesis was detected in 33% individuals >75 years old. Inactivation of one X chromosome probably occurs in the embryo when the total number of hemopoietic stem cell precursors reaches 14-16 (Tonon et al., 1998). There is evidence from monozygotic twin studies that there is a strong tendency of the same line to become predominant in different hemopoietic cells [$r=0.57$, $p= <0.01$.] suggesting that an X linked factor is responsible for clonal dominance (Christensen et al., 2000). A cleavage ratio of ≥3 in a HUMARA assay is usually taken as evidence of unbalanced X chromosome inactivation. It has been postulated by some that with age there is a stochastic loss of stem cell clones resulting from an accumulation of unbalanced divisions of the stem cells from which two maturing progeny cells are produced instead one stem cell and one differentiating cell. The hypothesis contends that one result of this process is that by chance one normal stem cell and its progeny become dominant. It has also been postulated that stress on stem cell (ie being used in an autotransplant) accelerates normal stem cell aging resulting in clonal dominance. One mechanism underlying these processes could be that the normal aging processes are associated with telomeric shortening leading to the inactivation of some clones (Gale et al., 1997). In fact, evidence for the rapid shortening of telomeres after stem cell transplantation is compatible with this concept (Lee J et al., 1999). In one study the absence of N-ras and c-fms mutations in the blood cells of 28 women in whom monoclonal hemopoiesis had been demonstrated was taken to indicate that the monoclonal hemopoiesis associated with aging is different from that which occurs after toxic exposure and is not associated with the appearance of MDS or AML (Gale et al., 1997).

On the other hand, clonal skewing may occur as a result of a genetic change in a stem cell which provides the cell and its progeny with a proliferative advantage over otherwise normal hemopoietic clones. In a study of clonality in an MDS patient in whom abnormalities of chromosome 9 or 11q23 were present in marrow cells, it was found that lymphoblastoid lines which were of the same clonal lineage as the myeloid MDS line did not carry either of these chromosomal abnormalities. These observations suggest that monoclonal hemopoiesis precedes the appearance of cytogenetic abnormalities and MDS (Raskind et al., 1984).

In another study of an elderly female with MDS, a mutation of the ALAS2 gene was found to be present in cells which were part of the clone responsible for the MDS. Studies of relatives of this woman led to the conclusion that the first step in the development of MDS was the appearance of monoclonal hemopiesis with the gene mutation occurring in one of the monoclonal stem cells resulting in the appearance of MDS (Cazzola et al., 2000).

Genetic Instability

The frequent evolutionary and nonevolutionary changes in chromosome pattern in secondary AML are testament to the high level of genetic instability which characterizes AML. The persistence of cytogenetic abnormalities and mutations of the ras and fms genes attest to the sequential nature of the development of secondary hematologic disorders. They also attest to the fact that these abnormalities in many cases occur prior to the development of AML. A variety of changes which occur in late MDS or at the MDS/AML interface undoubtedly play a role in the genetic instability of secondary AML.

There has been much speculation about the potential role of genetic instability in the genesis of myeloid disorders, perhaps being responsible for the first step in the disease process. This concept is supported by the high incidence of myeloid disorders in the inherited genetic instability syndromes and from the observed clonal evolutions of MDS and AML. One can use Fanconi's anemia perhaps as a model of the relationship between genetic instability and development of the secondary hematologic disorders (Shadduck, 2001). This autosomally recessive disease is characterized by bone marrow failure, a variety of other somatic abnormaities, and an increased incidence of cancer. Cultured FA cells have decreased DNA synthesis, a prolonged G2 phase, increased spontaneous chromosomal breakage, and increased sensitivity to bifunctional alkylating agents; the latter because the DNA interstrand cross links cannot be repaired. The most characteristic abnormality in FA are translocations between nonhomologous chromosomes.

There are at least 8 different complementation groups [FA-A to FA-H] which, when cells are fused together, correct the abnormality [therefore probably at least 8 different genes]. The protein products of all 8 genes may bind to each other to form a giant complex which carries out some important function in DNA replication or repair. The normal protein products of the FAA and FAC genes [FANCA and FANCC] bind to each other but mutant FAC fails to bind to FAA (Xie et al., 2000). The third cloned gene FANCG may be involved in post replication repair or cell cycle check point control.

Even if genetic instability were demonstrated to be present in MDS or AML one could always say that it is secondary to the reproductive stress being placed on the malignant cell populations which are already present when the illness becomes clinically apparent.

Significant genetic instability is associated with mutations of the p53 gene but mutations of this gene are rare before the appearance of AML.

Proliferative Advantage

Of the changes which have a positive effect on the ability of the leukemia clones to compete with and replace the founding MDS clones, the most significant appear to be the dysregulation of c-myc function [c-myc function has not been characterized in MDS cells so abnormal functions may appear prior to the transformation of MDS to AML and the increase in telomerase activity]. The effects of the dysregulation of myc expression are multifold: 1) inhibition of cell differentiation so that the leukemic cells remain primitive having a high proliferative potential and an extended life span, 2) the direct stimulation of telomerase activity, 3) suppression of the anti-proliferative effects of the p21 and p27 genes, 4) activation of cyclin D and cyclin E kinases, 5) the direct induction of cyclin E transcription, 6) an increase in cyclin D1 activity via a post-transcriptional effect, 7) the entry of cells into S phase even if the level of cyclin E/cdk2 activity is low, 8) generation of the means to bypass the cell cycle arrest normally associated with p16 expression, 9) stimulation of the transcription of the ODC gene, and 10)- stimulation the phosphatases Cdc 25 a,b,c. Clearly, the dysregulation of c-myc expression can have catastrophic consequences.

As described earlier in this chapter, the proliferative advantage which AML cells have over competing clones of cells is the result of a variety of phenomena: 1) those listed in the preceding paragraph, 2) the high IL1β/IL1ra activity ratio, 3) the high serum SCF levels,and 4) an insensitivity to TGFβ and perhaps to other mechanisms which come into play when proliferation is excessive.

Chromosomal Abnormalities (Cytogenetics)

The incidence of chromosomal abnormalities increases as the secondary hematologic disorders evolve into RAEB and RAEBt and AML (Michalova et al., 1991; White et al., 1992). Chromosomes 5 and 7 are the most common abnormalities in these disorders. Chromosomal abnormalities are less frequent in benign MDS [present in 41% of RA cases and as a single abnormality in 80%; present in 19.5% of RARS a single abnormality constituting 62.5% of the abnormalities; present in 51.4% of RAEB as a single abnormality in 47.4%; present in 88.9% RAEBt as a single abnormality in 50%; chronic myelomonocytic leukemia present in 23.5% and as a single abnormality in100%]. The distribution of abnormalities in primary MDS without a history of toxic exposure is: (1) del 5q - 27%; (2) tri 8 - 19%, (3) monosomy 7- 15%; and (4) del 7q- 4%. In contrast in secondary MDS with a history of toxic exposure the pattern of chromosomal abnormalities is different: -7 -41%; del 7q- 4%; 5q- 29%; -5- 11%; 7q- 8%; and +8- 8%.

While abnormalities of chromosomes 5 and 7 are inextricably tied to the secondary hematopoietic disorders in most patients with MDS or AML, abnormalities of these chromosomes are not present in all or even in most of the abnormal cells. In one study (Zhao et al., 1993) of AML patients in whom monosomy 7 had been detected by standard cytogenetic analysis, among 15 patients the proportion of interphase cells which contained monosomy 7 ranged from 7% to 83% while the comparable values for 6 MDS patients was a range of 6% to 89%. In this same report a group of 5 AML and 2 MDS patients were described in which there was a marker chromosome in addition to monosomy 7. Among 3 of these patients the frequency of monosomy 7 was 16-34% while in karyotypic analysis it was 88% to 100%. In a second study (Arif et al., 1996) in which 300-700 metaphases were evaluated, among 9 MDS marrows the % of cells with monosomy 7 ranged from 8.9% to 67.5% while among 25 de novo AML, 11 marrows had monosomy 7 with the range of cells affected varying from 10% to 58.5%.

The sequence of acquisition of chromosomal abnormalities described immediately above is consistent with the acquisition of cytogenetic abnormalities after the appearance of monoclonal hemopoiesis as described in a patient earlier in this chapter. While chromosomal abnormalities appear relatively early in the secondary hematologic disorders, in most cases the cytogenetic abnormality is not present in every metaphase though the marrow is clonal. Unless one can demonstrate that eventually all malignant cells have the same cytogenetic abnormality one cannot decide whether the appearance of the cytogenetic abnormality is part of a linear progression of the disease or is merely an epiphenomenon. If this were used as a guide, then one would conclude that chromosome 5 and 7 abnormalities in most cases are not etiologically involved in the genesis of the MDS or in its progression to AML. The basis for this statement are the observations that abnormalities of these chromosomes, while frequent in the secondary hematologic disorders, are not present in all of the abnormal cells (Table 4).

Table 4.

I.	the GADD45 gene which binds to PCNA blocking DNA replication;
II.	the p21 gene which binds to PCNA and inhibits cyclin dependent kinsases
III.	the BAX gene which promotes apoptosis
IV.	the ERCC3 gene which codes for an excision repair molecule which removes damaged DNA segments
V.	the MDM2 gene which blocks p53 targets, causes ubiquinization of p53 protein facilitating degradation of the p53 protein
VI.	the p19ARF gene which antagonizes MDM2 thus stabilizing p53 protein.

In vitro cloning studies were performed in leukemia in which both trisomy 8 and a ras mutation were present. The AML cells were cloned in vitro and the colonies picked and characterized for the presence or absence of tri 8 and/or N-ras mutations (Price et al., 1994). The following data were obtained: 1) tri 8 was present in 25/26 colonies, 2) 19/26 colonies contained a ras mutation and tri 8 and 3) 6/28 contained tri 8 without a ras mutation. The conclusion to be drawn from this elegant study is that tri 8 was acquired first and a subpopulation of these cells acquired a ras mutation. Additionally the latter population, at the time of the study, was in the process of replacing the founder tri 8/N-ras mut neg clone. These observations raise important questions regarding the interpretation of data which demonstrate the presence of N-ras mutations in a leukemia. When the presence of mutant ras gene or some other molecular or chromosomal abnormality are detected it is usually assumed that the abnormality is etiologically involved in the genesis of the AML. This supposition is based on the transforming ability of mutant ras genes in model systems (Bos 1989; Coghlan et al., 1994; Johannes, 1989). As indicated by the experiment described above, and by other studies described later in this chapter, ras mutations may not be primarily involved in the genesis of either MDS or AML.

Different cytogenetic evolutionary patterns are associated with transformation to AML (Heim, 1992). Among a combination of RA and RARS patients whose MDS was not characterized by cytogenetic abnormalities, only 2 of 12 developed AML. Secondary leukemic transformation occurred in 3/16 patients in whom abnormal clones were present at the time of diagnosis. By contrast leukemic transformation occurred in 8/29 patients in whom clonal evolution occurred. Additionally, AML developed in 4/13 patients in whom clonal evolution did not occur. For

CMMoL, there were no transformations among 3 patients who had normal karyotypes throughout. AML developed in 1/4 patients in whom an abnormality was present at the time of initial diagnosis and did not change upon transformation. Finally, clonal progression occurred in 2 patients with AML, developing a new abnormality in one. In another study of 6 MDS patients who illness transformed into AML (Michalova et al., 1991), 3 had the same abnormal karyotype at the time of evolution to AML as was present at the time of diagnosis of MDS. In the other 3 cases, additional chromosome abnormalities were present at the time of transformation. Thus clonal evolution in MDS appears to be associated with of leukemic transformation.

Clonal evolution also occurs during the course of AML. In one study of relapsed patients evolution occurred in 17 (Lawler et al., 1980; Testa et al., 1979). In 7 evolution was from a normal karyotype to an abnormal one. In ten, karyotypic abnormalities were detected at diagnosis and different abnormalities were present at the time of remission induction failure or at relapse. For patients who entered CR, 4 patients in whom normal cytogenetics were present at the time of initial diagnosis, abnormal karyotypes were present at relapse. For remission induction failures, 4 who were normal at diagnosis became abnormal after treatment and 5 patients with abnormal chromosomes at diagnosis had other changes after treatment. A gain of +8 was the most common abnormality occurring in 10/17 patients. In another report of 42 patients at diagnosis and relapse, clonal changes were detected in 21 cases at the time of relapse, in 4 an abnormal clone was present at relapse while the diagnostic karyotype had been normal, in 11 patients there was clonal evolution with new abnormalities superimposed on preexisting clones [in 8 patients a completely new subclone was present at relapse and in 3 patients completely new clones replaced the original ones]. In 6 patients there was the selection of a clone which had already been present at the time of diagnosis (Testa et al., 1979).

The consistent presence of chromosomal abnormalities and the acquisition of new abnormalities during disease evolution strongly suggest that genetic instability is indeed an important aspect of MDS as it evolves to AML.

Ineffective Hemopoiesis

Ineffective hemopoiesis is characteristic of both the myelodysplastic and acute leukemic phases of the secondary hematologic disorders. With respect to the former, recognition of the paradox of the simultaneous presence of a hypercellular marrow and peripheral blood cytopenia, in the absence of evidence of significant destruction of the peripheral blood cells, led to a search for the basis of this paradox (Raza et al., 1996a; Raza 1996b). Shortly thereafter the demonstration of substantial levels of apoptosis in the bone marrow, and especially apoptosis in the marrow stroma, led to the hypothesis that a "toxin" was responsible for the destruction of both marrow stroma and cells. Careful studies of the marrow environment demonstrated that there were increased levels of TNFα, TGFβ, and IL1β in the marrow and that the level of TNFα and the level of apoptosis were correlated (Raza, 1996b). Demonstration that anti-TNFα therapy can produce amelioration of the cytopenias in some patients provides resumptive evidence that this cytokine is involved in the production of apoptosis (Raza, 1995; Raza et al., 1996c).

On the other hand myelodysplastic syndrome is a clonal disorder of hemopoiesis and hence cannot be solely attributed to the presence of "toxic" cytokines in the bone marrow environment. Presumptive evidence for a "defect" in stem cell function in MDS has been found in the inability of MDS marrows to form normal hemopoietic colonies in vitro and by the inability of these cells to produce a normal stromal layers in vitro as well (Merchav, et al., 1989; Tennant et al., 1997). This "defect" is likely to be present because of the unsuitable in vitro conditions in which the cells are placed, since in vivo the cells grow quite well usually being associated with marrow hypercellularity. A comparison of the level of apoptosis in marrow CD34+ cells and in more mature cells of the MDS marrows have demonstrated that apoptosis is largely limited to maturing cells (Mundle et al., 1999).

Examination of the BM biospies of MDS patients simultaneously for cells in S phase and for cells undergoing apoptosis demonstrated that some cells were simultaneously engaged in both processes. The % cells engaged in this process was calculated by counting the double labeled cells and dividing by the number of single labeled cells [brown for cells undergoing apoptosis and blue for cells engaged in DNA syntheses]. While in normal marrow the % of double labeled cells is 1.3%, the value for MDS marrows is 53.5%. It is believed that this phenomenon is caused by "signal antonymy," that is the cells receiving two contradictory signals at the same time. Studies of the E2F1 transcription factor demonstrated that while in normal marrow specimens the mRNA for the E2F1 transcription factor is 380 bp, in 5/8 MDS marrow specimens a smaller [325 bp] RNA for the E2F1 factor was present. In 3 specimens both the large and small transcripts were present while in 2 specimens only the small transcript was present. Simultaneous apoptosis and DNA synthesis is significantly higher in marrows in which the small transcript is present than in marrows in which it is not (Mundle et al., 2000).

In contrast, significant levels of marrow apoptosis are not present in AML, rather ineffective hemopoisis in AML is the direct result of the replacement of normal hemopoietic elements by leukemia cells and by the secondary inhibition of normal hemopoiesis probably as a response to unregulated cytokine production with the negative feedback affects of elevated cytokine levels resulting in an inhibition of proliferation of normal elements [see below for additional details].

In contrast, in secondary AML significant levels of apoptosis in the marrow are very rare. The marrows of AML patients are usually densely populated with cells as a result of increased cell production in the absence of significant apotosis. This picture is not surprising when one considers the fact that the transition of MDS to AML is accompanied by significant block in the differentiation of marrow cells and that even in MDS, apoptosis is rarely detected in immature cells. Hence while ineffective hemopoiesis is characteristic of both MDS and AML, the pathophysiology of the ineffective hemopoiesis is quite different. This difference in etiology of pancytopenia between MDS and AML make it easy to understand why the blocking of TNFα effects improves hemopoiesis in MDS but not in AML.

Cytokines

Stem cell factor (SCF) levels in the blood and bone marrow serum of AML patients are 50% higher than that present in normal individuals while levels in MDS patients approximate the normal (Tao et al., 2000). The origin and significance of the elevation in SCF levels are unknown while the presence of equal levels in BM and PB serum suggests that at least most of the SCF comes from extra medullary sources.

As the secondary hematologic disorders evolve there is a fall in SCF and IL1ra transcript levels in bone marrow cells being fewer in MDS cells than in normal and still fewer in AML cells (Preisler, 1999). When these results were first obtained it was hypothesized that there was a fall in the production of these cytokines during the progression of these disorders. These conjectures proved to be incorrect since it was subsequently discovered, as described above, that SCF levels are actually 50% higher in the BM and PB serum of AML patients than they are in either MDS or normal individuals. While SCF transcripts fall to undetectable levels in aspirable marrow cells during the evolution of the secondary hematologic disorder, SCF transcripts are in fact present in the stromal cells of the BM cavity (Unpublished Observations). Taken together, these observations suggest that the fall in SCF transcript levels in BM aspirate cells which occurs during disease evolution is possibly a response to increasing SCF levels in the micro environment in which the cells reside.

As is the case with SCF transcripts, IL1ra transcript levels fall in marrow aspirate cells as the secondary hematologic disorders evolve from pre MDS to MDS to AML (Preisler et al., 1998). In contrast, IL1β transcript levels do not change or increase during disease evolution (Preisler et al., 1998). In fact, IL1β protein levels are higher in marrow leukemia cells than in normal marrow cells while IL1ra levels tend to be on the low normal side. Taken together, these abnormalities result in the IL1β: IL1ra protein ratio being 12 fold greater in AML cells than in normal marrow cells (Preisler, 2000). Given that in the normal situation IL1β stimulation triggers the production of IL1ra (Dinarello, 1996), the absence of this negative feedback loop in AML cells with the presence of the loop in normal cells results in the stimulation of proliferation of the leukemia cells while the proliferation of normal residual marrow cells is inhibited.

Telomerase Activity

A progressive increase in telomerase activity in bone marrow cells parallels the appearance of monoclonal hemopoiesis and evolution of preMDS to MDS and the latter to acute leukemia (Amundadottir et al., 1996). This increase in enzyme activity is not unexpected given that the proliferation potential of each successive clone exceeds that of its predecessors. This increase in telomerase activity could play a primary role in the development of these disorders or it might merely be a reflection of the evolution of cells with greater and greater self renewal capacity. The recent report that the constitutive expression of telomerase is associated with the immortalization of cells is compatible with a primary role for this gene in malignant transformation (Bodnar et al., 1998).

Until recently telomerase assays were based on the study of cell populations as a whole. While we could demonstrate a small increase in telomerase activity in monoclonal marrow cells vis a vis normal marrow cells, we could not determine whether there was an increase in telomerase activity within a subpopulation of cells or whether the number of bone marrow cells with telomerase activity increased with disease evolution. Our recent modification of an in situ telomerase assay will make it possible to obtain these data (Ohyashiki et al., 1997). In our modification, we have combined in situ telomerase assay with FISH so that we can now compare telomerase activity in different clones of abnormal cells as well in as cells without an abnormality detectable by FISH. The data to date demonstrate that the % cells with telomerase activity in normal marrow ranges from 2-4 % while in AML marrows the range is from 25% -100%.

Studies of the potential role of an increase in telomerase activity in facilitating the evolution of the secondary hematologic disorders are particularly important since we have demonstrated that telomerase activity in AML cells can be reduced in vivo in patients by the administration of amifostine and/or IL4 (Preisler, 2000).

MOLECULAR BIOLOGICAL ASPECTS OF THE SECONDARY HEMATOLOGIC DISORDERS

ras and fms

As noted earlier N-ras mutations are present in the bone marrows of 19.5% cured lymphoma patients, in 23.5% of patients with MDS, and in 28% of patients with AML [Figure 4A]. Similar numbers for fms are 9.5%, 5.9%, and 16% respectively (Cachia et al., 1993).

The assessment of N-ras mutations in the three major stages of the secondary hematologic disorders demonstrate that there may be a small increase in the proportion of marrows in which these mutations are found as these diseases evolve, accompanied by a small increase in the proportion of cells within the population which contain these mutations. Other investigators have also found that the proportion of cells in a leukemia cell population which contain ras mutations is substantially less than 100% (Bashey et al., 1992; Toksoz et al., 1987). With this being the case, can ras mutations be etiologically involved in the genesis of the secondary hematologic disorders? At first glance the answer would seem to be no, since if they were involved in the primary etiology of these diseases one would expect that 100% of the cells in a population would contain the mutated gene. Similarly, as described earlier, at the very least a ras mutation is not the last step in the genesis of AML since morphologically normal compete remission marrows obtained from treated AML patients can contain ras mutations. N-ras mutations are involved in the transmission of proliferation signals, being an essential part of one of the pathways which translates cell surface receptor binding by ligands into activity (Far and Der,1994). The c-fms gene codes for surface receptors for MCSF (Panterne et al., 1993). Thus mutations of either gene will result in the cell constantly bombarded with signals to proliferate. It has also been reported that in at least one system the introduction of mutant Ha-ras genes results in cellular production of growth factors such as IL1β, G-CSF, GM-CSF, and IL6 by virtue of the mutant genes effects on the rate of transcription and half life of the cytokines (Demetri et al.,1990). Inhibition of ras activity blocks normal growth factor dependent activation of G1 CDKs and prevents activation of the E1A genes and results in G1 arrest.

The presence of a mutant ras gene in an otherwise normal cell can result in permanent G1 arrest and apoptosis accompanied by increases in p53 and p16 expression (Serrano et al., 1997). In the absence of either gene, apoptosis does not occur. Mutant ras genes can cooperate with any one of the following to transform primary cells: 1) overexpression of the c-myc gene (Land et al., 1983), 2) the presence of a dominant-negative p53 mutation (Shimamura and Fisher 1996), 3) loss of a p53 gene, p16 function, or IRF1 function (Serrano et al., 1995), 4) overexpression of D type cyclins (Filmus et al., 1994), and 5) overexpression of cdc25a or cdc25b. Mutant ras genes can contribute to neoplastic formation by: 1)suppressing proteasome degradation of c-myc protein, 2) stabilizing myc protein and increasing myc expression during S phase and during the activation of the E2F transcription factor, 3) by cooperating with c-myc expression to activate the E2F transcription factor, and 4) perhaps by increasing the production of IL1β , GMCSF, GCSF, and IL6 (Beaupre et al., 1999). Parenthetically, however, our studies of human AML cells have failed to demonstrate a relationship between the presence or absence of ras mutations and cytokine production.

A Connection Between Chromosome 7 Abnormalities and Ras Mutations

Among 20 children with monosomy 7 or 7q- [13 MDS or AML], ras mutations were detected in 3 (Neubauer et al., 1991). In another study 48 patients were divided into different groups on the basis of the cytogenetic characteristics: group 1) among 9 patients in whom MDS had evolved to AML and in whom the 7th chromosome was abnormal, ras mutations were detected in 4; group 2) among 19 patients in whom MDS evolved to AML but in whom an abnormal chromosome 7 was not detected there were no ras mutations; group 3) among 5 patients with de novo AML with an abnormal chromosome 7, ras mutations were present in 1; group 4) of 18 patients with de novo AML without an abnormal chromosome 7, ras mutations were detected in 2. Thirteen patients who had been treated with rhG-CSF and who developed either MDS or AML, or a clonal cytogenetic abnormality, monosomy 7 was present in 10 marrows and 5 of these contained ras mutations as well. The % cells containing monosomy 7 ranged from 25-100% (Kalra et al., 1995).

Given that when present in an MDS or AML cell population neither chromosome 7 abnormalities or N-ras mutations are present in every cell (see above), the question is whether abnormalities of chromosome 7 or ras mutations are involved in the genesis of MDS and AML. Given the consistent independent association of these abnormalities with MDS and AML, as well as the apparent association of these two abnormalities in pediatric myeloid disease, it would seem highly unlikely that these abnormalities would not play an important role in the genesis and maintenance of these diseases.

One possible explanation for these observations is that the lesions are important but that whenever we detect them the cells carrying these lesions are in the process of being replaced by more malignant cells in which these abnormalities are not present. This seems highly unlikely. Another possibility is that these lesions are manifestations of genetic instability and thus are often present in diseased populations but do not have to be present in every cell. Nevertheless there has to be a reason for the persistence of these cell subpopulations.

The explanation which we prefer is that clones carrying an abnormal chromosome 7, with or without accompanying ras mutations, could initially have a proliferative advantage over competing clones without, however, the advantage falling with time. This situation would occur if the proliferative advantage of the monosomy 7 and/or ras mutations were the result of these cells producing growth factors which initially only stimulate their own proliferation. Whether the growth factors are released into the microenvironment or whether they are expressed on the cell surface it is possible that as the clone of cells producing these factors increases in size the factors become available to other leukemia cells, leukemia cells which are responsive to the factors but do not produce them. If this were the case, then an equilibrium would be reached in which the proportion of cells which make the growth factor would no longer increase in number relative to the cells which do not produce these factors but which are responsive to them.

p53 mutations

The p53 gene is mutated in over 50% of all malignant diseases in man with 85% of the mutations being missense mutations. Abnormalities of the p53 gene are likely to play a role in the genesis of secondary AML because of the steep rise in the incidence of such mutations between MDS and AML [figure 3a]. Loss of p53 function can play an important role in the genesis of chromosomal abnormalities since without normal p53 function excess centrioles appear which can result in abnormal mitoses with numerical chromosomal abnormalities (Miller and Therman, 1980). Additionally, loss of function of the p53 gene can be associated with an increase in the incidence of homologous chromosomal recombination and a defect in the repair of double stranded DNA damage.

The p53 gene also plays an important role in the maintenance of "genetic stability" by "sensing" DNA damage and delaying DNA synthesis so that DNA repair can occur (Lee S et al., 1995). In addition, the p53 gene can also "sense" proliferation abnormalities associated with the mutation of other genes and can reduce the rate of proliferation back to normal or can induce apoptosis in the abnormal cells (Levin et al., 1997; Soddu et al., 1996). Table 4 provides a list of some of the genes whose expression is affected by p53 expression.

Mice which are p53 -/- develop a variety of tumors at an early age. P53 -/- cells do not form spontaneous colonies in vitro nor do they produce tumors in animals. However infection with a ras retrovirus leads to spontaneous colony formation in vitro and tumor formation in mice. In the absence of p53 function, a mutant ras oncogene can cause neoplastic transformation.

Abnormalities of the IRF1 and IRF2 genes

The IRF1 gene is found on the long arm of chromosome 5. Del 5q is present in 30% of MDS cases and 50% of AMLs which occur after toxic exposure and in 15% of "spontaneous" AML. In a study of 13 leukemias or MDS with aberrations of 5q31, the IRF1 gene was found to be consistently deleted in one or both alleles. In fact, the loss of one IRF1 allele was shown to occur in 24% - 88% of leukemias with del [5q] or with translocations of 5q31 (Kalra et al., 1995; Willman et al., 1993). In another study of 12 MDS patients and 2 AML patients with 5q del, the loss of one allele was demonstrated in 12 of the 14 cases while in 2 cases there was a loss of both alleles (Boultwood et al., 1993). Nevertheless, the IRF1 gene is not located in the commonly deleted region of chromosome 5.

The IRF1 and IRF2 genes are interferon response genes which are complementary to each other in several ways (Harada et al., 1993; Tanaka et al., 1994b). IRF1 recognition elements on the promotors of IFN γ and other IFN inducible genes have been identified. The IRF1 gene turns on interferon response genes while the IRF2 gene turns them off (Birnbaum et al., 1997). The IRF1 gene is an anti-oncogene while the IRF2 gene is an oncogene (Lallemand et al., 1997). Further, the two genes are competitive inhibitors of each other with the protein product of each binding to the promotor of the other gene shutting off transcription. Based on these observations it seems likely that the ratio of expression between these two genes determines which genes effects are predominant (Harada et al., 1993; Tanaka et al., 1994b).

Expression of the IRF1 gene occurs early response in the myeloid pathway of differentiation and its expression is rapidly induced by IL6 or leukemia inhibitory factor (Bouchard et al., 1989). Expression of the IRF1 gene is associated with the inhibition of proliferation (Kirchhoff et al., 1992; Hochhaus et al., 1997). Expression of the IRF2 gene activates the transcription of cell cycle related histone gene (Vaugh et al., 1995). Overexpression of the IRF2 gene in NIH 3T3 cells results in neoplastic transformation with the ability of the cells to form tumors in nude mice. The introduction of an expression vector for the IRF1 gene suppresses the neoplastic formation. Adriamycin, 5-FU, and ionizing radiation cause apoptosis only in IRF1 +/+ cells and not in IRF1 -/- cells. DNA damage produced by ionizing irradiation results in cell cycle arrest in IRF1 +/+ cells but not in IFR1 -/- cells. This phenotype is similar to that of p53 -/- mice. The induction of p21 expression after irradiation requires the activity of both the IRF1 and the p53 genes. The apoptosis which occurs when cells containing constitutively expressed myc, E1A, or mutant ras genes are placed into medium containing low level of serum or when cells are placed into crowded conditions does not occur in IRF1 -/- cells (Abdollahi et al., 1991). Like p53 protein, IRF1 protein is stabilized in the presence of ras expressing embryo fibroblasts after ionizing irradiation (Abdollahi et al., 1991).

The IRF1:IRF2 expression ratio oscillates throughout the cell cycle in NIH 3T3 cells with IRF1 expression being highest when cells are growth arrested due to starving (Abdollahi et al., 1991). While IRF1 -/- animals will grow for one year without the spontaneous appearance of tumors, mutant Ha-ras is transforming in primary embryo fibroblasts obtained from IRF1-/- mice but not in IRF1 +/+ mice or IRF1 +/- mice. Ha-ras induced transformation is reversed by IRF1 expression (Abdollahi et al., 1991). In the presence of normal IRF1 genes the signaling of mutant ras genes results in the induction of apoptosis.

IRF1 and p53 promotors contain a sequence [IPCS] which increases the transcription of a reporter gene (Lallemand et al., 1997). A single nuclear factor extracted from U937 cells and from peripheral blood lymphocytes binds to this single peptide chain which then binds to DNA Additionally, there is some evidence that the promotors of the Bax, WT1, NN23h1, Rb, and WAF 1 genes may also contain a binding site for this protein. p53 and IRF1 null mice do not have identical characteristics. While the level of mutant ras expression is the same in cells from both types of animals, the absence of p53 expression results in the formation of colonies which are 3 times larger than that produced by cells from IRF1-/- mice and injection of the former cells into nude mice results in more rapid and larger tumor formation than when the latter cells are injected.

Some evidence has been presented that a significant proportion of IRF1 mRNA in normal hemopoietic cells and in tissue culture cell lines lack exons 2 and 3 as a result of exon skipping (Harada et al., 1994). Further, it has also been reported that in MDS cells or in secondary AML cells exon-skipped IRF1 mRNA can be detected but little intact IRF1 mRNA can be detected. These studies failed to demonstrate that mutation was the cause of exon skipping but did demonstrate that the exon skipped form does not bind to DNA and is not tumor suppressing .

The C-myc and C-myb Genes

At the time of diagnosis of AML more than 90% of the cells contain significant amounts of myc and myb protein while this is the case for only 20-30% of normal marrow cells (Banavali et al., 1991). Additionally, the level of myc protein in AML cells is higher than that in marrow cells in remission patients or in normal bone marrow cells (Preisler et al., 1987b). At the level of the bone marrow biopsy, myc protein containing cells are diffusely distributed in the marrows of AML patients while in early relapse the myc protein containing cells are found to be present in clones (Preisler, 1988). In normal marrows myc containing cells are found in clusters of 2-4 cells. It is of interest that an increase in myc expression can be seen in AML remission marrows just prior to leukemia relapse even though the marrow appears to still be in remission. Myc protein is always present in the nucleus when anti-myc antibodies are used to detect myc expression while p53 protein can be found in the nucleus, the cytoplast, or in both (Depinho et al., 1991).

High levels of expression of the myc or myb genes can prevent cell differentiation (Clark et al., 1988) while high levels of expression of the myc gene can force cells into S phase. Coexpression of mutated ras genes and moderate levels of myc expression can facilitate the activation of cyclin E/CdK and E2F. This process probably involves the suppression of p27 expression via cooperative effects between the two oncogenes.

While mutations in the myc gene are often present in lymphomas, it is not abnormal myc protein which is biologically important, rather the absolute level of expression and/or expression during an inappropriate phase of the cell cycle are responsible for the oncogenic effects of these genes. Myc/max can activate G1 cyclin/CDK complexes thereby stimulating cells to enter S phase without cytokine stimulation. Myc also induces S phase progression by increasing cyclin D/cdk4 and cyclin E/cdk2 activity (Steiner et al., 1995). When mice have been altered to contain constitutively expressed myc genes 10% of the mice develop tumors. When the same mice are constructed with mutant ras genes tumors develop in 40% of the animals. If animals are constructed containing both constitutively expressed myc genes and mutant ras genes tumors form in every animal and occur with a shorter lag period.

Campisi has reported that neoplastic transformation is associated with the deregulation of myc expression as manifested by the continued expression of myc in the absence of serum (Campisi et al., 1984). We have conducted similar studies of human myeloid leukemia cells (Venugopal et al., 1992b). When chronic myelogenous leukemia cells were placed into culture over night a decrease in myc expression occurred in 6 of 8 specimens whether or not serum was present in the culture medium. In one specimen myc expression was unchanged while in a second specimen myc expression rose. When myeloid blastic crisis cells were placed into culture over night myc expression was maintained. Similarly, myc expression fell in 4 of 5 normal marrow specimens placed into overnight culture. In contrast, when AML cells were placed into overnight culture there was no change in myc expression in 4 specimens, myc expression increased in 6 specimens, and fell in 5 specimens. Even in the latter specimens a subpopulation of leukemia cells were present in which myc expression did not fall during overnight culture.

As noted above, constitutive myc expression is present in the leukemia cells of many patients with AML. In model systems the constitutive expression of myc is associated with the inhibition of cell differentiation and with a high proliferative potential (Freytag et al., 1988). Similarly, high levels of myc expression in AML marrows prior to the initiation of remission induction therapy are associated with low levels of induced AML differentiation during remission induction therapy. In some studies high levels of myc and/or myb expression are associated with a poor prognosis in AML. The positive effects of these genes on cell proliferation and their negative effects on differentiation make it likely that overexpression or unregulated expression of either of these gene can directly contribute to a poor prognosis. Studies of myc and myb protein levels in individual leukemia cells demonstrate high levels of expression. In some sense, it doesn't matter whether or not changes in myc or myb expression are associated with the etiology of the disease because even if the abnormal expression is a secondary event, it will increase the malignant potential of the abnormal cells.

The P15 and P16 Genes

The $p16^{INK4a}$ and the $p15^{INK4b}$ genes are tumor suppressor genes which are located on chromosome 9p (Herman et al., 1995). The inactivation of the $p16^{INK4a}$ gene has been reported in many solid tumors including cancers of the breast, lung, kidney, and colon (Herman et al., 1995). The inactivation of this gene is usually the result of mutation or deletion (Williamson et al., 1995). Mice with a targeted deletion of the p16 gene, which eliminates both p16 and p19 ARF function, develop spontaneous tumors at an early age (Serrano et al., 1996). Primary fibroblasts from these animals proliferate rapidly in vitro and have a high cloning efficiency. The introduction of a mutant Ha-ras into $p16^{INK4a}$ deficient cells causes neoplastic transformation. In contrast, the introduction of a $p16^{INK4a}$ gene into cells bearing a mutant Ha-ras gene blocks the entry of cells into S phase (Serrano et al., 1995). The p16 gene also suppresses the transformation of primary rat embryo fibroblasts by Ha-ras/c-myc abnormalities but not by Ha-ras/E1a abnormalities (Serrano et al., 1997). Oncogenic ras can transform immortalized rodent cells requiring either a cooperating oncogene or the inactivation of a tumor suppressor gene like p16 or p15. If an oncogenic ras gene is introduced into a normal cell there is an increase in both $p16^{INK4a}$ and p53 expression resulting in permanent G1 arrest and apoptosis. If either $p16^{INK4a}$ or p53 are lacking apoptosis does not occur (Serrano et al., 1997).

The p19 ARF gene is coded for by the $p16^{INK4a}$ gene in a different reading frame from the $p16^{INK4a}$ protein. In the presence of abnormal proliferation signals, over expression of myc and E1a, presence of a mutant ras gene p19ARF is synthesized and its protein causes proliferation arrest in G1 and G2 by stablizing p53 protein by antagonizing MDM2 which blocks DNA transcription and facilitates the degradation of p53 protein (Faderl et al., 1999).

In acute leukemia, abnormal expression of the $p15^{INK4b}$ gene predominates with little evidence that abnormalities of the $p16^{INK4a}$ gene play a role in disease formation. In contrast to the mechanisms by which $p16^{INK4a}$ function is lost in solid tumors, $p15^{INK4b}$ function is lost in hemopoietic neoplasms via methylation of the promotor region of the gene. The inhibition of proliferation associated with the exposure of cells to TGFβ is mediated via the activity of the p15 gene. TGFβ increases p15 mRNA and protein stability with the inhibitory effects on cell proliferation being mediated by the displacement of cyclin D1 from its association with cdks and by preventing new cyclin/cdk complexes from forming (Sandhu et al., 1997). In TGFβ resistant cells p15 transcripts are increased but the protein is not stabilized and does not accumulate in the cell.

The Retinoblastoma Gene

The retinoblastoma gene functions as the switch which determines whether or not a cell will synthesize DNA. In nonreplicating cells and in cells which are not about to engage in DNA synthesis the Rb protein binds and inactivates the E2F transcription factors whose functioning is necessary for DNA synthesis to occur. Phosphorylation of the Rb protein results in the release of the transcription factors which activate several genes involved in cell cycle progression and DNA synthesis including cyclins A and E, DNA polymerase α, PCNA, Myc, thymidine kinase, thymidine synthetase and dihyorofolate reductase. Conversely the E2F/Rb complex can bind to and suppress the activity of these genes (Weinberg, 1995).

In kinetically quiescent cells Rb is not phosphorylated and the D cyclins are short lived with levels being low or absent in the absence of mitogens. The p16, p21, and p27 genes are also active in kinetically quiescent cells. If mitogens are removed from the environment cyclin D levels rapidly fall. In contrast the cyclin dependent kinases are long lived molecules. During the G1 phase of a cell which is going to synthesize DNA, cyclin dependent kinases 4 and 6 phosphorylate cyclin D which facilitates the activation of cyclin E-cdk complex which results in the phosphorylation of the Rb protein by cdk2 and the release of the E2F transcription factors. A loss of Rb function leads to deregulation of the E2F transcription factors and abnormal proliferation. The loss of both Rb and p53 function is probably usually required for neoplastic transformation (Weinberg, 1995).

As might be expected, the entire pathway extending from the initial activation of cyclin dependent kinases 4 and 6 to the phosphorylation of the Rb protein is under tight regulation. The cdc proteins a, b, and c are phosphatases which prevent the phosphorylation of the cyclins. The synthesis of these proteins is induced when cells are placed in serum-free media. The INK4 family of proteins, p15 and p16 block DNA synthesis by preventing cdk 4 and 6 from phopshorylating cyclin thereby ultimately preventing phosphorylation of the Rb protein. P16 protein increases in cells which are deficient of Rb, and in cells in which there is a mutant ras gene. Cells deficient in p16 protein proliferate rapidly and form colonies in vitro and are transformed by the introduction of a single mutant ras gene. A loss of Rb function results in the activation of the p19ARF tumor suppressor gene which in turn activates p53 transcription and which also prevents the degradation of p53 protein (Williams et al., 1994). The synthesis of p19ARF is also stimulated by the overexpression of c-myc, E1A, ras, and v-abl. The growth inhibitory effects of TGFβ are mediated via the activation of p15 and p27.

The cip/kip genes p21 and p27 inhibit all cyclin dependent kinases thereby preventing the activation of the cyclins.

There are multiple reports in the literature that the absence of Rb protein or a decrease in the level of protein is uncommon in MDS (Preudhomme et al., 1994) but is common in AML at a frequency ranging from 20-30% (Ahuja et al., 1991; Kornblau et al., 1994; Tang et al., 1992). It has also been reported that approximately one half of leukemia cell populations which lack Rb protein grow autonomously in vitro and that anti-sense Rb increases the proliferation of clonogenic AML blast cells (Herwig and Strauss, 1997). Further, it has also been reported that Rb is a transcription repressor of the IL6 gene and that a loss of Rb function is associated with the synthesis of IL6 by some AML cell populations.

APPEARANCE AND EVOLUTION OF THE SECONDARY HEMATOLOGIC DISORDERS

Pre MDS

Normal cells have effective surveillance systems to detect cells which have acquired a single mutation so that these cells can be induced into undergoing apoptosis. By contrast, in the presence of inactivated $p15^{INK4b}$ or $p16^{INK4a}$ even a single oncogene mutation can be transforming. As noted above, p15 methylation was found to be present in 9/10 pre MDS marrows studied, median level = 27% methylation. While we do not know if this level of methylation represents 100% methylation in 27% of the cells or 27% methylation in all of the cells, in studies described earlier, levels of p15 methylation as low as 10% were shown to be associated with extinction of expression of the p15 gene. Hence methylation of the $p15^{INK4B}$ gene may be a very early event in the development of preMDS.

The development of monoclonal hemopoiesis is likely to be an important milestone in the development of the secondary hematologic disorders since it is the manifestation of a single cell and its progeny acquiring a proliferative advantage over competing clones. This development has several implications: 1) that the cell mechanisms which control aberrant patterns of proliferation were either compromised or were insufficient to prevent the development of monoclonal hemopoiesis, and 2) the "strain" placed on the single stem cell and its progeny which are responsible for all of hemopoiesis probably increases the likelihood that additional molecular abnormalities will appear. Further, the very presence of ras and fms mutations and monoclonal hemopoiesis strongly suggests that some form of genetic instability in present in the marrows of some cured lymphoma patients. The exact molecular lesion[s] which permit the development of monoclonal hemopoiesis are not known nor do we have any information as to the role that aberrant cytokine production might play in the acquisition of a proliferative advantage of one clone over another.

Many of the changes which occur at the MDS/AML interface undoubtedly contribute to the greater genetic instability of AML vis a vis MDS. These changes include a significant increase in the incidence of p53 mutations, a further reduction in IRF1 function, an increase in p15 methylation and a reduction in its expression. The loss of p53 function is accompanied by a loss of several mechanisms by which genomic stability is usually maintained: 1) the induction of apoptosis in response to the appearance of new mutated oncogenes, 2) the lag in DNA synthesis which provides time for DNA repair to be conducted, 3) the production of enzymes which are involved in DNA repair function, and perhaps most importantly, and 4) the loss of centriole stability so that increased numbers are present. Losses of IRF1 function and p15 function increase the impact of these loses.

MDS

By the time that clinically apparent MDS has appeared a large number of changes have occurred at all levels. At the level of the patient, anemia and marrow hyperplasia are usually present. At the level of the cell a new clone has appeared and replaced the clone responsible for monoclonal hemopoiesis. The bone marrow is morphologically abnormal with evidence of dysmyelopoiesis. The marrow is hyperproliferative with significant levels of apoptosis being present in the marrow. The simultaneous presence of hyperproliferation and apoptosis is accompanied by an unusual situation in which cells are synthesizing DNA and undergoing apoptosis at the same time.

Disorders of cytokine production are present along with evidence of increasing abnormalities at the molecular biological level.

While a primary stem cell disorder is undoubtedly present, a significant number of the clinical symptoms appear to be the result of the production of cytokines to abnormal levels. Increased levels of TNFα, IL1β, and TGFβ are found in the marrow. The increased levels of TNFα undoubtedly play a role in the increases in proliferation and apoptosis which are going on in the marrow since the levels of apoptosis and TNFα in the marrow are roughly correlated. Additionally TNFα has been shown to stimulate the proliferation of MDS and AML cells (Elbaz and Mahmoud, 1994; Munker and Koeffler, 1987). The significance of the increase in IL1β levels is not understood but TNFα and IL1β levels in AML patients are correlated. The important role of cytokines in the production of the clinical manifestations of MDS is also demonstrated by the fact that anti-TNFα therapy can alleviate the cytopenias in some cases.

To what may we attribute these significant changes in cell biology? During the MDS phase direct evidence for genomic instability becomes apparent, the appearance and evolution of chromosomal abnormalities. The relationship between a change in abnormality [evolution] and disease evolution attests to the importance of this new feature. It should be noted that the transfection of a mutant ras gene into normal hemopoietic stem cells produces dysplastic changes and in some cases a slight increase in the % of blast cells which are present.

The extent of methylation of the p15 gene is greater in MDS than in preMDS and p15 expression is lower as well. An abnormally low IRF1/IRF2 expression ratio has also been found to be present in MDS marrows but, as with p15 methylation, it is not known if all of the marrow cells are affected or only in a small proportion. The consequences of both of these abnormalities can be significant in terms of further disease evolution since both are tumor suppressor genes. The greater telomerase activity in MDS as compared to pre MDS is of interest for several reasons: 1) increased activity could contribute to the proliferative advantage which MDS cells enjoy over preMDS cells, 2) constitutive telomerase activity can be transforming, and 3) the increase in telomerase activity could be evidence of aberrant c-myc expression

The basis for the abnormal production of cytokines in MDS has not been defined as yet, but there are reports that some oncogene abnormalities can be associated with aberrant cytokine production as can a loss of Rb function (Zhu et al., 1994). In fact, abnormal cytokine production may represent the host attempting to destroy clones of abnormal cells. Further, the presence of large numbers of macrophages, cells which make many cytokines, in the marrows of MDS patients may contribute to or be the result of abnormal cytokine production.

AML

At the level of cell, apoptosis which is present in MDS marrows is not present in AML marrows. These cells have a marked proliferative advantage over MDS cells and usually have replaced virtually all MDS elements. As noted in the section on MDS, apoptosis was much greater in maturing cells than in primitive cells so the absence of apoptosis might be expected in AML. TNFα nevertheless, appears to play an important role in AML in that there is a correlation between the % leukemia cells in S phase and the level of TNFα mRNA in the leukemia cells themselves (Munker and Koeffler,1987) TNFα has also been demonstrated to stimulate the production of colony formation by AML cells in vivo (Elbaz and Mahmoud,1994). Further, high BM levels of TNFα at the end of remission induction therapy are associated with early relapse. Hence, the proliferation stimulatory effects are preserved but the apoptosis inducing effects are not apparent in AML.

The initiation of DNA synthesis and cell division are dependent upon the activities of the E2F transcription factors which, in proliferating cells are bound to and are inactivated by Rb protein. Release of the E2F transcription factors is dependent upon the phosphorylation of the Rb protein by the activation of the cdk/cyclin system. Rb protein levels are reduced or absent from 20-40% of AML cell populations. Given that the Rb protein is situated at a critical cross section in the regulatory system that controls cell proliferation, a loss of Rb function removes a critical regulator of cell proliferation. Malignant transformation occurs if both Rb and p53 function are lost. Further, the introduction of anti sense Rb RNA leads to cell proliferation. It has also been reported that cells begin to synthesize IL6 when Rb function is lost.

Taking all of the above into consideration, there are 3 genes which play critical roles in the control of cell proliferation and which are frequently abnormal in AML: the p53 gene, c-myc, and the Rb gene. The inactivation of these genes either play a role in the transition of MDS to AML or occur just after AML appears. The author favors the former. The location of the genes in the pathways that control proliferation and differentiation make them not only critical targets for agents which cause malignant transformation, but also provide excellent targets for therapeutic intervention.

FUTURE DIRECTIONS:

As noted earlier, the incidence of monoclonal hemopoiesis, myelodysplastic syndrome, and acute myelogenous leukemia all increase with age. This relationship suggests that as with the secondary hematologic disorders, the monoclonality which occurs with increasing age may be the first step in the development of MDS and AML. Given the low incidence of spontaneous monoclonal hemopiesis and the still lesser incidences of MDS and secondary AML which occur after the monoclonal hemopoiesis that often follows toxic exposure, if the same were the case for the MDS and AML which occur subsequent to spontaneous monoclonal hemopoiesis then it would be financially impossible to prospectively screen a sufficiently large number of women to determine whether or not such a relationship existed.

One possible approach to this problem could be taken by collaboration with the Women's Health Initiative. In this government-sponsored study, over 150,000 women are being studied prospectively for cardiovascular disease. At the start of the trial both peripheral blood cells and serum are obtained from every participant and stored for future study. Given that it is already known that more than 60 participants in the Women's Health Initiative have already developed a myeloid leukemia it should be possible to collect cells obtained from the women who developed AML or CML and determine the incidence of monoclonal hemopoiesis among these women. A similar or larger sized matched control group could be studied for the possible relationship between the spontaneous monoclonal hemopoiesis, which occurs with advancing age and the development of myeloid leukemia.

ACKNOWLEDGEMENTS

This work has been supported by NIH grant POI CA 75606 and the Coleman Foundation.

REFERENCES

Abdollahi, A., Lord, K.A., Hoffman, R., Liebermann, B., Liebermann, D.A. (1991) Interferon regulatory factor 1 is a myeloid differentiation primary response gene induced by interleukin 6 and leukemia inhibitory factor: role in growth inhibition. *Cell Growth and Differentiation*, **2**, 401-407.

Adams, J.M., Harris, A.W., Pinkert, C.A., Corcoran, L.M., Alexander, W.S., Cory, S., Palmiter R.D., Brinster, R.L. (1985) The c-myc oncogene driven by immunoglobulin enhancers induces lymphoid malignancy in transgenic mice. *Nature*, **318**, 533-538.

Ahuja, H.G., Jat, P.S., Foti, A., Bar-Eli, M., Cline, M.J. (1991) Abnormalities of the retinoblastoma gene in the pathogenesis of acute leukemia. *Blood*, **78**, 3259-3268.

Amundadottir, L.T., Merlino, G., Dickson, R.B. (1996) Transgenic mouse models of breast cancer. Breast Cancer Research, 119-135.

Arif, M., Tanaka, K., Damodaran, C., Asou, H., Kyo, T., Dohy, H., Kamada, N. (1996) Hidden monosomy 7 in acute myeloid leukemia and myelodysplastic syndrome detected by interphase fluorescence in situ hybridization. *Leukemia Research*, **20**, 709-716.

Banavali, S.D., Silvestry, F.F., Pavelic, K., Pavelic, Z.P., Smith, P.L., Preisler, H.D. (1991) Studies of the geographic patterns of c-myc expression in bone marrow. *Cell Proliferation*, **24**, 529-542.

Bashey, A., Gill, R., Levi, S., Farr, C.J., Clutterbuck, R., Millar, J.L., Pragnell, I.B., Marshall, C.J. (1992) Mutational activation of the N-ras oncogene assessed in primary clonogenic culture of acute myeloid leukemia (AML): Implications for the role of N-ras mutation in AML pathogenesis. *Blood*, **79**, 981-989.

Beaupre, D.M., Talpaz, M., Marini, III F.C., Cristiano, R.J., Roth, J.A., Estrov, Z., Albitar, M., Freedman, M.H., Kurzrock, R. (1999) Autocrine interleukin-1β production in leukemia: Evidence for the involvement of mutated ras[1]. *Cancer Research,* **59**, 2971-2980.

Benchimo, S., Minden, M.D. (1987) "Viruses, Oncogenes, and tumor suppressor genes." The basic science of Oncology. Ian F. Tannck and Richard P. Hill, McGraw-Hill, 79-105.

Bi, S., Horvath, E., Yang, J., Gao, X-Z., Chopra, H., Raza, A., Shahidi, H., Gregory, S., Kaizer, H., Preisler, H.D. (1997) Molecular biologic studies in premyelodysplasia, myelodysplasia, and AML. *Proceedings of the American Society of Clinical Oncology*,**16**:542a, Abstract #1952.

Birnbaum, M.J., van Zundert, B., Vaughan, P.S., Whitmarsh, A.J., van Wijnen, A.J., Davis, R.J., Stein, G.S., Stein, J.L. (1997) Phosphorylation of the oncogenic transcription factor interferon regulatory factor 2 (IRF2) in vitro and in vivo. *Journal of Cellular Biochemistry*, **66**, 175-183.

Bodnar, A.G., Ouellette, M., Frolkis, M., Holt, S.E., Chiu, C.P., Morin, G.B., Harley, C.B., Shay, J.W., Lichtsteiner, S., Wright, W.E. (1998) Extension of life-span by introduction of telomerase into normal human cells. *Science*, **279**, 349-352.

Boultwood, J., Fidler, C., Lewis, S., MacCarthy, A., Sheridan, H., Kelly, S., Oscier, D., Buckle, V.J., Wainscoat, J.S. (1993) Allelic loss of IRF-1 in myelodysplasia and acute myeloid leukemia: retentionof IRF1 on the 5q- chromosome in some patients with the 5q-syndrome. ***Blood***, **82**, 2611-1616.

Bos, J.L., Verlaan-deVries, M., van der, E.B. A.J., Janssen, J.W.G., Delwel, R., Lowenberg, B., Colly, L.P. (1987) Mutations in N-ras predominate in acute myeloid leukemia. *Blood*, **69**, 1237-1241.

Bos, J.L. (1989). Ras oncogenes in human cancer: a review. *Cancer Research*, **49**, 4682-4689.

Bouchard, L., Lamarre, L., Tremblay, P.J., Jolicoeur, P. (1989) Stochastic appearance of mammary tumors in transgenic mice carrying the MMTV/c-neu oncogene. *Cell*, **57**,931-936.

Busque, L., Mio, R., Mattioli, J., Brais, E., Blais, N., Lalonde, Y., Maragh, M., Gilliland, D.G. (1996) Nonrandom x-inactivation patterns in normal females: Lyonization ratios vary with age. *Blood*, **88**, 59-65.

Cachia, P.G., Culligan, D.J., Clark, R.E., Whittaker, J.A., Jacobs, A., Padua, R.A. (1993) Clonal Haemopoiesis following cytotoxoic therapy for lymphoma. *Leukemia*, **7**, 795-800.

Campisi, J., Gray, H.E., Pardee, A.B., Sonenshein, G.E. (1984) Cell-cycle control of c-myc but not c-ras expression is lost following chemical transformation. *Cell*, **36**, 241-247.

Carter, G., Hughes, D.C., Clark, R.E., McCormick, F., Jacobs, A., Whittaker, J.A., Padua, R.A. (1990) RAS mutations in patients following cytotoxic therapy for lymphoma. *Oncogene*, **5**, 411-416.

Cazzola, M., May, A., Bergamaschi, G., Cerani, P., Rosti, V., Bishop, D.F. (2000) Familial-skewed x-chromosome inactivation as a predisposing factor for late-onset x-linked sideroblastic anemia in carrier females. *Blood*, **15**,4363-4365.

Champion, K.M., Gilbert, J.G., Asimakopoulos, F.A., Hinshelwood, S., Green, A.R. (1997) Clonal haemopoiesis in normal elderly women: implications for the myeloproliferative disorders and myelodysplastic syndromes. *British Journal of Haematology*, **97**, 920-926.

Christensen, K., Kristiansen, M., Hagen-Larsen, H., Skytthe, A., Bathum, L., Jeune, B., Andersen-Ranberg, K., Vaupel, J.W., Orstavik, K.H. (2000) X-linked genetic factors regulate hematopoietic stem-cell kinetics in females. *Blood*, **95**, 2449-2451.

Clark, M.F., Kukowska, J.F., Westin, E., Smith, M., Prochownik, E.V. (1988) Constitutive expressionof a c-myc cDNA blocks friend murine erythroleukemia cell differentiation. *Molecular & Cellular Biology*, **8**, 884-892.

Coghlan, D.W., Morley, A.A., Matthews, J.P., Bishop, J.F. (1994) The incidence and prognostic significance of mutations in codon 13 of the N-ras gene in acute myeloid leukemia. *Leukemia*, **8**, 1682-1687.

Darrington, D.L., Voss, J.M., Anderson, J.R., Bierman, P.J., Bishop, M.R., Chan, W.C., Morris, M.E., Reed, E.C., Sanger, W.G., Tarantolo, S.R., Weisenburger, D.D., Kessinger, A., Armitage, J.O. (1994) Incidence and characterization of secondary myelodysplastic syndrome and acute myelogenous leukemia following high-dose chemoradiotherapy and autologous stem-cell transplantation for lymphoid malignancies. *Journal of Clinical Oncology*, **12**, 2527-2534.

Demetri, G.D., Ernst, T.J., Pratt, E.X., Zenzie, B.W., Rheinwald, J.G., Griffin, J.D. (1990) Expressionof ras oncogenes in cultured human cells alters the transcriptional and posttranscriptional regulation of cytokine genes. *Journal of Clinical Investigation*, **86**,1261-1269.

Depinho, R.A., Schreiber-Agus, N., Alt, F.W. (1991) My family oncogenes in the development of normal and neoplastic cells. *Advances in Cancer Research*, **57**,1-46.

Dinarello, C.A. (1996). Biologic basis for interleukin-1 in disease. *Blood*, **87,** 2095-2147.

Elbaz, O., Mahmoud, L.A. (1994) Tumor necrosis factor and human acute leukemia. *Leukemia and Lymphoma* ,**12**,191-195.

Faderl, S., Kantarjian, H.M., Estey, E., Manshouri, T., Chan, C.Y., Elsaied, A.R., Kornblau, S.M., Cortes, J., Thomas, D.A., Pierce, S., Keating, M.J., Estrov, Z., Albitar, M. (1999) The prognositc significance of p16INKa/P14ARF locus deletion and MDM-2 protein expressionin adult acute myelogenous leukemia. *Blood*, **94**, 74a.

Far, R.K., Der, C.J. (1994) The ras signal transduction pathway. *Cancer and Metastasis Reviews*, **13**, 67-89.

Filmus, J., Robles, A.I., Shi, W., Wong, M.J., Colombo, L.L., Cont, C.J. (1994) Induction of cyclin D1 overexpression by activated ras. *Oncogene*, **9**, 3627-3633.

Freytag, S.O. (1988) Enforced expression of the c-myc oncogene inhibits cell differentiation by precluding entry into a distinct predifferentiation state in G0/G1. *Molecular and Cellular Biology*, **8**, 1614-1624.

Gale, R.E., Bunch, C., Moir, D.J., Patterson, K.G., Goldstone, A.H., Linch, D.C. (1996) Demonstration of developing myelodysplasia/acute myeloid leukaemia in haematologically normal patients after high-dose chemotherapy and autologous bone marrow transplantation using X-chromosome inactivation patterns. *British Journal of Haematology*, **93**, 53-58.

Gale RE, Fielding AK, Harrison CN, Linch DC. (1997) Acquired skewing of X-chromosome inactivation patterns in myeloid cells of the elderly suggests stochastic clonal loss with age. *British Journal of Haematology* **17**, 512-519.

Harada, H., Kitagawa, M., Tanaka, N., Yamamoto, H., Harada, K., Ishihara, M., Taniguchi, T. (1993) Anti-oncogenic and oncogenic potentials of interferon regulatory factors -1 and -2. *Science*, **259**, 971-974.

Harada, H., Kondo, T., Ogawa, S., Tamura, T., Kitagawa, M., Tanaka, N., Lamhier, M.S., Hrai, H., Taniguchi, T. (1994) Accelerated exon skipping of Irf-1 mRNA in human myelodysplasia/ leukemia; a possible mechanism of tumor suppressor inactivation. *Oncogene*, **9**, 3313-3320.

Heim, S. (1992) Cytogenetic findings in primary and secondary MDS. *Leukemia Research*, **16**, 43-46.

Herman, J.G., Merlo, A., Mao, L., Lapidus, R.G., Issa, J.P., Davidson, N.E., Sidransky, D., Baylin, S.B. (1995) Inactivation of the CDKN2/p16/MTS1 gene is frequently associated with aberrant DNA methylation in all common human cancers. *Cancer Research*, **55**, 4525-4230.

Herwig, S., Strauss, M. (1997) The retinoblastoma protein: a master regulator of cell cycle, differentiation and apoptosis. *European Journal of Biochemistry*, **246**, 581-601.

Hochhaus, A., Yan, X.H., Willer, A., Hehlmann, R., Gordon, M..Y., Goldman, J.M., Melo, J.V. (1997). Expression of interferon regulatory factor (IRF) genes and response to interferon-γ in chronic myeloid leukaemia. *Leukemia*, **11**, 933-939.

Hunter, T. (1991) Cooperation between oncogenes. Cell, 64, 249-270.

Johannes, L.B. (1989) Ras oncogenes in human cancer: A Review[1]. *Cancer Research*, **49**, 4682-4689.

Jonveaux, P.H., Fenaux, P., Quiquandon, I., Pignon, J.M., Lai, J.L., Loucheux-Lefebvre, M.D., Goossens, M., Bauters, F., Berger, R. (1991) Mutations in the p53 gene in myelodysplastic syndromes. *Oncogene*, **6**, 2243-2247.

Kalra, R., Dale, D., Freedman, M., Bonilla, M.A., Weinblatt, M., Ganser, A., Bowman, P., Abish, S., Priest, J., Oseas, R.S. (1995) Monosomy 7 and activating RAS mutations accompany malignant transformation in patients with congenital neutropenia. *Blood*, **86**, 4579-4586.

Kassar, N.E., Hetet, G., Briere, J., Grandchamp, B. (1998) X-chromosome inactivation inhealthy females: incidence of excessive lyonization with age and comparison of assay involving DNA methylation and transcript polymorphism. *Clinical Chemistry*, **44**, 61-67.

Kataoka, H., Tahara, H., Watanable, T., Sugawara, M., Ide, T., Goto, M., Furuichi, Y., Sugimoto, M. (1997) Immortalization of immunologically committed Epstein-Barr virus-transformed human B-lymphoblastoid cell lines accompanied by a strong telomerase activity. *Differentiation*, **62**, 203-211.

Kirchhoff, S., Schaper, F., Hauser, H. (1992) Interferon regulatory factor 1 (IRF-1) mediates cell growth inhibition by transactivation of downstream target genes. *Nucleic Acids Research*, **21**,2881-2889.

Kornblau, S.M., Xu, H.J., Zhang, W., Hu, S.X., Beran, M., Smith, T.L., Hester, J., Estey, E., Benedict, W.F., Deisseroth, A.B. (1994) Levels of retinoblastoma protein expression in newly diagnosed acute myelogenous leukemia. *Blood*, **84**, 256-261.

Lallemand, C., Bayat-Sarmadi, M., Blanchard, B., Tovey, M.G. (1997) Identificationof a novel transcriptional regulatory element common to the p53 and interferon regulatory factor 1 genes. *Journal of Biological Chemistry*, **272**, 29801-29809.

Land, H., Parada, L.F., Weinberg, R.A. (1983) Cellular oncogenes and multistep carcinogenesis. Science, **222**, 771-778.

Lawler, S.D., Summersgill, B., Clink, H.M., McElwain, T.J. (1980) Cytogenetic follow-up study of acute non-lymphocytic leukaemia. *British Journal of Haematology*, **44**, 395-405.

Le Beau, M.M., Albain, K.S., Larson, R.A., Vardiman, J.W., Davis, E.M., Blough, R.R., Golomb, H.M., Rowley, J.D. (1986) Clinical and cytogenetic correlations in 63 patients with therapy-related myelodysplastic syndromes and acute nonlymphocytic leukemia: Further evidence for characteristic abnormalities of chromosomes NO. 5 and 7. *Journal of Clinical Oncology*, **4**, 325-345.

Lee, J., Kook, H., Chung, I., Kim, H., Park, M., Kim, C., Nah, J., Hwang, T. (1999) Telomere length changes in patients undergoing hematopoietic stem cell transplantation. *Bone Marrow Transplantation*, **24**, 411-415.

Lee, S., Elenbaas, B., Levine, A., Griffith, J. (1995) p53 and its 14 kDa C-terminal domain recognize primary DNA damage in the form of insertion/deletion mismatches. *Cell*, 81, 1013-1020.

Levin, A.J. (1997) P53, the cellular gatekeeper for growth and division. *Cell*, **88**,323-331.

Li, B., Yang, J., Andrews, C., Chen, Y-X., Toofanfard, P., Huang, R-W., Horvath, E., Chopra, H., Raza, A., Preisler, H.D. (2000) Telomerase activity in preleukemia and acute myelogenous leukemia. *Leukemia and Lymphoma*, **36**, 579-587.

Loew, S.W., Ruley, H.E., Jacks, T., Housman, D.E. (1993) p53-dependent apoptosis modulates the cytotoxicity of anticancer agents. *Cell*, **76**, 957-67.

Lubbert, M., Oster, W., Knopf, H.P., McCormick, F., Mertelsmann, R., Herrmann, F. (1993) N-ras gene activation in acute myeloid leukemia: Association with expression of interleukin-6. *Leukemia*, **7**, 1948-1954.

Mach-Pascual, S., Legare, R.D., Lu, D., Kroon, M., Neuberg, D., Tantravahi, R., Stone, R.M., Freedman, A.S., Nadler, L.M., Gribben, J.G., Gilliland, D.G. (1998) Predictive value of clonality assays in patients with non-Hodgkin's lymphoma undergoing autologous bone marrow transplant: A single institution study. *Blood*, **91**, 4496-4503.

Mayani, H., Baines, P., Bowen, D.T., Jacobs, A. (1989) In vitro growth of myeloid and erythroid progenitor cells from myelodysplastic patients in response to recombinant human granulocyte-macrophage colony-stimulating factor. *Leukemia*, **3**, 29-32.

Merchav, S., Nagler, A., Fleischer-Kurtz, G., Tatarsky, I. (1989) Regulatory abnormalities in the marrow of patents with myelodysplastic syndromes. *British Journal of Haematology* **73**, 158-164.

Michalova, K., Musilova, J., Zemanova, Z. (1991) Consecutive chromosomal studies in patients with myelodysplastic syndrome (MDS). *Czechoslovak MDS Cooperative Group. Annales de Genetique*, **34**, 212-218.

Miller, O.J., Therman, E. (1980) "Genome destabilization and multistep progression to cancer."Human Chromosomes, Springer-Verlag, New York , USA.

Mundle, S. Venugopal, P., Shetty, V., Ali., A., Chopra, H., Rose, S., Mativi, B.Y., Gregory, S., Preisler, H. & Raza, A. (1999) The relative extent and propensity of $CD34^+$ vs. $Cd34^-$ cells to undergo apoptosis in myelodysplastic marrows. *International Journal of Hematology*, **69**, 152-159.

Mundle, S.D., Mativi, B.Y., Cartlidge, J.D., Dangerfield, B., Robinson, L.B., Li, B., Shetty, V., Venugopal, P., Gregory, S.A., Preisler, H.D., Raza, A. (2000) Signal antonymy unique to myelodysplastic marrows correlates with altered expression of E2F1. *British Journal of Haematology*, **109**, 376-381.

Munker, R., Koeffler, P. (1987) In vitro action of tumor necrosis factor on myeloid leukemia cells. *Blood*, **69**, 1102-1108.

Neubauer, A., Greenberg, P., Negrin, R., Ginzton, N., Liu, E. (1994) Mutations in the ras proto-oncogenes in patients with myelodysplastic syndromes. *Leukemia*, **8**, 638-641.

Neubauer, A., Shannon, K., Liu, E. (1991) Mutations of the ras proto-oncogenes in childhood monosomy 7. *Blood*, **77**, 594-598.

Ohmori, M., Ohmori, S., Ueda, Y., Yoshida, Y., Okuma, M. (1991) Ineffective hemopoiesis in the myelodysplastic syndromes (MDS) as studied by daily in situ observation of colony-cluster formation. *International Journal of Cell Cloning*, **9**, 521-530.

Ohyashiki, K., Ohyashiki, J.H., Nishimaki, J., Toyama, K., Ebihara, Y., Kato, H., Wright, W.E., Shay, J.W. (1997) Cytological detection of telomerase activity using an in situ telomeric repeat amplification protocol assay. *Cancer Research*, **57**, 2100-2103.

Panterne, B., Zhou, Y.Q., Hatzfeld, J., Li, M.L., Levesque, J.P., Clark, S.C., Hatzfeld, A. (1993) CSF-1 control of C-FMS expression in normal human bone marrow progenitors. *Journal of Cellular Physiology*, **155**, 282-289.

Paquete, R.L., Landaw, E.M., Pierre, R.V., Kahan, J., Lubbert, M., Lazcano, O., Isaac, G., McCormick, F., Koeffler, P. (1993) N-ras mutations are associated with poor prognosis and increased risk of leukemia in myelodysplastic syndrome. *Blood*, **82,** 590-599.

Parker, J., Mufti, G.J. (1996) Ras and myelodysplasia: Lessons from the last decade. *Seminars in Hematology*, **33**, 206-224.

Pedersen-Bjergaard, J., Philip, P., Larsen, S.O., Andersson, M., Daugaard, G., Ersboll, J., Hansen, S.W., Hou-Jensen, K., Nielsen, D., Sigsgaard, T.C., Specht, L., Osterlind, K. (1993) Therapy-related myelodysplasia and acute myeloid leukemia. Cytogenetic characteristics of 115 Consecutive cases and risk in seven cohorts of patients treated intensively for malignant diseases in the Copenhagen series. *Leukemia*, **7**, 1975-1986.

Preisler, H.D., Raza, A. (1987a) Proto-oncogene transcript levels and acute nonlymphocytic leukemia. *Seminars in Oncology*, **14**, 207-216.

Preisler, H.D., Kinniburgh, A.J., Wei-Don, G., Khan, S. (1987b) Expression of the protooncogenes c-myc, c-fos, and c-fms in acute myelocytic leukemia at diagnosis and in remission. *Cancer Research*, **47**, 874-880.

Preisler, H.D. (1988) Hypothesis regarding the development of acute myeloid leukemia from preleukemic disorders: The role of proto-oncogenes. *Cancer Genetic Cytogenetics*, **32**, 133-142.

Preisler, H.D., Raza, A., Larson, R., LeBeau, M., Browman, G., Goldberg, J., Grunwald, H., Volger, R., Verkh, L., Singh, P., Block, A.M., Sandberg, A. (1989) Proto-oncogene expression and the clinical characteristics of acute nonlymphocytic leukemia: A Leukemia Intergroup Pilot Study. *Blood*, **73**, 255-262.

Preisler, H.D., Raza, A., Larson, R., Goldberg, J., Tricot, G., Browman, G., Bennett, J. (1994a) The relationship of the in vivo cells cycle characteristics and treatment outcome in acute myelogenous leukemia to the expression of the Fms, and Myc Photo-Oncogenes. *Leukemia and Lymphoma,* **14**, 273-278.

Preisler, H.D., Venugopal, P. (1994b) Regrowth resistance in leukemia and lymphoma: The need for a new system to classify treatment failure and for new approaches to treatment. *Leukemia Research,* **18**, 149-160.

Preisler, H.D. (1995a) Resistance to cytotoxic therapy: A speculative overview. *Annals of Oncology*, **6**, 651-657.

Preisler, H.D. (1995b) Multidrug resistance is more than MDR1 activity. *Leukemia Research*, **19**, 429-431.

Preisler, H.D., Gao, X-Z., Chopra, H., Devemy, E., Venugopal, P., Bi, S. (1998) Control of leukemia proliferation in vivo in patients: In vivo cytokine production. Acute Leukemia VII Symposium, Published in Acute Leukemias VII, Experimental Approaches and Novel Therapies. Hiddeman W, Buchner T, Wormann B, Ritter J, Creutzig U, Keating M, Plunkett W (eds). Springer Verlag Berlin Heidelberg, 307-316.

Preisler, H.D., Gao, X-Z., Tao, M., Li, B., Bi, S., Devemy, E., Loew, J., Raza, A. (1999) Marrow cytokine transcripts and the secondary hematologic disorders. *Leukemia and Lymphoma*, **35**, 297-302.

Preisler, H.D., Li, B., Yang, J., Huang, R-W., Devemy, E., Venugopal, P., Tao, M., Chopra, H., Gregory, S.A., Adler, S., Sivaraman, S., Toofanfard, P., Jajeh, A., Galvez, A., Robin, E. (2000) Suppression of telomerase activity, cytokine mRNA level in acute myelogenous leukemia cells in vivo in patients by amifostine and IL-4. *Clinical Cancer Research*, **6**, 807-812.

Preisler, H.D., Li, B., Chen, H., Fisher, L., Nayini, J., Raza, A., Creech, S., Venugopal, P. (2001) $P15^{INK4B}$ gene methylation and expression in normal, myelodysplastic, and acute myelogenous leukemia cells and in the marrow cells of cured lymphoma patients. In Press, *Leukemia*.

Price, C.M., Marshall, C.J., Bashey, A. (1994) Sequential acquisition of trisome 8 and N-ras mutation in acute myeloid leukaemia demonstrated by analysis of isolated leukaemic colonies. *British Journal of Haematology*, **88**, 338-342.

Preudhomme, C., Vachee, A., Lepelley, P., Vanrumbeke, M., Zandecki, M., Quesnel, B., Cosson, A., Fenaux, P. (1994) Inactivationof the retinoblastoma gene appears to be very uncommon in myelodysplstic syndromes. *British Journal of Haematology*, **91**, 61-67.

Radich, J.P., Kopecky, K.J., Willman, C.L., Weick, J., Head, D., Appelbaum, F., Collins, S.J. (1990) N-ras mutations in adult De Novo acute myelogenous leuekmia: Prevalence and clinical significance. *Blood*, **76**, 801-807.

Raskind, W.H., Tirumali, N., Jacobson, R., Singer, J., Fialkow, P.J. (1984) Evidence for a multistep pathogenesis of a myelodysplastic syndrome. *Blood*, **63**, 1318-1323.

Raza, A., Preisler, H.D., Li, Q.U., Larson, R.A., Goldberg, J., Browman, G., Bennett, J., Grunwald, H., Vogler, R., Kukla, C. (1993) Biological characteristics of newly diagnosed poor prognosis acute myelogenous leukemia. *American Journal of Hematology,* **42**, 359-366.

Raza A, Rifkin S, Showel J, Gregory S, Gezer S, Parcharidou A, Mundle A, Shetty V, Alvi S, Borok R, Loew J, Preisler H: Novel treatment of myelodysplastic syndromes (MDS) by suppression of high apoptotic intramedullary cell death (1995) *American Society of Clinical Oncology* **14**:78, Abstract #17.

Raza, A., Mundle, S., Shetty, V., Alvi, S., Chopra, H., Span, L., Parcharidou, A., Dar, S., Venugopal, P., Borok, R., Gezer, S., Showel, J., Loew, J., Rifkin, S., Alston, D., Hernandez, B., Shah, R., Kaizer, H., Gregory, S., Preisler, H.D. (1996a) A paradigm shift in myelodysplastic syndromes. *Leukemia*, **10**, 1648-1652.

Raza, A., Mundle, S.. Shetty, V., Alvi, S., Chopra, H., Span, L., Parcharidou, A., Dar, S., Venugopal, P., Borok, R., Gezer, S., Showel, J., Loew, J., Robin, E., Rifkin, S., Alston, D., Hernandez, B., Shah, R., Kaizer, H., Gregory, S. (1996b) Novel insights into the biology of myelodysplastic syndromes: excessive apoptosis and the role of cytokines. *International Journal of Hematology*, **63**, 265-278.

Raza, A. Gezer, S. Gregory, S.A. Venugopal, P., Kaizer, H., Dong, L.M., Span, L., Hines, C., Thomas, R., Alvi, S., Mundle, S.D., Shetty, V., Borok, R., Loew, J., Reza, S., Robin, E.L., Rifkin, S.D., Alston, D., Hernandez, B.M., Shah, R., Preisler, H.D. (1996c) Anti-cytokine therapy produces responses in patients with myelodysplastic syndromes (MDS). *Blood*, **88**, 580a, Abstract # 2310.

Sandhu, C., Garbe, J., Bhattacharya, N., Daksis, J., Pan, C.H., Yaswen, P., Koh, J., Slingerland, J.M., Stampfer, M.R. (1997) Transforming growth factor B stabilizes $p15^{INK4B}$ protein, increases $p15^{INK4B}$-cdk4 complexes, and inhibits cyclin D1-cdk4 association in human mammary epithelial cells. *Molecular and Cellular Biology*, **17**, 2458-2467.

Serrano, M., Gomez-Lahoz, E., DePinho, R., Beach, D., Bar-Sagi, D. (1995) Inhibition of Ras-induced proliferation and cellular transformation by p16^{INK4}. *Science*, **267**, 249-252.

Serrano, M., Lee, H.W., Chin, L., Cordon-Cardo, C., Beach, D., DePinho, R.A. (1996) Role of the INK4a locus in tumor suppression and cell mortality. *Cell*, **85**, 27-37.

Serrano, M., Li, A.W., McCurrach, M.E., Beach, D., Lowe, S.W. (1997) Oncogenic ras provokes premature cell senescence associated with a accumulation of p53 and p16^{INK4a}. *Cell*, **88**, 593-602.

Shadduck, R.K (2001) "Aplastic anemia" Williams Hematology, Sixth Edition, Beutler E, Lichtman MA, Coller BS, Kipps TJ, Seligsohn U. McGraw Hill Companies. New York.

Shimamura, A., Fisher, D.E. (1996) P53 in life and death. *Clinical Cancer Research*, **2**, 435-440.

Soddu, S., Blandino, G., Scardigli, R., Coen, S., Marchetti, A., Rizzo, M.G., Bossi, G., Cimino, L., Crescenzi, M., Sacchi, A. (1996) Interference with p53 protein inhibits hematopoietic and muscle differentiation. *Journal of Cellular Biology*, **134**, 193-204.

Steiner, P., Philipp, A., Lukas, J., Godden-Kent, D., Pagano, M., Mittnacht, S., Bartek, J., Eilers, M. (1995) Identification of a myc-dependent step during the formation of active G1 cyclin-cdk complexes. *European Journal of Molecular Biology and Biochemistry*, **14**, 4814-4826.

Stone, R.M. (1994) Myelodysplastic syndrome after autologous transplantation for lymphoma: the price of progress. *Blood*, **83**, 3437-3440.

Sugimoto, K., Hirano, N., Toyoshima, H., Chiba, S., Mano, H., Takaku, F., Yazaki, Y., Hirai, H. (1993) Mutations of the p53 gene in myelodysplastic syndrome (MDS) and MDS-derived leukemia. *Blood*, **81**, 3022-3026.

Tanaka, N., Ishihara, M., Taniguchi, T. (1994a) Suppression of c-myc or fosB-induced cell transformation by the transcription factor IRF-1. *Cancer letters*, **83**, 194-196.

Tanaka, N., Ishihara, M., Kitagawa, M., Harada, H., Kimura, T., Matsuyama, T., Lamphier, M.S., Aizawa, S., Mak, T.W., Taniguchi, T. (1994b) Cellular commitment to oncogene-induced transformation or apoptosis is dependent n the transcription factor IRF-1. *Cell*, **77**, 829-835.

Tanaka, N., Ishihara, M., Lamphier, M.S., Nozawa, H., Matsuyama, T., Mak, T.W., Aizawa, S., Tokino, T., Oren, M., Taniguchi, T. (1996) Cooperationof the tumour suppressors IRF-1 and p53 in response to DNA damage. *Nature*, **382**, 816-818.

Tang, J.L., Yeh, S.H., Chen, P.J., Lin, M.T., Tien, H.F., Chen, Y.C. (1992) Inactivation of the retinoblastoma gene in acute myelogenous leukaemia. *British Journal of Haematology*, **82**, 502-507.

Tao, M., Li, B., Nayini, J., Andrews, C.B., Huang, R-W., Yang, J., Devemy, E., Song, S., Venugopal, P., Preisler, H.D. (2000) SCF, IL1β, IL1ra and GMCSF in the bone marrow and serum of normal individuals and of AML and CML patients. *Cytokine*, **12**, 699-707.

Tennant, G.D., Truran, L.N., Kell, W.J., Burnett, A.K. (1997) Myelodysplastic bone marrow stroma is defective in its ability to sustain normal stem cell growth. *Blood*, **90**, 582a, Abstract #2588.

Testa, J.R., Mitz, U., Rowley, J.D., Vardiman, J.W., Golomb, H.M. (1979) Evolution of karyotypes in acute nonlymphocytic leukemia. *Cancer Research*, **39**, 3619-3627.

Toksoz, D., Farr, C.J., Marshall, C.J. (1987) ras gene activation in a minor proportion of the blast population in acute myeloid leukemia. *Oncogene*, **1**, 409-413.

Tonon, L., Bergamaschi, G., Dellavecchia, C., Rosti, V., Lucotti, C., Malabarba, L., Novella, A., Vercesi, E., Frassoni, F., Cazzola, M. (1998) Unbalanced x-chromosome inactivation in haemopoietic cells from normal women. *British Journal of Haematology*, **102**, 996-1003.

Traweek, T.S., Slovak, L., Nademanee, A.P., Bynes, R.K., Niland, J.C., Forman, S.J. (1994) Clonal karyotypic hematopoietic cell abnormalities occurring after autologous bone marrow transplantation for Hodgkin's Disease and Non-Hodgkin's Lymphoma. *Blood*, **84**, 957-963.

Vaugh, P.S., Aziz, F., van Wijnen, A.J., Wu, S., Harada, H., Taniguchi, T., Soprano, K.J., Stein, J.L., Stein, G.S. (1995) Activation of a cell-cycle-regulated histone gene by the oncogenic transcription factor IRF-2. *Nature*, **377**, 362-364.

Vaziri, H., Benchimo, S. (1998) Reconstitution of telomerase activity in normal human cells leads to elongation of telomeraes and extended replicative life span. *Current Biology*, **8**,279-282.

Venugopal, P., Kadam, P., Preisler, H.D., Hulette, B., Li, Y.Q., Steele, P., Freeman, J., Banavali, S. (1992a) Abnormal regulation of the MYC gene in myeloid leukemia. *Medical Oncology and Tumor Pharmacotherapy*, **9**, 139-147.

Venugopal, P., Hulette, B., Li, Y.Q., Kuvelkar, R., Raza, A., Larson, R., Goldberg, J., Tricot, G., Bennett, J., Preisler, H.D. (1992b) c-MYC and c-MYB expression in acute myelogenous leukemia. *Leukemia Research*, **16**, 1003-1011.

Vogelstein, B., Kinzler, K.W. (1993) The multistep nature of cancer. *TIG*, **9**, 138-141.

Weinberg, R.A. (1995) The retinoblastoma protein and cell cycle control. *Cell*, **81**, 323-330.

White, A.D., Culligan, D.J., Hoy, T.G., Jacobs, A. (1992). Extended cytogenetic follow-up of patietns with myelodysplastic syndrome (MDS). *British Journal of Haematology*, **81**,499-502.

Williams, B.O., Remington, L., Albert, D.M., Mukai, S., Bronson, R.T., Jacks, T. (1994) Cooperative tumorigenic effects of germline mutations in Rb and p53. *Nature Genetics*, **7**, 480-484.

Williamson, M.P., Elder, P.A., Shaw, M.E., Devlin, J., Knowles, M.A. (1995) p16 (CDKN2) is a major deletion target at 9p21 in bladder cancer. *Human Molecular Genetics*, **4**, 1569-1577.

Willman, C.L., Sever, C.E., Pallavicini, M.G., Harada, H., Tanaka, N., Slovak, M.L., Yamamto, H., Harada, K., Meeker, T.C., List, A.F. (1993) Deletion of IRF-1, mapping to chromosome 5q31.1, in human leukemia and preleukemic myelodysplasia. *Science*, **259**, 968-971.

Xie, Y., DeWinter, J.P., Waisfisz, Q., Nieuwint, A.W., Scheper, R.J., Arwert, F., Hoatling, M.E., Ossenkoppele, G.J., Schuurhuis, G., Joenje, H. (2000) Aberrant fanconi anaemia protein profiles in acute myeloid leukaemia cells. *British Journal of Haematology*, **111**, 1057-1064.

Yunis, J.J., Boot, A.J.M., Mayer, M.G., Bos, J.L. (1989) Mechanisms of ras mutation in myelodysplastic syndrome. *Oncogene*, **4**, 609-614.

Zhao, L., van Oort, J., Cork, A., Liang, J.C. (1993) Comparison between interphse and metaphase cytogenetics in detecting chromosome 7 defects in hematological neoplasias. *American Journal of Hematology*, **43,** 205-211.

Zhu, Y.M., Bradbury, D., Russell, N. (1994) Decreased retinoblastoma protein expression in acute myeloblastic leukaemia is associated with the autonomous proliferation of clonogenic blasts. *British Journal of Haemtology*, **86**, 533-539.

12

THE IMPACT OF BIOLOGY ON THE TREATMENT OF SECONDARY AML

Ivana Gojo and Judith E. Karp
University of Maryland School of Medicine, and
Marlene and Stewart Greenebaum Cancer Center, Baltimore, MD

INTRODUCTION

Secondary, or therapy-related, acute myeloid leukemia (AML) developing after exposure to genotoxic agents accounts for approximately 10-20% of all AML cases. The prototype "induced AML" was described almost half a century ago in the setting of environmental exposures to DNA-damaging toxins including benzene, organic solvents, arsenicals and ionizing radiation (Golomb et al., 1982; Mitelman et al., 1978). The emergence of AML after cytotoxic therapy was initially recognized in patients with Hodgkin's disease, one of the first malignancies cured with cytotoxic therapy. In the case of Hodgkin's disease, the leukemia arises from the background of multi-agent cytotoxic therapy that includes alkylating agents, often in combination with radiation (Levine & Bloomfield, 1992; Pedersen-Bjergaard & Larsen, 1982). Recent reports of therapy-related myelodysplastic syndromes (MDS) and AML encountered in patients with Hodgkin's and non-Hodgkin's lymphoma following high-dose chemotherapy and autologous bone marrow transplantation (ASCT) have confirmed a positive relationship between the cumulative dose of alkylating agents and the risk of developing secondary AML (Andre et al., 1998; Darrington et al., 1994; Harrison et al., 1999; Milligan et al., 1999; Pedersen-Bjergaard et al., 2000; Traweek et al., 1994). In several studies, the cumulative risk of secondary MDS/AML has varied widely from 1.1% at 20 months to 24.3% 43 months after ASCT

(Pedersen-Bjergaard et al., 1997; Taylor et al., 1997). Although the alkylating agents are incorporated in the most of myeloablative regimens, it is likely that hematopoietic stem cell damage may occur earlier, during prolonged pre-transplant cytotoxic chemotherapy. The AMLs arising after exposure to diverse environmental toxins and the AMLs caused by DNA-damaging chemotherapeutic agents are similar on both the genetic and biologic levels, and are characterized by deletions of all or part of chromosomes 5 and/or 7, evolution through a myelodysplastic prodrome, and poor response to antileukemic chemotherapy (Golomb et al., 1982; Mitelman et al., 1978; Pedersen-Bjergaard & Rowley, 1994).

A distinct form of secondary AML related to prior treatment with epipodophyllotoxins and other topoisomerase II (topo-II) inhibitors has been recognized in the mid-80's in children who developed secondary AML following treatment with etoposide for acute lymphoblastic leukemia, and in men treated for testicular cancer with etoposide (Bokemeyer & Schmoll, 1995; Kollmannsberger et al., 1998; Pui et al., 1991). This form of secondary AML is characterized by translocations, in particular those involving chromosome band 11q23 and disrupting the MLL gene (mixed lineage or myeloid-lymphoid leukemia; also known as ALL1 and HRX), with resultant formation of different leukemogenic fusion proteins (Hunger et al., 1993; Pedersen-Bjergaard & Rowley, 1994; Super et al., 1993). As with alkylating agents, the highest rates of secondary AML after treatment with epipodophyllotoxins are reported in patients who receive high cumulative doses of these agents (Pui et al., 1991; Sugita et al., 1993). However, it appears that a weekly or twice-weekly schedule of administration carries a higher-risk for development of secondary AML than daily administration of these drugs. Secondary AML arising after exposure to alkylating agents and the topoisomerase-associated secondary AML are two very distinct genotypic and clinical entities, as summarized in "Table 1" (Karp & Sarkodee-Adoo, 2000; Karp & Smith, 1997; Pedersen-Bjergaard & Rowley, 1994). Understanding the molecular pathogenesis of each is of extreme importance in order to develop new therapeutic strategies for the prevention and treatment of these disorders.

Secondary AML is of increasing concern, because of the increasing armentarium of genotoxic drugs that, used alone or in combination or at higher dose intensities, may lead to substantial DNA damage in a variety of ways. Improved survival of patients treated for a variety of malignancies will increase the numbers of those who, following curative therapy for this primary malignancy, will go on to develop secondary leukemias. Our deeper understanding of molecular events that precipitate the development of these highly incurable diseases will hopefully lead to the design of effective therapeutic options in the New Millenium. Below we discuss possible mechanisms that underlie the etiology and pathogenesis of these devastating diseases and that, in turn, can be exploited for the purpose of devising new treatment approaches, some of which have already entered clinical arena.

Table 1. *Secondary AML.*

Alkylating Agents	***Topoisomerase II Directed Agents***
Clinical Presentation	
4-8 years latency (range 1-20)	1-3 years latency (range 0.5-4.5)
Gradual onset; antecedent MDS	Abrupt onset; high blast count
M6, M7 with myelofibrosis common	M4, M5 (monocytic) common
Genetic Abnormalities	
Segmental losses, deletions: (-5, -7)	Translocations: 11q23-based, t(8;21), t(15;17)

MOLECULAR EPIDEMIOLOGY: THE FOUNDATION FOR PATHOGENESIS-BASED TREATMENT

Stem Cells As Target For Toxins

Over the last decade, extensive efforts have been made in order to characterize the leukemic stem cell (LSC) and to differentiate it from its normal counterpart. Recognition of various chromosomal abnormalities and translocations associated with different types of AML has resulted in identification of multiple oncogenes and tumor suppressors that may play an important role in the clonal evolution of this disease. However, the existence of extensive clinical, phenotypic and genotypic diversity in AML has made it difficult to define the target cell at which process of leukemogenesis begins. The main issue for years was whether the degree of commitment of the target cell determines the subsequent characteristics of the leukemic blasts, or the process of leukemogenesis starts at the level of the primitive pluripotent stem cell.

The most important set of data on LSCs came from the studies on irradiated non-obese diabetic mice with severe combined immunodeficiency syndrome (NOD/SCID mice) which led to identification of SCID-leukemia initiating cell (SL-IC), a $CD34^+CD38^-$ cell with extensive self-renewal capabilities and the ability to give a rise to a large number of $CD34^+CD38^+$ cells, AML-colony forming units (CFUs) and well-defined leukemic blasts when transplanted in the NOD/SCID recipients (Bonnet & Dick, 1997; Lapidot et al., 1994). Subsequent studies in the same model system and in vitro assay systems resulted in further delineation of the LSC phenotype as being $CD34^+CD71^-HLADR^-CD38^-$, which is shared with normal stem cells (Blair et al., 1998). Furthermore, recognition that the chromosomal aberrations in LSCs are also present in the leukemic blasts and in differentiated cells in multiple lineages in patients with AML further supports idea that initial leukemogenic insult occurs at the level of primitive stem cell (Haase et al., 1995; Mehrotra et al., 1995; Nilsson et al., 2000). The unique susceptibility of the primitive stem cell to the genotoxic insult was recently examined by direct exposure of the $CD34^+CD19^-$ cells to the benzene metabolite, hydroquinone (HQ) in vitro (Stillman et al., 2000). HQ was not only able to induce AML-specific cytogenetic damage such as –7 and selective deletion of 5q31 in these cells, but did so at the significantly lower concentrations than previously reported for other cell types. Thus, the primitive stem cell represents a unique target for genotoxic insult conferred by DNA-damaging environmental toxins and cytotoxic agents that induce secondary AML. It is likely that the nature of the initial insult and the stem cell's inherent ability to counteract it through a panoply of protective mechanisms (e.g., DNA-repair mechanisms, cell cycle arrest, induction of apoptosis) will determine if the process of leukemogenesis will start immediately or if the multiple subsequent insults will be required for the full expression of leukemic phenotype (multi-step carcinogenesis).

Persistence of clonal chromosomal abnormalities in the stem cell compartment of patients with AML in morphological complete remission (minimal residual disease, MRD) suggests that these primordial leukemic stem cells can survive intensive chemotherapy and, therefore, may be responsible for subsequent relapse (Feuring-Buske et al., 1999). Thus, the development of strategies which specifically target LSCs may provide a more effective treatment for AML patients. Recent discovery of selective interleukin-3 receptor alpha chain (CD123) expression on $CD34^+CD38^-$ cells from AML patients brings more excitement to this area (Jordan et al., 2000). The identification of unique phenotypic markers for the LSCs may have an important implication for the development of new therapeutic approaches for this disease such as a targeted monoclonal antibody therapy, effective purging of stem cells for ASCT, and monitoring of MRD.

Chromosome 7: Home of Many Tumor Suppressors

The abnormalities of chromosome 7, either the loss of a whole chromosome 7 (-7) or a deletion of its long arm del(7q-), are frequently encountered in patients with myeloid malignancies suggesting that these regions contain novel tumor suppressor gene(s) whose loss of function may play a role in leukemia initiation, progression, and full leukemic transformation. More than 50% of patients with secondary AML/MDS and approximately 10% of patients with AML/MDS arising de novo carry one or more of these abnormalities (1984; Le Beau et al., 1986; Mitelman et al., 1978). In addition, leukemias arising in patients with constitutional disorders such as neurofibromatosis 1 (NF1), Fanconi anemia or congenital neutropenia frequently carry –7/del(7q) cytogenetic abnormalities (Luna-Fineman et al., 1995). Extensive efforts have been made to delineate the most commonly involved regions, but, so far, no single tumor suppressor gene has been identified as a potential candidate. Initial chromosomal banding analysis suggested the presence of two critical regions, one in band q22 and another in bands q32-q35 (Johansson et al., 1993; Le Beau et al., 1996; Neuman et al., 1992; Velloso et al., 1996). Subsequent fluorescence in situ hybridization (FISH) analysis of both regions on blood or bone marrow (BM) samples of patients with AML/MDS/chronic myeloid leukemia (CML) reveals the existence of extensive heterogeneity in the translocation and deletion breakpoints. In some cases of chronic phase CML, a narrow segment in band 7q22 has been found to be deleted in the region containing the genes encoding plasminogen activator inhibitor (PLANH1) and the human homologue of the Drosophila homeobox gene cut-like 1 (CUTL1, CCAAT displacement protein) (Fischer et al., 1997). For AML and MDS, two regions appear to be important, one encompassing the terminal part of band 7q22 and entire band 7q31, and another commonly deleted region of 4-5 megabasepairs in bands7q35-q36 (Dohner et al., 1998; Fischer et al., 1997). The proximal region is characterized by scattering of deletion breakpoints along the large region extending from band 7q11 to 7q22, suggesting the existence of multiple genes that may be important in pathogenesis of myeloid leukemias (Fischer et al., 1997). Specific genes localized to that area are the erythropoeitin (EPO) gene, PLANH1, genes for elastin (ELN) and collagen 1 α 2 (COL1A2), the cell cycle control enzyme asparagine synthetase gene (ASNS) and others. Furthermore, the proto-oncogene MET at band 7q31 was found to be deleted in some patients, as well as T-cell receptor β (TCRB) gene at band 7q35 (Kere et al., 1989; Lewis et al., 1996). The gene encoding *ras* homologue enriched in brain 2 (RHEB) has been mapped to the 7q35-q36 region (Mizuki et al., 1996). To date, it is still not clear which gene or genes are going to be critical to the leukemogenic process associated with chromosome 7 abnormalities, and it is important to note that no consistent mutations have been detected in any of the previously mentioned genes. Also, there is no direct evidence suggesting that functional inactivation of both alleles of a putative tumor suppressor gene is necessary in leukemogenesis in monosomy 7 and it remains to be determined if the loss of function of only one allele (haploinsufficiency) is sufficient to cause disease. The entire 7q gene segment may be intrinsically unstable and the deletion of one or more of these genes may be in itself sufficient to disrupt the balance between the growth and differentiation leading to dysmyelopoiesis and differentiation arrest. Furthermore, the presence of *ras* mutations in the leukemic blasts from some children with monosomy 7 and constitutional predisposition to leukemia suggests that aberrant *ras*-mediated signaling and chromosome 7 deletions may cooperate in leukemogenesis by disrupting different pathways important in myelopoiesis (Bollag et al., 1996; Luna-Fineman et al., 1995; Shannon et al., 1994). An interesting observation is the high frequency of an inactivating polymorphism of NAD(P)H:quinone oxidoreductase (NQO1), an enzyme important in conversion of benzene-derived quinines to less toxic HQS, in patients with therapy-related AML with chromosome 5 or 7 abnormality (Larson et al., 1999). This finding represents an important step in identifying patients who may have an increased susceptibility to the genotoxic and leukemogenic effect of cytotoxic agents.

11q23 Fusion Proteins: Loss of Regulation of Gene Expression and Chromatin Remodeling

Chromosomal translocations involving the MLL gene on chromosome 11q23 are among the most common in humane acute leukemias, and some of them, such as t(11;16) and t(9;11), are frequently encountered in secondary AML (Karp & Sarkodee-Adoo, 2000; Thirman et al., 1993). The predilection of topoisomerase II-directed agent-induced DNA cleavage for 11q23 has been demonstrated in vitro and topoisomerase II consensus binding segments have been found to be clustered in exon 9 of chromosome 11q23 (Aplan et al., 1996; Broeker et al., 1996). Epipodophyllotoxins exert their cytotoxic effects by stabilizing the DNA/topo-II covalent linkage, and their ability to increase the frequency of illegitimate chromosomal breaks may be related to their cytotoxic and leukemogenic effects (Chen et al., 1996; Karp & Smith, 1997).

MLL is the human homologue of the Drosophila tritorax gene which has an important role in regulation of embryonic differentiation in Drosophila and appears to have a role in controlling differentiation in primitive hematopoietic stem cells (Djabali et al., 1992; Hunger et al., 1993). Recent studies in mice revealed that MLL-deficiency in mice results in embryonic lethality while MLL+/- heterozygotes have numerous developmental skeletal abnormalities and abnormal hematopoiesis, suggesting that MLL is an important mammalian developmental regulator (Yu et al., 1995). This is consistent with MLL's role in the positive regulation of the highly conserved homeobox (HOX) genes, which serve critical roles as transcriptional activators of genes important in both axial organization and hematopoietic differentiation (Lawrence & Largman, 1992). Therefore, it seems likely that disruption of MLL and the creation of fusion genes as a result of translocations could lead to chimeric proteins that result in inappropriate transcription.

While the MLL gene is a more than 100 kb long and contains 23 exons, nearly all of the rearrangements occur in a 8.5-kB region of genomic DNA that span exons 5 to 11 (Thirman et al., 1993). More than 30 different translocation partner genes for MLL have been identified so far and, for some of them, transforming potential has been demonstrated in retroviral transduction systems and in knock-in mice (Corral et al., 1996; Dobson et al., 1999; Slany et al., 1998). The amino terminus of MLL contains an AT–hook important for binding to the minor grove DNA, and a region that shares homology with the regulatory domain of DNA methyltransferase which, in turn, may be important in chromatin structure recognition (Ma et al., 1993; Reeves & Nissen, 1990). In addition, it appears that the carboxyterminal protein interaction domain of MLL known as a SET domain may play an important role in chromatin remodeling. It is known that the SET domain interacts with 2 proteins, INI1 and SNR1, which are homologous to members of the SWI/SNF complex that participates in ATP-dependent chromatin remodeling (Rozenblatt-Rosen et al., 1998). Thus, through its SET domain, MLL may engage the SWI/SNF complex with resultant changes in nucleosomal structure leading to an open chromatin conformation. Interestingly, in all MLL chromosomal translocations, the SET domain is lost, likely resulting in disruption of MLL regulatory function on gene expression. In this regard, it is provocative that two of MLL-fusion partners, AF9 in t(9;11) and ENL in t(11;19), share homology with the SWI/SNF complex, suggesting that loss of MLL regulatory function may be replaced by fusion proteins that constitutively activate the SWI/SNF complex and therefore result in aberrant expression of MLL target genes, for example, HOX genes (Cairns et al., 1996). Furthermore, recent laboratory studies suggest that MLL proteins interact with the GADD34 protein which leads to apoptosis following irradiation-induced DNA damage. Three different MLL-fusion proteins (MLL-AF9, MLL-AF4, MLL-ENL) inhibited GADD34-mediated apoptosis, therefore implicating that at least part of their leukemogenic effect may occur through inhibition of post-DNA damage induced apoptosis (Adler et al., 1999). Observation that GADD34 associates with SNF5/INI1, a member of the SWI/SNF complex, further underscores the importance of altered chromatin remodeling mechanisms in leukemogenesis.

Another pathway that fusion proteins may use to affect chromatin remodeling is through constitutive activation of histone acetyltransferase (HAT) or through the engagement of other components of HAT containing coactivator complex. Two known MLL-fusion partners that could preferentially use this pathway to affect chromatin remodeling and therefore gene transcription are the CREB binding protein (CBP) in t(11;16) and p300 in t(11;22). Both CBP and p300 retain their HAT-catalytic sites and binding sites for coactivator complex upon fusion with MLL (Ida et al., 1997; Redner et al., 1999; Sobulo et al., 1997). It is clear that further studies are needed in order to clarify the avenues that diverse MLL-fusion proteins may use to affect gene expression. However, the realization that abnormalities in chromatin remodeling mechanisms may be responsible for leukemogenic effect of such fusion proteins opens the gate for development and exploration of new therapeutic agents, such as inhibitors of SWI/SNF complexes or specific modulators of HAT.

Stromal Damage: Activation of Angiogenesis

Orderly proliferation and differentiation of hematopoietic stem cells in the BM is tightly regulated by the BM microenvironment, in which reciprocal interaction between the BM stromal cells and hematopoietic progenitors is achieved through direct cellular contact via adhesion molecules as well as by paracrine secretion of cytokines. It is reasonable to speculate that clonal hematopoiesis in secondary AML/MDS does not occur solely as a result of the genotoxic insult to hematopoietic progenitor cells. Instead, an altered BM microenvironment arising in the setting of cytotoxic damage is likely to play a significant role in the initiation and propagation of malignant hematopoiesis.

In this light, angiogenesis, a multi-step process of new blood vessel formation from an existing vasculature and diverse angiogenic factors, may play pivotal roles in the pathogenesis and survival of diverse hematologic malignancies, including the acute leukemias. Recent studies further support this notion. For instance, vascular endothelial growth factor (VEGF) is a heparin-binding cytokine that promotes the proliferation and survival of endothelial cells and multipotential hematopoietic stem cells (Bautz et al., 2000; Bertolini et al., 2000; Kennedy et al., 1997). Indeed, the compartment of truly pluripotent hematopoietic stem cells that gives rise to lineage-restricted precursors expresses both CD34 and VEGF receptor-2 (known as KDR), with KDR expression being lost in the process of lineage commitment (Ziegler et al., 1999). A significant proportion of both de novo and secondary AML blast cell populations express VEGF mRNA and produce and secrete VEGF protein, with the amount of VEGF secreted by cultured leukemic blasts exceeding that secreted by cultured normal BM counterparts (Fiedler et al., 1997). In addition to promoting angiogenesis in the marrow (Hussong et al., 2000; Padro et al., 2000), the secreted VEGF may provoke marrow stromal production and release of cytokines such as basic fibroblast growth factor (bFGF) and granulocyte-macrophage colony stimulating factor (GM-CSF), both of which may drive leukemic cell (Fiedler et al., 1997; Gabrilove et al., 1994) and endothelial cell proliferation (Bikfalvi & Han, 1994; Bussolino et al., 1993) in paracrine fashion. Studies comparing BM microvasculature in AML and normal marrows demonstrate increased amounts of angiogenesis in leukemia, with a striking reduction in microvessel density (MVD) observed at the time of chemotherapy-induced marrow aplasia in patients who ultimately achieve complete remission (CR) but not in those who fail to respond to therapy (Hussong et al., 2000; Padro et al., 2000). Along this line, other investigators have demonstrated that, at least in patients who present with high blast counts, the amount of VEGF produced by AML cells is inversely related to the duration of CR and survival (Aguayo et al., 1999). Taking all of these findings together, it is reasonable to postulate that VEGF may act as a pivotal growth and survival factor in AML and may contribute to net drug resistance, as manifested by the link between VEGF expression and adverse clinical outcome. A logical outgrowth of this hypothesis is the clinical testing of agents that could interfere with the process of angiogenesis in the setting of de novo and secondary AML. A variety of agents targeting this process are entering the clinical arena, and selected novel compounds and their mechanisms of action will be discussed further below.

Epigenetic Control of Gene Transcription: p15 Methylation

A number of molecular mechanisms responsible for altered gene expression may play pivotal roles in the process of leukemogenesis. Some of these mechanisms affect the primary structure of the gene, such as chromosomal deletions or translocations, while others lead to aberrant gene expression without affecting gene structure per se. In this regard, hypermethylation of the regulatory sequences of various genes will lead to their transcriptional silencing through altered nucleosomal configuration that renders them inaccessible to transcription factors (Davey et al., 1997; Razin & Cedar, 1991). The MeCP2 (methyl-CpG-binding protein), a chromatin-associated protein which binds to methylated regions of DNA, directly associates with Sin3/histone deacetylase 1 (HDAC1) complex. In turn, this MeCP2-binding results in a transcriptionally-repressed chromatin structure of the methylated DNA (Jones et al., 1998; Nan et al., 1997; Nan et al., 1998). Thus, MeCP2 may prove to be a key contributor to the transcriptional silencing effect of DNA methylation.

In this context, hypermethylation of CpG (cytosine-phospho-guanine) dinucleotides in the promoter region of p15INK4B gene, frequently encountered in patients with AML/MDS, suggests that the resultant loss of p15 function may be an important step in the leukemogenic process (Aoki et al., 2000; Quesnel et al., 1998; Uchida et al., 1997; Wong et al., 2000). p15INK4B is a cyclin-dependent kinase (CDK) inhibitor that associates with and blocks the activation of CDK4, CDK6, and cyclinD-CDK4/6 complexes. Such inhibition, in turn, leads to cell cycle arrest at the G1/S boundary (Hannon & Beach, 1994). In orderly hematopoiesis, as the process of differentiation progresses, the proliferative capability of the cells decreases. Thus, it is not surprising that p15INK4B, a potent cell cycle inhibitor, is upregulated during the normal granulo-monocytic and megakaryocytic differentiation (Teofili et al., 2000). Loss of p15 function may allow genetically damaged cells to escape DNA repair or recognition and destruction through pathways that would otherwise occur at an intact G1 checkpoint. Such escape, would allow the damaged cell to enter S phase, replicate, and accumulate. The resultant survival of the abnormal cell could be an important step in the initiation and propagation of a leukemic clone in secondary AML.

It appears that hypermethylation of the p15INK4B gene is associated with increasing numbers of blasts in MDS, occuring as a late event at the time of progression to full-blown AML (Quesnel et al., 1998; Uchida et al., 1997). However, recent identification of this epigenetic abnormality in cells more differentiated than blasts in patients with MDS raises the question as to whether or not p15 hypermethylation is really a late event (Aoki et al., 2000). More than 50% of patients with AML harbor hypermethylated p15INK4B gene in their bone marrow and peripheral blood cells, and loss of p15 function appears to be associated with shortened overall survival for these patients (Wong et al., 2000). Furthermore, many other genes including calcitonin, estrogen receptor, E-cadherin, p16 and retinoblastoma have been found to be hypermethylated in AML. The full significance of the silencing of one or more of these genes is not yet clear.

Novel agents that interfere with the activity of DNA methyltransferase appear capable of reversing the process of hypermethylation and, as such, may prove to be useful therapeutic agents in AML. One such agent, 5-aza-2'deoxycytidine, a cytidine methyltansferase inhibitor, is currently undergoing clinical testing in patients with AML in combination with other modulators of gene expression, such as phenylbutyrate (discussed below in the context of histone deacetylase inhibition). When tested as a single agent in elderly patients with MDS, the response rate of approximately 50% was achieved. However, it is unclear whether its cytotoxic or differentiation effect or both were responsible for observed responses (Wijermans et al., 2000).

TARGETING MOLECULAR LESIONS

Signaling Pathways As Therapeutic Targets: Farnesyltransferase Inhibitors

The process of signal transduction from cell membrane to nucleus provides a panoply of molecular targets that can be exploited for therapeutic purposes (Ito & May, 1996; Rebollo & Martinez, 1999; Reuter et al., 2000). At least two pivotal cell surface and intracellular components are activated during the early steps of cellular response to environmental signals: 1) protein tyrosine kinases (PTKs), some forming the internal domains of many membrane-spanning growth factor receptors and others acting within the cytoplasm; and 2) membrane-associated G proteins encoded by the *ras* family of oncogenes. Ras proteins, which participate in a crucial early step in transmitting biochemical signals from the cell membrane through the cytoplasm and into the nucleus, play a key role in proliferation and malignant transformation of hematopoietic cells (Rebollo & Martinez, 1999; Sasaoka et al., 1994). Upon ligand binding to extracellular domains of receptor tyrosine kinases or cytokine receptors, receptor dimerization and phosphorylation of its tyrosine residues occurs. These phosphotyrosine residues represent docking sites for various signaling molecules, including adapter protein Grb2 (growth factor receptor bound protein 2) which, in turn, activates Ras by binding to guanine nucleotide exchange factor known as SOS (son of sevenless) (Egan et al., 1993; Li et al., 1993; Sasaoka et al., 1994). Therefore, Ras appears to be a convergence point for several types of biochemical signals, which underscores its important role in oncogenesis.

The constitutive activation of Ras protein is an important event in the clonal evolution of MDS/AML. Mutations and abnormal expression of *ras*, especially N-*ras*, are detected in roughly 10-15% of MDS (mainly in transformation to full-blown leukemia) and AMLs (especially those associated with exposures to occupational mutagens) (Bartram, 1996; Paquette et al., 1993; Taylor et al., 1992). *ras* mutations, either in the gene or in the promoter region, have been detected in 15-25% of AML studied to date (Bos et al., 1987; Neubauer et al., 1994; Thorn et al., 1995). The potential linkage between *ras* mutations (or at least net Ras activation) and the presence of chromosome 7 abnormalities, makes Ras an ideal target for therapeutic manipulations, not only in de novo but also in secondary AMLs (Bollag et al., 1996; Luna-Fineman et al., 1995; Neubauer et al., 1994; Shannon et al., 1994). In addition, the coupling of Ras proteins and receptor PTKs through Grb2 raises the possibility that PTK-driven malignancies may be susceptible to Ras inhibition even if *ras* is not mutated, e.g. CML or AML with activating mutations in receptor TK genes.

In this regard, extensive efforts have been made to develop selective inhibitors of Ras-signaling pathway. Recognition that full biologic function of Ras depends upon its binding to the cell membrane, which is accomplished through the post-translational modification of Ras known as isoprenylation, led to the development of a novel class of agents known as farnesyl transferase inhibitors (FTIs) (Gelb, 1997; Khosravi-Far et al., 1992; Reuter et al., 2000). The enzyme farnesyltransferase (FT) catalyzes the critical post-translational modification of Ras. FTIs were developed on the premise that FT inhibition would prevent the post-translational modification of Ras and, therefore, transduction of proliferative signals (Beaupre & Kurzrock, 1999; End, 1999). However, cell biology studies suggest that the cytotoxic actions of these agents are much more complex and may involve non-Ras prenylated polypeptides as well, including RhoB and the phosphoinositide 3-OH kinase (PI3K)/AKT pathway (Du et al., 1999; Jiang et al., 2000; Lebowitz & Prendergast, 1998).

R115777, a selective competitive inhibitor of the CAAX peptide-binding site of FT, has been already tested in phase I clinical study in patients with recurrent or refractory leukemias. Preliminary data are encouraging, since 30% of these heavily pretreated patients achieved either partial remission (PR) or CR. R115777 effects were noted mainly in AML variants and CML in myeloid blast crisis, and it appeared that responsive patients had lower percentage of marrow blasts than non-responders. Interestingly, in this small group of patients clinical responses to R115777 were achieved in the absence of detectable *ras* mutations. The finding that 3 of the 5 AMLs associated with abnormalities of chromosome 7 were responsive to R115777 and the known (but poorly understood) link between abnormalities of chromosome 7 and aberrant Ras expression also suggests that R115777 exerts its antileukemic effects, at least in part, by interrupting Ras function. Further testing of R115777 in newly diagnosed patients with poor-risk AML and MDS (including age > 60 and secondary AML or MDS), as a chronic suppressive or maintenance therapy following remission induction, or in combination with already known antileukemic agents such as ara-C, anthracyclines or etoposide is warranted. At least for now, it appears that FTIs may become a part of therapeutic armentarium employed in treatment of AML patients.

Histone Deacetylase Inhibitors

Development of histone deacetylase inhibitors (HDIs) as a potential modulators of chromatin remodeling came from recognition that local remodeling of chromatin plays an important role in transcriptional activation of genes and that the proteins involved in this process are frequently disrupted in various chromosomal translocations associated with acute leukemias and other malignancies (Marks et al., 2000; Redner et al., 1999; Zwiebel, 2000). Two pivotal chromatin remodeling mechanisms that are frequently disrupted in leukemias include 1) histone acetylation; and 2) ATPase-mediated DNA-histone dissociation (the SWI/SNF complex) (Bazett-Jones et al., 1999; Redner et al., 1999; Stopka et al., 2000). As discussed previously, the constitutive activation of SWI/SNF complex appears to be a key modulator of altered gene expression encountered in leukemias associated with the chromosomal translocations involving the MLL gene. On the other hand, certain leukemogenic fusion proteins such as PML-RARα in t(15;17), PZLF-RARα in t(11;17), AML1-ETO in t(8;21), and diverse MLL translocations may exert their leukemogenic potential by altering the state of chromatin acetylation to a non-transcriptional state (Gelmetti et al., 1998; Grignani et al., 1998; Guidez et al., 1998; Lin et al., 1998; Lutterbach et al., 1998; Redner et al., 1999). Such alterations relate to the recruitment of a nuclear receptor corepressor (N-CoR)/Sin3/HDAC1 complex which, by virtue of inhibiting histone acetylation and increasing the affinity between histones and DNA, modifies chromatin to a non-transcriptional conformation. The resultant transcriptional repression may lead to abrogation of orderly differentiation. The net effects of this histone deacetylation are similar to the transcriptional silencing caused by hypermethylation of key genes encountered in various MDS/AMLs (Jones et al., 1998; Lorincz et al., 2000; Tycko, 2000).

Agents that inhibit or reverse HDA activity may reconstitute normal differentiation programs and, as such, could have important roles in the therapy of diverse leukemias, including secondary AMLs and MDS (DiGiuseppe et al., 1999; Kosugi et al., 1999; Redner et al., 1999; Warrell et al., 1998). In support of this notion are findings obtained in AML cell lines with (myeloid HL-60, retinoid-resistant progranulocytic NB4) or without (monocytic U937, megakaryocytic MEG-01) leukemia-related fusion proteins, where exposure to the HDIs trichostatin A or trapoxin A resulted in upregulation of expression of the CDK inhibitors p21 and p16, with resultant evidence for myeloid differentiation (Kosugi et al., 1999). Similarly, HDIs induced maturation, as measured by morphology and immunophenotype, in roughly 1/3 of fresh AML marrow populations (M0-M7) (Kosugi et al., 1999). This concept has been tested recently in the clinic by adding sodium phenylbutyrate to all-trans retinoic acid (ATRA) to achieve complete clinical, cytogenetic and molecular remission in a patient with retinoid-refractory progranulocytic leukemia (APL) (Warrell et al., 1998). Pertinently, the clinical and genetic response to sodium phenylbutyrate and ATRA was accompanied by induction of histone acetylation. While sodium phenylbutyrate per se has weak HDI activity, its synergism with ATRA suggests that the HDI activity of both drugs together may have an important clinical effect that warrants further studies. Furthermore, laboratory observation of synergism between the DNA demethylation agent decitabine and HDA inhibitor Trichostatin A in re-expression of trancriptionally silenced genes in cancer, has led to the design of a clinical trial that employs both 5-azacytidine and phenylbutyrate (Cameron et al., 1999; Zwiebel, 2000). Recently, several more potent HDIs have been identified and some of them, such as depsipeptide and the new benzamide derivative MS-275 are entering phase I clinical trials in patients with diverse hematologic malignancies including acute leukemias, MDS, and multiple myeloma (Marks et al., 2000; Saito et al., 1999). While results of these trials remain to be seen, currently available pre-clinical and clinical data suggests that HDIs, either alone or in combination with other antileukemic agents, may find an important place in the treatment of leukemias in a near future.

"Anti-Angiogenesis" Agents

A large amount of preclinical and clinical data have accumulated which suggest that the process of angiogenesis plays an important role in development of diverse hematologic malignancies. The detection of increased VEGF production by leukemic blasts, increased bone marrow MVD, and the potential inverse correlation with response to treatment suggest that development of agents that interfere with net angiogenesis could have therapeutic efficacy in these diseases (Aguayo et al., 1999; Fiedler et al., 1997; Hussong et al., 2000; Padro et al., 2000). A large number of drugs interfering with different steps that are critical for process of angiogenesis have been developed, for example, metalloprotease inhibitors (e.g., Marimastat), inhibitors of endothelial cell migration and proliferation (e.g., TNP-740, endostatin), inhibitors of angiogenic growth factors (GF) (monoclonal antibodies) and GF receptors (selected TK inhibitors such as SU5416 and SU6668) and others (Bertolini et al., 2000; Brem, 1999). Some of the currently used drugs that exhibit anti-angiogenic activities include thalidomide and interferon α. While it is still not clear in which way these drugs interfere with the process of angiogenesis, responses observed in patients with multiple myeloma, MDS and myeloproliferative disorders (MPD) treated with thalidomide are encouraging (Raza et al., 1999; Singhal et al., 1999; Thomas et al., 1999). Daily thalidomide treatment in patients with MDS and long-standing refractory anemias resulted in significant hematologic improvement (transfusion independence and improvement in platelet count) in 17 of 25 evaluable patients and was associated with decrease in bone marrow MVD (Raza et al., 1999). Similar results were observed in approximately 2/3 of patients with MPD treated with thalidomide, in whom decreases in VEGF, bFGF and tumor necrosis factor α (TNF-α) levels during treatment were noted (Thomas et al., 1999). The potential role of VEGF as a pivotal growth and survival factor in AML suggests that agents that directly interfere with its function may lead to inhibition of leukemic cell growth by interrupting the existing autocrine and paracrine loops for VEGF activity in the BM. Various VEGF inhibitors have been synthesized such as monoclonal antibodies that block the ability of VEGF to bind to its cognate receptor (e.g., bevacizumab) and anti-KDR molecules that specifically inhibits VEGF signaling through the FLk-1/KDR receptor (e.g., SU5416), and these agents are currently undergoing clinical testing in acute leukemias (Asano et al., 1995; Bertolini et al., 2000; Fong et al., 1999; Zwiebel, 2000). Bevacizumab has been shown to inhibit the growth of diverse epithelial and hematopoietic cell lines, including AML, in vitro and in vivo in nude mouse xenograft models, and to synergize with cytotoxic chemotherapy (Brekken et al., 2000; Dias et al., 2000; Wild et al., 2000). Early data from clinical trials of this agent in various solid tumors suggest that bevacizumab can exert anti-tumor effects, particularly when combined with cytotoxic drugs, with evidence of possible tumor necrosis resulting from blockade of VEGF-based signaling and a consequent disruption of the vascular supply (Bergsland et al., 2000; DeVore et al., 2000). The leukemias provide a fertile testing ground for this monoclonal antibody, and clinical trials with laboratory correlates to examine the effects of bevacizumab on AML and stromal cell VEGF production and activity are imminent.

FUTURE DIRECTIONS

Secondary AMLs remain a therapeutic challenge and provide a fertile testing ground for the development of novel agents and the concomitant molecular dissection of the mechanisms by which these agents induce growth inhibition, differentiation and eventual cell death. There are many more novel molecular targeted agents that remain to be tested in this disease, such as protein kinase inhibitors (e.g., bryostatin, UCN-01), cell cycle inhibitors (e.g., flavopiridol) and others. For many of these agents, the optimal effective dose that has desired pharmacologic and biologic effects remains to be established. Another strategy under investigation relies upon antisense constructs and ribozymes directed against unique fusion gene products. Newly developed models in the SCID mouse that permit engraftment of human leukemia cells provide preclinical models for testing of novel agents against cells with specific translocations. In the future, it will be important to see how these agents could be effectively combined with already-established antileukemic agents to improve clinical responses and patient survival. After many years of therapeutic frustration and darkness in secondary AML, the ability to target specific molecular lesions brings excitement and encouragement to this therapeutic challenge. "Eppur si muove!" (It is moving!)

REFERENCES

(1984). The Fourth International Workshop on Chromosomes in Leukemia: a prospective study of acute nonlymphocytic leukemia. Chicago, Illinois, U.S.A., September 2-7, 1982. *Cancer Genet Cytogenet*, **11,** 249-360.

Adler, H.T., Chinery, R., Wu, D.Y., Kussick, S.J., Payne, J.M., Fornace, A.J., Jr. & Tkachuk, D.C. (1999). Leukemic HRX fusion proteins inhibit GADD34-induced apoptosis and associate with the GADD34 and hSNF5/INI1 proteins. *Molecular and Cellular Biology*, **19,** 7050-60.

Aguayo, A., Estey, E., Kantarjian, H., Mansouri, T., Gidel, C., Keating, M., Giles, F., Estrov, Z., Barlogie, B. & Albitar, M. (1999). Cellular vascular endothelial growth factor is a predictor of outcome in patients with acute myeloid leukemia. *Blood*, **94,** 3717-21.

Andre, M., Henry-Amar, M., Blaise, D., Colombat, P., Fleury, J., Milpied, N., Cahn, J.Y., Pico, J.L., Bastion, Y., Kuentz, M., Nedellec, G., Attal, M., Ferme, C. & Gisselbrecht, C. (1998). Treatment-related deaths and second cancer risk after autologous stem-cell transplantation for Hodgkin's disease. *Blood*, **92,** 1933-40.

Aoki, E., Uchida, T., Ohashi, H., Nagai, H., Murase, T., Ichikawa, A., Yamao, K., Hotta, T., Kinoshita, T., Saito, H. & Murate, T. (2000). Methylation status of the p15INK4B gene in hematopoietic progenitors and peripheral blood cells in myelodysplastic syndromes. *Leukemia*, **14,** 586-93.

Aplan, P.D., Chervinsky, D.S., Stanulla, M. & Burhans, W.C. (1996). Site-specific DNA cleavage within the MLL breakpoint cluster region induced by topoisomerase II inhibitors [see comments]. *Blood*, **87,** 2649-58.

Asano, M., Yukita, A., Matsumoto, T., Kondo, S. & Suzuki, H. (1995). Inhibition of tumor growth and metastasis by an immunoneutralizing monoclonal antibody to human vascular endothelial growth factor/vascular permeability factor121. *Cancer Research*, **55,** 5296-301.

Bartram, C.R. (1996). Molecular genetic aspects of myelodysplastic syndromes. *Seminars in Hematology*, **33,** 139-49.

Bautz, F., Rafii, S., Kanz, L. & Mohle, R. (2000). Expression and secretion of vascular endothelial growth factor-A by cytokine-stimulated hematopoietic progenitor cells. Possible role in the hematopoietic microenvironment. *Experimental Hematology*, **28,** 700-6.

Bazett-Jones, D.P., Cote, J., Landel, C.C., Peterson, C.L. & Workman, J.L. (1999). The SWI/SNF complex creates loop domains in DNA and polynucleosome arrays and can disrupt DNA-histone contacts within these domains. *Molecular and Cellular Biology*, **19,** 1470-8.

Beaupre, D.M. & Kurzrock, R. (1999). RAS and leukemia: from basic mechanisms to gene-directed therapy. *Journal of Clinical Oncology*, **17,** 1071-9.

Bergsland, E., Hurwitz, H., Fehrenbacher, L., Meropol, N.J., Novotny, W.F., Gaudreault, J., Lieberman, G. & Kabbinavar, F. (2000). A randomized phase II trial comparing rhuMAb VEGF (recombinant humanized monoclonal antibody to vascular endothelial cell growth factor) plus 5-fluorouracil/leucovorin (FU/LV) to FU/LV alone in patients with metastatic colorectal cancer. *Proceedings of ASCO*, **19,** 242a:939 (abstr).

Bertolini, F., Mancuso, P., Gobbi, A. & Pruneri, G. (2000). The thin red line. Angiogenesis In normal and malignant hematopoiesis. *Experimental Hematology*, **28,** 993-1000.

Bikfalvi, A. & Han, Z.C. (1994). Angiogenic factors are hematopoietic growth factors and vice versa. *Leukemia*, **8,** 523-9.

Blair, A., Hogge, D.E. & Sutherland, H.J. (1998). Most acute myeloid leukemia progenitor cells with long-term proliferative ability in vitro and in vivo have the phenotype CD34(+)/CD71(-)/HLA-DR. *Blood*, **92,** 4325-35.

Bokemeyer, C. & Schmoll, H.J. (1995). Treatment of testicular cancer and the development of secondary malignancies. *Journal of Clinical Oncology*, **13,** 283-92.

Bollag, G., Clapp, D.W., Shih, S., Adler, F., Zhang, Y.Y., Thompson, P., Lange, B.J., Freedman, M.H., McCormick, F., Jacks, T. & Shannon, K. (1996). Loss of NF1 results in activation of the Ras signaling pathway and leads to aberrant growth in haematopoietic cells. *Nature Genetics*, **12,** 144-8.

Bonnet, D. & Dick, J.E. (1997). Human acute myeloid leukemia is organized as a hierarchy that originates from a primitive hematopoietic cell. *Nature Medicine*, **3,** 730-7.

Bos, J.L., Verlaan-de Vries, M., van der Eb, A.J., Janssen, J.W., Delwel, R., Lowenberg, B. & Colly, L.P. (1987). Mutations in N-ras predominate in acute myeloid leukemia. *Blood*, **69,** 1237-41.

Brekken, R.A., Overholser, J.P., Stastny, V.A., Waltenberger, J., Minna, J.D. & Thorpe, P.E. (2000). Selective inhibition of vascular endothelial growth factor (VEGF) receptor 2 (KDR/Flk-1) activity by a monoclonal anti-VEGF antibody blocks tumor growth in mice. *Cancer Research*, **60,** 5117-24.

Brem, S. (1999). Angiogenesis and Cancer Control: From Concept to Therapeutic Trial. *Cancer Control*, **6,** 436-458.

Broeker, P.L., Super, H.G., Thirman, M.J., Pomykala, H., Yonebayashi, Y., Tanabe, S., Zeleznik-Le, N. & Rowley, J.D. (1996). Distribution of 11q23 breakpoints within the MLL breakpoint cluster region in de novo acute leukemia and in treatment-related acute myeloid leukemia: correlation with scaffold attachment regions and topoisomerase II consensus binding sites. *Blood*, **87,** 1912-22.

Bussolino, F., Colotta, F., Bocchietto, E., Guglielmetti, A. & Mantovani, A. (1993). Recent developments in the cell biology of granulocyte-macrophage colony-stimulating factor and granulocyte colony-stimulating factor: activities on endothelial cells. *International Journal of Clinical and Laboratory Research*, **23,** 8-12.

Cairns, B.R., Henry, N.L. & Kornberg, R.D. (1996). TFG/TAF30/ANC1, a component of the yeast SWI/SNF complex that is similar to the leukemogenic proteins ENL and AF-9. *Molecular and Cellular Biology*, **16,** 3308-16.

Cameron, E.E., Bachman, K.E., Myohanen, S., Herman, J.G. & Baylin, S.B. (1999). Synergy of demethylation and histone deacetylase inhibition in the re-expression of genes silenced in cancer. *Nature Genetics*, **21,** 103-7.

Chen, C.L., Fuscoe, J.C., Liu, Q., Pui, C.H., Mahmoud, H.H. & Relling, M.V. (1996). Relationship between cytotoxicity and site-specific DNA recombination after in vitro exposure of leukemia cells to etoposide [see comments]. *Journal of the National Cancer Institutes*, **88,** 1840-7.

Corral, J., Lavenir, I., Impey, H., Warren, A.J., Forster, A., Larson, T.A., Bell, S., McKenzie, A.N., King, G. & Rabbitts, T.H. (1996). An Mll-AF9 fusion gene made by homologous recombination causes acute leukemia in chimeric mice: a method to create fusion oncogenes. *Cell*, **85,** 853-61.

Darrington, D.L., Vose, J.M., Anderson, J.R., Bierman, P.J., Bishop, M.R., Chan, W.C., Morris, M.E., Reed, E.C., Sanger, W.G., Tarantolo, S.R. & et al. (1994). Incidence and characterization of secondary myelodysplastic syndrome and acute myelogenous leukemia following high-dose chemoradiotherapy and autologous stem-cell transplantation for lymphoid malignancies. *Journal of Clinical Oncology*, **12,** 2527-34.

Davey, C., Pennings, S. & Allan, J. (1997). CpG methylation remodels chromatin structure in vitro. *Journal of Molecular Biology*, **267,** 276-88.

DeVore, R.F., Fehrenbacher, L., Herbst, R.S., Langer, C.J., Kelly, K., Gaudreault, J., Holmgren, E., Novotny, W.F. & Kabbinavar, F. (2000). A randomized phase II trial comparing Rhumab VEGF (recombinant humanized monoclonal antibody to vascular endothelial growth factor) plus carboplatin/paclitaxel (CP) to CP alone in patients with stage III/IV NSCLC. *Proceedings of ASCO*, **19,** 485a:1896 (abstr).

Dias, S., Zhu, Z., Wu, Y., Witte, L., Hicklin, D.J. & Raffi, S. (2000). Expression of VEGF and its receptor VEGF-2 by human leukemia cells generate an autocrine loop that mediates cell growth and migration. *Proceedings of American Association for Cancer Research*, **41,** 792 (abstr).

DiGiuseppe, J.A., Weng, L.J., Yu, K.H., Fu, S., Kastan, M.B., Samid, D. & Gore, S.D. (1999). Phenylbutyrate-induced G1 arrest and apoptosis in myeloid leukemia cells: structure-function analysis. *Leukemia*, **13,** 1243-53.

Djabali, M., Selleri, L., Parry, P., Bower, M., Young, B.D. & Evans, G.A. (1992). A trithorax-like gene is interrupted by chromosome 11q23 translocations in acute leukaemias [published erratum appears in Nat Genet 1993 Aug;4(4):431]. *Nature Genetics*, **2,** 113-8.

Dobson, C.L., Warren, A.J., Pannell, R., Forster, A., Lavenir, I., Corral, J., Smith, A.J. & Rabbitts, T.H. (1999). The mll-AF9 gene fusion in mice controls myeloproliferation and specifies acute myeloid leukaemogenesis. *Embo Journal*, **18,** 3564-74.

Dohner, K., Brown, J., Hehmann, U., Hetzel, C., Stewart, J., Lowther, G., Scholl, C., Frohling, S., Cuneo, A., Tsui, L.C., Lichter, P., Scherer, S.W. & Dohner, H. (1998). Molecular cytogenetic characterization of a critical region in bands 7q35-q36 commonly deleted in malignant myeloid disorders. *Blood*, **92,** 4031-5.

Du, W., Lebowitz, P.F. & Prendergast, G.C. (1999). Cell growth inhibition by farnesyltransferase inhibitors is mediated by gain of geranylgeranylated RhoB. *Moecular and Cellular Biology*, **19,** 1831-40.

Egan, S.E., Giddings, B.W., Brooks, M.W., Buday, L., Sizeland, A.M. & Weinberg, R.A. (1993). Association of Sos Ras exchange protein with Grb2 is implicated in tyrosine kinase signal transduction and transformation [see comments]. *Nature*, **363,** 45-51.

End, D.W. (1999). Farnesyl protein transferase inhibitors and other therapies targeting the Ras signal transduction pathway. *Investigational New Drugs*, **17,** 241-58.

Feuring-Buske, M., Haase, D., Buske, C., Hiddemann, W. & Wormann, B. (1999). Clonal chromosomal abnormalities in the stem cell compartment of patients with acute myeloid leukemia in morphological complete remission. *Leukemia*, **13,** 386-92.

Fiedler, W., Graeven, U., Ergun, S., Verago, S., Kilic, N., Stockschlader, M. & Hossfeld, D.K. (1997). Vascular endothelial growth factor, a possible paracrine growth factor in human acute myeloid leukemia. *Blood*, **89,** 1870-5.

Fischer, K., Frohling, S., Scherer, S.W., McAllister Brown, J., Scholl, C., Stilgenbauer, S., Tsui, L.C., Lichter, P. & Dohner, H. (1997). Molecular cytogenetic delineation of deletions and translocations involving chromosome band 7q22 in myeloid leukemias. *Blood*, **89,** 2036-41.

Fong, T.A., Shawver, L.K., Sun, L., Tang, C., App, H., Powell, T.J., Kim, Y.H., Schreck, R., Wang, X., Risau, W., Ullrich, A., Hirth, K.P. & McMahon, G. (1999). SU5416 is a potent and selective inhibitor of the vascular endothelial growth factor receptor (Flk-1/KDR) that inhibits tyrosine kinase catalysis, tumor vascularization, and growth of multiple tumor types. *Cancer Research*, **59,** 99-106.

Gabrilove, J.L., White, K., Rahman, Z. & Wilson, E.L. (1994). Stem cell factor and basic fibroblast growth factor are synergistic in augmenting committed myeloid progenitor cell growth. *Blood*, **83,** 907-10.

Gelb, M.H. (1997). Protein prenylation, et cetera: signal transduction in two dimensions [comment]. *Science*, **275,** 1750-1.

Gelmetti, V., Zhang, J., Fanelli, M., Minucci, S., Pelicci, P.G. & Lazar, M.A. (1998). Aberrant recruitment of the nuclear receptor corepressor-histone deacetylase complex by the acute myeloid leukemia fusion partner ETO. *Molecular and Cellular Biology*, **18,** 7185-91.

Golomb, H.M., Alimena, G., Rowley, J.D., Vardiman, J.W., Testa, J.R. & Sovik, C. (1982). Correlation of occupation and karyotype in adults with acute nonlymphocytic leukemia. *Blood*, **60,** 404-11.

Grignani, F., De Matteis, S., Nervi, C., Tomassoni, L., Gelmetti, V., Cioce, M., Fanelli, M., Ruthardt, M., Ferrara, F.F., Zamir, I., Seiser, C., Lazar, M.A., Minucci, S. & Pelicci, P.G. (1998). Fusion proteins of the retinoic acid receptor-alpha recruit histone deacetylase in promyelocytic leukaemia. *Nature*, **391,** 815-8.

Guidez, F., Ivins, S., Zhu, J., Soderstrom, M., Waxman, S. & Zelent, A. (1998). Reduced retinoic acid-sensitivities of nuclear receptor corepressor binding to PML- and PLZF-RARalpha underlie molecular pathogenesis and treatment of acute promyelocytic leukemia. *Blood*, **91,** 2634-42.

Haase, D., Feuring-Buske, M., Konemann, S., Fonatsch, C., Troff, C., Verbeek, W., Pekrun, A., Hiddemann, W. & Wormann, B. (1995). Evidence for malignant transformation in acute myeloid leukemia at the level of early hematopoietic stem cells by cytogenetic analysis of CD34+ subpopulations. *Blood*, **86,** 2906-12.

Hannon, G.J. & Beach, D. (1994). p15INK4B is a potential effector of TGF-beta-induced cell cycle arrest [see comments]. *Nature*, **371,** 257-61.

Harrison, C.N., Gregory, W., Hudson, G.V., Devereux, S., Goldstone, A.H., Hancock, B., Winfield, D., MacMillan, A.K., Hoskin, P., Newland, A.C., Milligan, D. & Linch, D.C. (1999). High-dose BEAM chemotherapy with autologous haemopoietic stem cell transplantation for Hodgkin's disease is unlikely to be associated with a major increased risk of secondary MDS/AML. *British Journal of Cancer*, **81,** 476-83.

Hunger, S.P., Tkachuk, D.C., Amylon, M.D., Link, M.P., Carroll, A.J., Welborn, J.L., Willman, C.L. & Cleary, M.L. (1993). HRX involvement in de novo and secondary leukemias with diverse chromosome 11q23 abnormalities [see comments]. *Blood*, **81,** 3197-203.

Hussong, J.W., Rodgers, G.M. & Shami, P.J. (2000). Evidence of increased angiogenesis in patients with acute myeloid leukemia. *Blood*, **95,** 309-13.

Ida, K., Kitabayashi, I., Taki, T., Taniwaki, M., Noro, K., Yamamoto, M., Ohki, M. & Hayashi, Y. (1997). Adenoviral E1A-associated protein p300 is involved in acute myeloid leukemia with t(11;22)(q23;q13). *Blood*, **90,** 4699-704.

Ito, T. & May, W.S. (1996). Drug development train gathering steam. *Nature Medicine*, **2,** 403-4.

Jiang, K., Coppola, D., Crespo, N.C., Nicosia, S.V., Hamilton, A.D., Sebti, S.M. & Cheng, J.Q. (2000). The phosphoinositide 3-OH kinase/AKT2 pathway as a critical target for farnesyltransferase inhibitor-induced apoptosis. *Molecular and Cellular Biology*, **20,** 139-48.

Johansson, B., Mertens, F. & Mitelman, F. (1993). Cytogenetic deletion maps of hematologic neoplasms: circumstantial evidence for tumor suppressor loci. *Genes Chromosomes and Cancer*, **8,** 205-18.

Jones, P.L., Veenstra, G.J., Wade, P.A., Vermaak, D., Kass, S.U., Landsberger, N., Strouboulis, J. & Wolffe, A.P. (1998). Methylated DNA and MeCP2 recruit histone deacetylase to repress transcription. *Nature Genetics*, **19,** 187-91.

Jordan, C.T., Upchurch, D., Szilvassy, S.J., Guzman, M.L., Howard, D.S., Pettigrew, A.L., Meyerrose, T., Rossi, R., Grimes, B., Rizzieri, D.A., Luger, S.M. & Phillips, G.L. (2000). The interleukin-3 receptor alpha chain is a unique marker for human acute myelogenous leukemia stem cells [In Process Citation]. *Leukemia*, **14,** 1777-84.

Karp, J.E. & Sarkodee-Adoo, C.B. (2000). Therapy-related acute leukemia. *Clinical and Laboratory Medicine*, **20,** 71-81, ix.

Karp, J.E. & Smith, M.A. (1997). The molecular pathogenesis of treatment-induced (secondary) leukemias: foundations for treatment and prevention. *Seminars in Oncology*, **24,** 103-13.

Kennedy, M., Firpo, M., Choi, K., Wall, C., Robertson, S., Kabrun, N. & Keller, G. (1997). A common precursor for primitive erythropoiesis and definitive haematopoiesis. *Nature*, **386,** 488-93.

Kere, J., Donis-Keller, H., Ruutu, T. & de la Chapelle, A. (1989). Chromosome 7 long-arm deletions in myeloid disorders: terminal DNA sequences are commonly conserved and breakpoints vary. *Cytogenetics and Cell Genetics*, **50,** 226-9.

Khosravi-Far, R., Cox, A.D., Kato, K. & Der, C.J. (1992). Protein prenylation: key to ras function and cancer intervention? *Cell Growth and Differentiation*, **3,** 461-9.

Kollmannsberger, C., Beyer, J., Droz, J.P., Harstrick, A., Hartmann, J.T., Biron, P., Flechon, A., Schoffski, P., Kuczyk, M., Schmoll, H.J., Kanz, L. & Bokemeyer, C. (1998). Secondary leukemia following high cumulative doses of etoposide in patients treated for advanced germ cell tumors. *Journal of Clinical Oncology*, **16,** 3386-91.

Kosugi, H., Towatari, M., Hatano, S., Kitamura, K., Kiyoi, H., Kinoshita, T., Tanimoto, M., Murate, T., Kawashima, K., Saito, H. & Naoe, T. (1999). Histone deacetylase inhibitors are the potent inducer/enhancer of differentiation in acute myeloid leukemia: a new approach to anti-leukemia therapy. *Leukemia*, **13,** 1316-24.

Lapidot, T., Sirard, C., Vormoor, J., Murdoch, B., Hoang, T., Caceres-Cortes, J., Minden, M., Paterson, B., Caligiuri, M.A. & Dick, J.E. (1994). A cell initiating human acute myeloid leukaemia after transplantation into SCID mice. *Nature*, **367,** 645-8.

Larson, R.A., Wang, Y., Banerjee, M., Wiemels, J., Hartford, C., Le Beau, M.M. & Smith, M.T. (1999). Prevalence of the inactivating 609C-->T polymorphism in the

NAD(P)H:quinone oxidoreductase (NQO1) gene in patients with primary and therapy-related myeloid leukemia. *Blood*, **94,** 803-7.

Lawrence, H.J. & Largman, C. (1992). Homeobox genes in normal hematopoiesis and leukemia. *Blood*, **80,** 2445-53.

Le Beau, M.M., Albain, K.S., Larson, R.A., Vardiman, J.W., Davis, E.M., Blough, R.R., Golomb, H.M. & Rowley, J.D. (1986). Clinical and cytogenetic correlations in 63 patients with therapy-related myelodysplastic syndromes and acute nonlymphocytic leukemia: further evidence for characteristic abnormalities of chromosomes no. 5 and 7. *Journal of Clinical Oncology*, **4,** 325-45.

Le Beau, M.M., Espinosa, R., 3rd, Davis, E.M., Eisenbart, J.D., Larson, R.A. & Green, E.D. (1996). Cytogenetic and molecular delineation of a region of chromosome 7 commonly deleted in malignant myeloid diseases. *Blood*, **88,** 1930-5.

Lebowitz, P.F. & Prendergast, G.C. (1998). Non-Ras targets of farnesyltransferase inhibitors: focus on Rho. *Oncogene*, **17,** 1439-45.

Levine, E.G. & Bloomfield, C.D. (1992). Leukemias and myelodysplastic syndromes secondary to drug, radiation, and environmental exposure. *Seminars in Oncology*, **19,** 47-84.

Lewis, S., Abrahamson, G., Boultwood, J., Fidler, C., Potter, A. & Wainscoat, J.S. (1996). Molecular characterization of the 7q deletion in myeloid disorders. *British Journal of Haematology*, **93,** 75-80.

Li, N., Batzer, A., Daly, R., Yajnik, V., Skolnik, E., Chardin, P., Bar-Sagi, D., Margolis, B. & Schlessinger, J. (1993). Guanine-nucleotide-releasing factor hSos1 binds to Grb2 and links receptor tyrosine kinases to Ras signalling [see comments]. *Nature*, **363,** 85-8.

Lin, R.J., Nagy, L., Inoue, S., Shao, W., Miller, W.H., Jr. & Evans, R.M. (1998). Role of the histone deacetylase complex in acute promyelocytic leukaemia. *Nature*, **391,** 811-4.

Lorincz, M.C., Schubeler, D., Goeke, S.C., Walters, M., Groudine, M. & Martin, D.I. (2000). Dynamic analysis of proviral induction and De Novo methylation: implications for a histone deacetylase-independent, methylation density-dependent mechanism of transcriptional repression. *Molecular and Cellular Biology*, **20,** 842-50.

Luna-Fineman, S., Shannon, K.M. & Lange, B.J. (1995). Childhood monosomy 7: epidemiology, biology, and mechanistic implications. *Blood*, **85,** 1985-99.

Lutterbach, B., Westendorf, J.J., Linggi, B., Patten, A., Moniwa, M., Davie, J.R., Huynh, K.D., Bardwell, V.J., Lavinsky, R.M., Rosenfeld, M.G., Glass, C., Seto, E. & Hiebert, S.W. (1998). ETO, a target of t(8;21) in acute leukemia, interacts with the N-CoR and mSin3 corepressors. *Molecular and Cellular Biology*, **18,** 7176-84.

Ma, Q., Alder, H., Nelson, K.K., Chatterjee, D., Gu, Y., Nakamura, T., Canaani, E., Croce, C.M., Siracusa, L.D. & Buchberg, A.M. (1993). Analysis of the murine All-1 gene reveals conserved domains with human ALL-1 and identifies a motif shared with DNA methyltransferases. *Proceedings of the National Academy of Sciences, U S A*, **90,** 6350-4.

Marks, P.A., Richon, V.M. & Rifkind, R.A. (2000). Histone deacetylase inhibitors: inducers of differentiation or apoptosis of transformed cells. *Journal of the National Cancer Institutes*, **92,** 1210-6.

Mehrotra, B., George, T.I., Kavanau, K., Avet-Loiseau, H., Moore, D., 2nd, Willman, C.L., Slovak, M.L., Atwater, S., Head, D.R. & Pallavicini, M.G. (1995). Cytogenetically aberrant cells in the stem cell compartment (CD34+lin-) in acute myeloid leukemia. *Blood*, **86,** 1139-47.

Milligan, D.W., Ruiz De Elvira, M.C., Kolb, H.J., Goldstone, A.H., Meloni, G., Rohatiner, A.Z., Colombat, P. & Schmitz, N. (1999). Secondary leukaemia and myelodysplasia after autografting for lymphoma: results from the EBMT. EBMT Lymphoma and Late Effects Working Parties. European Group for Blood and Marrow Transplantation. *British Journal of Haematology*, **106,** 1020-6.

Mitelman, F., Brandt, L. & Nilsson, P.G. (1978). Relation among occupational exposure to potential mutagenic/carcinogenic agents, clinical findings, and bone marrow chromosomes in acute nonlymphocytic leukemia. *Blood*, **52,** 1229-37.

Mizuki, N., Kimura, M., Ohno, S., Miyata, S., Sato, M., Ando, H., Ishihara, M., Goto, K., Watanabe, S., Yamazaki, M., Ono, A., Taguchi, S., Okumura, K., Nogami, M., Taguchi, T., Ando, A. & Inoko, H. (1996). Isolation of cDNA and genomic clones of a human Ras-related GTP-binding protein gene and its chromosomal localization to the long arm of chromosome 7, 7q36. *Genomics*, **34,** 114-8.

Nan, X., Campoy, F.J. & Bird, A. (1997). MeCP2 is a transcriptional repressor with abundant binding sites in genomic chromatin. *Cell*, **88,** 471-81.

Nan, X., Ng, H.H., Johnson, C.A., Laherty, C.D., Turner, B.M., Eisenman, R.N. & Bird, A. (1998). Transcriptional repression by the methyl-CpG-binding protein MeCP2 involves a histone deacetylase complex [see comments]. *Nature*, **393,** 386-9.

Neubauer, A., Dodge, R.K., George, S.L., Davey, F.R., Silver, R.T., Schiffer, C.A., Mayer, R.J., Ball, E.D., Wurster-Hill, D., Bloomfield, C.D. & et al. (1994). Prognostic importance of mutations in the ras proto-oncogenes in de novo acute myeloid leukemia. *Blood*, **83,** 1603-11.

Neuman, W.L., Rubin, C.M., Rios, R.B., Larson, R.A., Le Beau, M.M., Rowley, J.D., Vardiman, J.W., Schwartz, J.L. & Farber, R.A. (1992). Chromosomal loss and deletion are the most common mechanisms for loss of heterozygosity from chromosomes 5 and 7 in malignant myeloid disorders. *Blood*, **79,** 1501-10.

Nilsson, L., Astrand-Grundstrom, I., Arvidsson, I., Jacobsson, B., Hellstrom-Lindberg, E., Hast, R. & Jacobsen, S.E. (2000). Isolation and characterization of hematopoietic progenitor/stem cells in 5q-deleted myelodysplastic syndromes: evidence for involvement at the hematopoietic stem cell level. *Blood*, **96,** 2012-21.

Padro, T., Ruiz, S., Bieker, R., Burger, H., Steins, M., Kienast, J., Buchner, T., Berdel, W.E. & Mesters, R.M. (2000). Increased angiogenesis in the bone marrow of patients with acute myeloid leukemia. *Blood*, **95,** 2637-44.

Paquette, R.L., Landaw, E.M., Pierre, R.V., Kahan, J., Lubbert, M., Lazcano, O., Isaac, G., McCormick, F. & Koeffler, H.P. (1993). N-ras mutations are associated with poor prognosis and increased risk of leukemia in myelodysplastic syndrome. *Blood*, **82,** 590-9.

Pedersen-Bjergaard, J., Andersen, M.K. & Christiansen, D.H. (2000). Therapy-related acute myeloid leukemia and myelodysplasia after high-dose chemotherapy and autologous stem cell transplantation. *Blood*, **95,** 3273-9.

Pedersen-Bjergaard, J. & Larsen, S.O. (1982). Incidence of acute nonlymphocytic leukemia, preleukemia, and acute myeloproliferative syndrome up to 10 years after treatment of Hodgkin's disease. *New England Journal of Medicine*, **307,** 965-71.

Pedersen-Bjergaard, J., Pedersen, M., Myhre, J. & Geisler, C. (1997). High risk of therapy-related leukemia after BEAM chemotherapy and autologous stem cell transplantation for previously treated lymphomas is mainly related to primary chemotherapy and not to the BEAM-transplantation procedure. *Leukemia*, **11,** 1654-60.

Pedersen-Bjergaard, J. & Rowley, J.D. (1994). The balanced and the unbalanced chromosome aberrations of acute myeloid leukemia may develop in different ways and may contribute differently to malignant transformation. *Blood*, **83,** 2780-6.

Pui, C.H., Ribeiro, R.C., Hancock, M.L., Rivera, G.K., Evans, W.E., Raimondi, S.C., Head, D.R., Behm, F.G., Mahmoud, M.H., Sandlund, J.T. & et al. (1991). Acute myeloid leukemia in children treated with epipodophyllotoxins for acute lymphoblastic leukemia. *New England Journal of Medicine*, **325,** 1682-7.

Quesnel, B., Guillerm, G., Vereecque, R., Wattel, E., Preudhomme, C., Bauters, F., Vanrumbeke, M. & Fenaux, P. (1998). Methylation of the p15(INK4b) gene in myelodysplastic syndromes is frequent and acquired during disease progression. *Blood*, **91,** 2985-90.

Raza, A., Lisak, L., Andrews, C., Little, L., Muzammil, M., Alvi, S., Mazzoran, L., Zorat, F., Akber, A., Ekbal, M., Razvi, S. & Venugopal, P. (1999). Thalidomide produces transfusion independence in patients with long-standing refractory anemias and myelodysplastic syndromes. *Blood*, **94,** 661a (abstr).

Razin, A. & Cedar, H. (1991). DNA methylation and gene expression. *Microbiology Reviews*, **55,** 451-8.

Rebollo, A. & Martinez, A.C. (1999). Ras proteins: recent advances and new functions. *Blood*, **94,** 2971-80.

Redner, R.L., Wang, J. & Liu, J.M. (1999). Chromatin remodeling and leukemia: new therapeutic paradigms. *Blood*, **94,** 417-28.

Reeves, R. & Nissen, M.S. (1990). The A.T-DNA-binding domain of mammalian high mobility group I chromosomal proteins. A novel peptide motif for recognizing DNA structure. *Journal of Biological Chemistry*, **265,** 8573-82.

Reuter, C.W., Morgan, M.A. & Bergmann, L. (2000). Targeting the Ras signaling pathway: a rational, mechanism-based treatment for hematologic malignancies? *Blood*, **96,** 1655-69.

Rozenblatt-Rosen, O., Rozovskaia, T., Burakov, D., Sedkov, Y., Tillib, S., Blechman, J., Nakamura, T., Croce, C.M., Mazo, A. & Canaani, E. (1998). The C-terminal SET domains of ALL-1 and TRITHORAX interact with the INI1 and SNR1 proteins, components of the SWI/SNF complex. *Proceedings of National Academy of Sciences, U S A*, **95,** 4152-7.

Saito, A., Yamashita, T., Mariko, Y., Nosaka, Y., Tsuchiya, K., Ando, T., Suzuki, T., Tsuruo, T. & Nakanishi, O. (1999). A synthetic inhibitor of histone deacetylase, MS-27-275, with marked in vivo antitumor activity against human tumors. *Proceedings of National Academy of Sciences, U S A*, **96,** 4592-7.

Sasaoka, T., Rose, D.W., Jhun, B.H., Saltiel, A.R., Draznin, B. & Olefsky, J.M. (1994). Evidence for a functional role of Shc proteins in mitogenic signaling induced by insulin, insulin-like growth factor-1, and epidermal growth factor. *Journal of Biological Chemistry*, **269,** 13689-94.

Shannon, K.M., O'Connell, P., Martin, G.A., Paderanga, D., Olson, K., Dinndorf, P. & McCormick, F. (1994). Loss of the normal NF1 allele from the bone marrow of children with type 1 neurofibromatosis and malignant myeloid disorders [see comments]. *New England Journal of Medicine*, **330,** 597-601.

Singhal, S., Mehta, J., Desikan, R., Ayers, D., Roberson, P., Eddlemon, P., Munshi, N., Anaissie, E., Wilson, C., Dhodapkar, M., Zeddis, J. & Barlogie, B. (1999). Antitumor activity of thalidomide in refractory multiple myeloma [see comments] [published erratum appears in N Engl J Med 2000 Feb 3;342(5):364]. *New England Journal of Medicine*, **341,** 1565-71.

Slany, R.K., Lavau, C. & Cleary, M.L. (1998). The oncogenic capacity of HRX-ENL requires the transcriptional transactivation activity of ENL and the DNA binding motifs of HRX. *Molecular and Cellular Biology*, **18,** 122-9.

Sobulo, O.M., Borrow, J., Tomek, R., Reshmi, S., Harden, A., Schlegelberger, B., Housman, D., Doggett, N.A., Rowley, J.D. & Zeleznik-Le, N.J. (1997). MLL is fused to CBP, a histone acetyltransferase, in therapy-related acute myeloid leukemia with a t(11;16)(q23;p13.3). *Proceedins of National Academy of Sciences, U S A*, **94,** 8732-7.

Stillman, W.S., Varella-Garcia, M. & Irons, R.D. (2000). The benzene metabolite, hydroquinone, selectively induces 5q31- and -7 in human CD34+CD19- bone marrow cells. *Experimental Hematology*, **28,** 169-76.

Stopka, T., Zakova, D., Fuchs, O., Kubrova, O., Blafkova, J., Jelinek, J., Necas, E. & Zivny, J. (2000). Chromatin remodeling gene SMARCA5 is dysregulated in primitive hematopoietic cells of acute leukemia. *Leukemia*, **14,** 1247-52.

Sugita, K., Furukawa, T., Tsuchida, M., Okawa, Y., Nakazawa, S., Akatsuka, J., Ohira, M. & Nishimura, K. (1993). High frequency of etoposide (VP-16)-related secondary leukemia in children with non-Hodgkin's lymphoma [see comments]. *American Journal of Pediatric Hematology and Oncology*, **15,** 99-104.

Super, H.J., McCabe, N.R., Thirman, M.J., Larson, R.A., Le Beau, M.M., Pedersen-Bjergaard, J., Philip, P., Diaz, M.O. & Rowley, J.D. (1993). Rearrangements of the MLL gene in therapy-related acute myeloid leukemia in patients previously treated with agents targeting DNA-topoisomerase II. *Blood*, **82,** 3705-11.

Taylor, J.A., Sandler, D.P., Bloomfield, C.D., Shore, D.L., Ball, E.D., Neubauer, A., McIntyre, O.R. & Liu, E. (1992). ras oncogene activation and occupational exposures in acute myeloid leukemia [see comments]. *Journal of the National Cancer Institutes*, **84,** 1626-32.

Taylor, P.R., Jackson, G.H., Lennard, A.L., Hamilton, P.J. & Proctor, S.J. (1997). Low incidence of myelodysplastic syndrome following transplantation using autologous non-cryopreserved bone marrow. *Leukemia*, **11,** 1650-3.

Teofili, L., Morosetti, R., Martini, M., Urbano, R., Putzulu, R., Rutella, S., Pierelli, L., Leone, G. & Larocca, L.M. (2000). Expression of cyclin-dependent kinase inhibitor p15(INK4B) during normal and leukemic myeloid differentiation. *Experimental Hematology*, **28,** 519-26.

Thirman, M.J., Gill, H.J., Burnett, R.C., Mbangkollo, D., McCabe, N.R., Kobayashi, H., Ziemin-van der Poel, S., Kaneko, Y., Morgan, R., Sandberg, A.A. & et al. (1993). Rearrangement of the MLL gene in acute lymphoblastic and acute myeloid leukemias with 11q23 chromosomal translocations [see comments]. *New England Journal of Medicine*, **329,** 909-14.

Thomas, D.A., Aguayo, A., Giles, F.J., Albitar, M., O'Brien, S.O., Cortes, J., Faderl, S., Bivins, C., Zeldis, J., Keating, M.J., Barlogie, B. & Kantarijan, H.M. (1999). Thalidomide anti-angiogenesis therapy in Phyladelphia-negative myeloproliferative disorders and myelofibrosis. *Blood*, **94,** 702a (abstr).

Thorn, J., Molloy, P. & Iland, H. (1995). SSCP detection of N-ras promoter mutations in AML patients. *Experimental Hematology*, **23,** 1098-103.

Traweek, S.T., Slovak, M.L., Nademanee, A.P., Brynes, R.K., Niland, J.C. & Forman, S.J. (1994). Clonal karyotypic hematopoietic cell abnormalities occurring after autologous bone marrow transplantation for Hodgkin's disease and non-Hodgkin's lymphoma. *Blood*, **84,** 957-63.

Tycko, B. (2000). Epigenetic gene silencing in cancer. *Journal of Clinical Investigation*, **105,** 401-7.

Uchida, T., Kinoshita, T., Nagai, H., Nakahara, Y., Saito, H., Hotta, T. & Murate, T. (1997). Hypermethylation of the p15INK4B gene in myelodysplastic syndromes. *Blood*, **90,** 1403-9.

Velloso, E.R., Michaux, L., Ferrant, A., Hernandez, J.M., Meeus, P., Dierlamm, J., Criel, A., Louwagie, A., Verhoef, G., Boogaerts, M., Michaux, J.L., Bosly, A., Mecucci, C. & Van den Berghe, H. (1996). Deletions of the long arm of chromosome 7 in myeloid disorders: loss of band 7q32 implies worst prognosis. *British Journal of Haematology*, **92,** 574-81.

Warrell, R.P., Jr., He, L.Z., Richon, V., Calleja, E. & Pandolfi, P.P. (1998). Therapeutic targeting of transcription in acute promyelocytic leukemia by use of an inhibitor of histone deacetylase [see comments]. *Journal of the National Cancer Institutes*, **90,** 1621-5.

Wijermans, P., Lubbert, M., Verhoef, G., Bosly, A., Ravoet, C., Andre, M. & Ferrant, A. (2000). Low-dose 5-aza-2'-deoxycytidine, a DNA hypomethylating agent, for the treatment of high-risk myelodysplastic syndrome: a multicenter phase II study in elderly patients. *Journal of Clinical Oncology*, **18,** 956-62.

Wild, R., Dhanabal, M., Olson, T.A. & Ramakrishnan, S. (2000). Inhibition of angiogenesis and tumour growth by VEGF121-toxin conjugate: differential effect on proliferating endothelial cells [In Process Citation]. *British Journal of Cancer*, **83,** 1077-83.

Wong, I.H., Ng, M.H., Huang, D.P. & Lee, J.C. (2000). Aberrant p15 promoter methylation in adult and childhood acute leukemias of nearly all morphologic subtypes: potential prognostic implications. *Blood*, **95,** 1942-9.

Yu, B.D., Hess, J.L., Horning, S.E., Brown, G.A. & Korsmeyer, S.J. (1995). Altered Hox expression and segmental identity in Mll-mutant mice. *Nature*, **378,** 505-8.

Ziegler, B.L., Valtieri, M., Porada, G.A., De Maria, R., Muller, R., Masella, B., Gabbianelli, M., Casella, I., Pelosi, E., Bock, T., Zanjani, E.D. & Peschle, C. (1999). KDR receptor: a key marker defining hematopoietic stem cells. *Science*, **285,** 1553-8.

Zwiebel, J.A. (2000). New agents for acute myelogenous leukemia. *Leukemia*, **14,** 488-90.

13

SPECIAL CLINICAL CONCERNS/ PROBLEMS IN THE MANAGEMENT OF MDS AND SEDONDARY ACUTE MYELOID LEUKEMIAS

Parameswaran Venugopal, Sharon Manson and Harvey D. Preisler
Rush Cancer Institute,
Rush Presbyterian St. Luke's Medical Center, Chicago, IL

INTRODUCTION

Management of patients with myelodysplastic syndromes (MDS) and acute myeloid leukemias arising from pre-existing MDS (Secondary AML, sAML) presents many unique problems to the treating physician. These patients are often elderly and are at high risk for life threatening complications of treatment. Recurrent infections and a history of multiple blood product transfusions complicate the clinical management and compromise their ability to tolerate therapy. Drug resistance and the frequent occurrence of cytogenetic abnormalities result in lower remission rates and decreased long term responses. This chapter will review these unique aspects of management of these patients.

CHEMOTHERAPY OF sAML

What Is Currently Available?

Standard treatment for AML consists of chemotherapy that includes an anthracycline and cytarabine. While this can provide a complete remission (CR) rate of 70-80% in patients under the age of 60 years, in older adults the rate drops to approximately 50%. Despite the relatively good CR rate in young patients, only about 40% are alive without disease at the end of 5 years. In patients over 60 years age, the 5-year disease-free survival is only 15%. Analysis of our own data (Preisler et al, 2000a) reveals that age alone may not have such a dramatic influence on the outcome of the patients if they have a good performance status, do not have cytogenetic abnormalities, or prior history of myelodysplastic syndromes. The influence of cytogenetics on the outcome of AML therapy has been well documented. Data including large numbers of patients, published by the UK Medical Research Council (MRC), have demonstrated the influence of cytogenetics on outcome in the favorable, standard and unfavorable subgroups (Mauritzon et al 2000). A study by the Southwest Oncology Group (SWOG) has indicated that favorable cytogenetics is a good prognostic factor irrespective of age (Mayer et al, 1994).

Problems in delivering chemotherapy

The mainstays of chemotherapy in the treatment of AML are cytosine arabinoside and an anthracycline. Anthracyclines appear to be important in overcoming disease resistance however are well known for their cardiac toxicity.

a. ***Compromised organ function:*** cardiac dysfunction remains the major side effect of anthracyclines. Toxicity increases steeply beyond daunorubicin dose of 550 mg/m2. Mitoxantrone may have less cardiac adverse effects. cardioprotective agents like doxerzine have not been successful in AML. Rigorous monitoring of cardiac function during chemotherapy helps in identifying early dysfunction. Neurologic side effects of cytosine arabinoside is unpredictable but the use of routine neurochecks prior to administration of each dose of high dose ara-C helps in early recognition of these adverse effects.
b. ***Infections:*** bacterial, viral, fungal and other opportunistic infections occurring during therapy: Empiric therapy with broadspectrum antibiotics should be instituted at the onset of fever in a neutropenic patient. Work up

should simultaneously be initiated to find out the source of infection. Fungal infections have been a major problem after chemotherapy. Intensive prophylaxis with amphotericin nasal spray and early institution of intravenous amphotericin therapy are helpful in preventing or treating the fungal infection which otherwise could prove fatal.

c. ***Bleeding*****:** Prophylactic platelet transfusions help in preventing bleeding complication following therapy. Recent data support lowering of threshold for platelet transfusion to $10{,}000\text{x}10^6$ without increasing the risk of bleeding. Pooled platelets may be used in place of single donor platelets with no increase in allo immunization.

d. ***Poor response / Lack of response to blood product transfusions (repeated prior transfusions; allo-antibodies).*** In many cases, this results from peripheral destruction of platelets either from sensitization to alloantibodies or excessive reticulo-endothelial activity and hypersplenism. The use of intravenous immunoglobulins may be useful in improving the platelet counts transiently for an acute episode of bleeding or in preparation for a surgical procedure, but the high cost prohibits its routine use. The use of HLA-matched platelets may be useful in patients who are heavily allo-immunized. The availability and cost are limiting factors.

e. *Other supportive measures*:

1. Neutropenia & Thrombocytopenia precautions: Reverse Isolation: Washing hands in between examining patients and the use of disposable gloves are necessary during the period of neutropenia. Thrombocytopenia precautions include avoidance of intramuscular injections and fall precautions.

2. Nutrition: Oral intake is usually poor not only because of nausea and vomiting, but also secondary to mucositis causing pain and alteration in taste induced by chemotherapy. If the calorie intake is suboptimal, parenteral nutrition should be instituted.

3. Care of skin and mucous membranes: oral hygiene, prevention of infection, dental care, sinuses: Dental caries is a common source of infection and prophylaxis is essential. Frequent mouth rinses reduces bacterial count and help reduce infections.

4. Pain control: Pain from mucositis can be severe and may require effective analgesics like continuous infusion of morphine sulfate.

5. Psychosocial; support groups play a vital role in the management of these patients by helping them to cope with the situation.

Response to Chemotherapy

Majority of patients who are able to receive chemotherapy in adequate doses on schedule do respond to therapy. While complete remissions are obtained in only 50-60% of patients with sAML with intensive induction regimens, vast majority of patients achieve significant cytoreduction.

Short Duration of Remission

Chemotherapy of sAML is associated with short duration of remission. Duration of first remission is an important prognostic factor for response to subsequent therapy. This has been confirmed in many studies. Longer first CRs have been associated with a significantly higher response rate (Walters et al, 1998) and longer DFS (Burnett et al, 1998) following subsequent therapy. In view of the short duration of remission in sAML, conventional salvage regimens may not be useful and this calls for novel approaches to manage these patients. The major problems in the treatment of these patients today include induction failure, intrinsic resistance to therapy, the toxicity of anti-leukemia therapy, and relapse.

NOVEL APPROACHES TO THERAPY

a. ***Increase response rates***: dose intensification

b. ***Reduce Toxicity of Regimens***: Cytoprotective agents (amifostine); growth factors (GCSF, GMCSF, EPO, SCF)

c. ***Use of Bioactive Agents to reduce Leukemia regrowth in between chemotherapy cycles***: e.g., Interferon, Retinoic Acid, Interleukin-4, Interleukin-10.

Intensive chemotherapy courses with the use of bioactive agents in between the courses of chemotherapy to suppress the regrowth resistance offers the best chance of reducing the probability of leukemia regrowth (Preisler et al 1999).

d. ***Anti-cytokine therapy***: Recent studies by our group have shown substantial differences in cytokine levels between AML and normal (Preisler et al 2000c). Stem cell factor levels in AML blood and marrow serum are almost 2x >normal (2506 pg/ml vs. 1565 pg/ml). The ratio of interleukin-1 (IL-1) levels to Interleukin-1 receptor antagonist (IL1-ra) in normal BM cell is 0.002 while it is 0.12 in AML cells. This indicates that the restriction of IL1 stimulation of AML and other cells by IL1ra is markedly reduced in AML. These are consistent within vitro effects of IL1beta ra as already shown by our group (Yin et al 1992). The effects of IL1ra in vivo is currently being studied by our group (Preisler et al 2000b). The altered levels of IL1ra in myeloid leukemias have been shown by others as well (Rambaldi et al, 1991, Extrov et al 1991)

e. ***Therapy aimed at correcting abnormal gene functions***: The p15 gene is methylated in 82% of AMLs and not in normal marrow. Methylation abrogates p15 expression thereby removing a normal negative regulator of progression through G1 and in this way, facilitates the phophorylation of rb, release of E2F and entry into S phase. Demethylation of op15 can be produced by 5-azacytidine; this is currently being tried at our institution.

The IRF1 and IRF2 genes regulate the transcription of many genes. The IRF1 gene inhibits and IRF2 gene stimulates proliferation. Recent studies by our group demonstrated that the IRF1/IRF2 ratio is abnormally low in 75% of AMLs suggesting that expression of IRF2 is dominant in most AMLs. Studies by our group have shown that the IRF1/IRF2 abnormalities can be corrected by administration of Interleukin-4 (Preisler et al 2000b).

f. ***Newer approaches to remission induction in AML***:Remission induction therapy for AML remains a problem especially for elderly patients and for patients whose AML was preceded by MDS and / or toxic exposure. We have developed a remission induction regimen consisting of 2 doses of araC at 2 gm/m2 at t=0 and t=12 hrs with mitoxantrone 30 mg/m2 administered immediately after the second dose of araC. The same chemotherapy is administered 96 hours later. After the second "pulse" of therapy, amifostine (ami) is administered until treatment outcome is known. Ami was administered with 3 goals: to accelerate BM recovery, to reduce toxicity, and to reduce the regrowth of residual leukemia after the second pulse of therapy by reducing telomerase activity in the AML cells which survived therapy. 16 patients with standard prognosis AML (<70 years old, no history of MDS or toxic exposure; median age 49) were treated with 15 CRs (94%). 27 patients with poor prognosis disease were treated (age >70 years and/or history of MDS and/or toxic exposure). Among these patients, there were 9 CRs, 3 returns to prior MDS (CR + RMDS=44%), 4 incomplete remissions (ICR=CR BM but failure of ANC and / or platelets to normalize), 7 resistant disease (RD) failures, and 4 deaths. Considering the patients 70 years old or greater who were included in the poor prognosis disease category because of old age, there were 5 CRs (71%). Considering these patients together with standard prognosis patients, the CR rate is 87% (20/23). These data demonstrate that this regimen is highly effective in remission induction in AML including patients over 70 years old. The regimen is much less effective for AML with a history of MDS or toxic exposure with resistant disease remaining a significant cause of treatment failure in the latter group of patients (Preisler et al 2000a).

g. ***Incorporation of novel agents into the therapeutic regimen***:
Targeted Therapy: One of the promising new approaches to antileukemic treatment is targeted therapy, in which a number of exciting molecules are becoming available. These include antisense oligonucleotides, inhibitors of DNA repair, oncogenes and the cell cycle, differentiation inducers, tyrosine kinase inhibitors, and fusion toxins, including CMA-676 (gemtuzumab ozogamicin) which is targeted to the leukemic cell using a monoclonal antibody against CD33 antigen. AML is an ideal target for monoclonal antibody therapy because the leukemia cells are easily accessible to an antibody given intravenously. Anti-CD33 antibodies have been identified as the most suitable carrier for an anti-ANL agent because of the characteristics and distribution of this antigen. The CD33 is an integral membrane protein with extracellular domain that is expressed on >80% of AML cells.. Its expression is restricted to hemapoietic cells; specifically it is absent from pluripotent stem cells and also non-hematopoietic tissues. Following antibody binding, the CD33 antigen is internalized and therefore could act as a carrier that will deliver the toxin effectively into the cell. The number of antigen molecules required for the latter may be much lower than what is necessary for detection by flow cytometry. We have shown that subcutaneous administration of Interleukin-10 (IL-10) can significantly increase the CD33 antigen expression on AML cells (Mamani et al 200). We have administered this cytokine to patients with AML with minimal or no side effects (Unpublished Observation). Thus pretreatment of leukemia cells with appropriate cytokines may enhance the response to monoclonal antibody. Cytokines like IL-10 may have other beneficial effects in these patients (Tao et al 2000) which could potentially augment the therapeutic benefit.

Although Mylotarg has not been studied well in the setting of sAML, results of the three phase II studies on 142 patients in untreated first relapse with CD33 positive AML indicate an overall response rate of 30%. The responses were equally divided between CR and CRp (CR with incomplete platelet recovery). There was no significant difference in the response rates between patients aged <60 years or >60 years (34% versus 26%, respectively). These results are encouraging and call for the use of this antibody in sAML either as single agent or in combination with chemotherapy (Sievers et al 1999a, Sievers et al 1999b). Trials at our institution are currently evaluating the effects of this antibody on the clinical and biological characteristics of sAML.

Thalidomide is an oral agent that can be administered easily with tolerable side effects. Very little data is available on its use in AML. Preliminary results from ongoing studies at our institution show that this agent may be useful in reducing the transfusion requirements in some sAML patients (Unpublished Observations). Data published from our institution by Raza et al indicate 50% response in low-risk MDS using thalidomide as a single agent (Raza et al 1999).

h. ***Stem Cell Transplantation***

1. Autologous stem cell transplantation: This procedure has no curative role because the stem cells which are given back to the patient are contaminated by leukemic stem cells. The relapse rate of this kind of transplantation is high although the mortality rate is lower than allogenic transplantation (Burnett et al 1998).
2. Allogeneic transplantation: Most patients with MDS and sAML are ineligible because of age, co-morbid conditions and lack of HLA-matched donors (Gamberi et al 1994). In the few patients who are eligible, excessive transplant-related morbidity and mortality has been a major problem. Large cooperative group and single institution studies have indicated a 50% long-term survival rate following HLA-identical allogeneic BMT. The relapse rate following this is reasonably low at 15-20% but the treatment related mortality remains high at 15-25%. The rate of infectious complications during post-transplant period is very high.
3. Non-myeloablative stem cell transplantation (NST): Neither autologous nor allogeneic transplantation is generally a treatment option for older patients with AML, primarily because of the treatment related toxicity. In an attempt to reduce the toxicity from high dose therapy prior to transplant, non-myeloablative doses of chemotherapy are used. The use of lower doses of chemotherapy may have the risk of leaving behind a significant leukemic cell mass. This novel approach relies upon the ability of graft versus leukemia effect of allogeneic transplant to gradually eliminate the minimal residual disease. Although the concept of NST appears to be very attractive,

its utility in this group of patients is yet to be proven. However, it may have a role in combination with biologic therapy.

i. ***Vaccines against leukemia*:**

Attempts to develop effective vaccination strategies against the leukemic blasts are in progress. One of the approaches include the development of viral vectors that will specifically target leukemic blasts, delivering the foreign antigen that would then be processed to induce an effective endogenous immune response, complete with memory. Another approach that is being actively pursued is to better characterize the leukemia-associated antigens and their presentation and to use currently-existing vaccination approaches to induce an effective immune response against such antigens, in an attempt to eliminate the minimal residual disease. Autologous tumor cells enzymatically treated to express alpha gal epitopes is being developed for autologous vaccination (Galili et al 1998). This program is being set up at the Rush Cancer Institute, Chicago. In vivo targeting of the autologous tumor vaccine by the natural anti-Gal antibody to antigen presenting cells enhances the immunogenecity of these vaccines.

REFERENCES:

Burnett AK, Goldstone AH, Stevens RM (1998) Randomized comparison of addition of autologous bone-marrow transplantation to intensive chemotherapy for acute myeloid leukemia in first remission: Results of MRC AML 10 trial. UK Medical Research Council Adult and Children's Leukemia Working Parties. *Lancet*, **351**:700-708.

Extrov Z, Kurzrock R, Wetzler M, Kantarjian H, Blake M, Harris D, Gutterman J, Talpaz M (1991) Suppression of chronic myelogenous leukemia colony growth by interleukin-1 (IL1) receptor antagonist and soluble IL-1 receptors; a novel application for inhibitors of IL-1 activity. *Blood*, **78** (6):1476.

Galili U, LaTemple DC, Radic MZ (1998) A sensitive assay for measuring alpha-gal expression on cells by a monoclonal angi-Gal antibody. *Transplantation*, **65**:1129.

Gamberi B, Bandini G, Visani G (1994) Acute Myeloid Leukemia from diagnosis to bone marrow transplantation: experience from a single center. *Bone Marrow Transplant,* **14**:69-72.

Mamani, D, Venugopal P, Coon J, Preisler H (2001): Immunophenotypic profile of leukemic cells from acute myeloid leukemia (AML) patients at diagnosis and after a three-day course of cytokine administration. Proceedings of the American Society of Clinical Oncology.

Mayer RJ, Davis RB, Schiffer CA (1994) Intensive postremission chemotherapy in adults with acute myeloid leukemia. *New England Journal of Medicine*, **331**:896-903.

Preisler H, Venugopal P, Sivaraman S, Manson S (2000b) Abnormalities of Poliferation control in AML: *Blood*, **96**: abstract #4428.

Preisler H, Larson RA, Goldberg J, Tricot G, Raza A, Venugopal P, Gregory S, Adler A(1999) The administration of retinoic acid/alpha-interferon between courses of cemotherapy results in very long remissions and a high proportion of apparent cures in AML: *Blood*, **95**: abstract # 1306 .

Rambaldi A, Torcia M, Bettoni S, Vannier E, Barbui T, Shaw A, Dinarello C, Cozzolino (1991) Modulation of cell proliferation and cytokine production in acute myeloblastic leukemia by interleukin-1 receptor antagonist and the lack of its expression by leukemic cells. *Blood*, **78**: 3248.

Raza A, Lisam L, Andrews C, Little L, Muzammil M, Alvi S, Mazzoran L, Zorat F, Akber A, Ekbal M, Razvi S, Venugopal P (1999) Thalidomide produces transfusion independence in patieints with long-standing refractory anemias and myelodysplastic syndromes (MDS). *Blood*, **94**:661a, abstract #2935.

Sievers EL, Applebaum FR, Spielberger RT, Forman SJ, Flowers D, Smith FO, shannon-Dorcy K, Berger MS, Bernstein ID (1999a) Selective ablation of acute myeloid leukemia using antibody-targetsd chemotherap: a phase I Study of an anti-CD33 calicheamicin immunocojugate. *Blood*, **93**: 3678-3684.

Sievers EL, Larson RA, Estery E, Stadtmauer EA, Erba HP, Roy DC, Tarantolo S, Spielberger R, Berger MS, Eten C, Manley L, Stone A, Bernstein I, Applebaum FR (1999b): Efficacy and safety of CMA-676 inpatients with AML in first relapse. *Blood*, **94**:abst#307a.

Tao M, Li B, Nayini J , Sivaraman S, Song S, Larson A, Toofanfard M, Chen H, Venugopal P, Preisler H (2000) Regulation of serum cytokines following IL-4 and IL-10 therapy in patients with acute myelogenous leukemia. *Blood*, **96**:abstract #1403.

Walters RS, Kantarjian HM, Keating MJ (1998) Mitoxantrone and high-dose cytosine arabinoside in refractory acute myelogenous leukemia. *Cancer*, **15**:677-82.

Yin M, Venugopal P, Banavali SD, Gartside P, Preisler HD (1992) Effects of an IL-1beta receptor antagonist on acute myeloid leukemia cell. *Leukemia*, **6**:898-901.

14

MDS AND SECONDARY AML : AN EVOLUTIONARY PERSPECTIVE

M. William Audeh
University of California, Los Angeles
And Division of Hematology/Oncology, Cedars-Sinai Medical Center, Los Angeles, CA

"...in Biology, nothing makes sense except in the light of Evolution"
Dobzhansky (1970)

" Evolutionary Biology is the foundation for all Biology, and Biology is the foundation for all Medicine"
Nesse and Williams (1994)

INTRODUCTION

The way in which medicine explains disease determines, to a great extent, the approach that is taken to treatment and prevention (Thagard, 1999). Myelodysplastic Syndrome (MDS) and its frequent sequela, secondary Acute Myeloid Leukemia (AML), have been explained as clonal disorders of hematopoietic stem cells, which arise as the result of exposure to genotoxic agents, particularly cancer therapies such as chemotherapy and radiation (Lichtman and Brennan, 2001). Treatment has until recently been guided by viewing MDS as a disorder of differentiation, or an incipient malignancy requiring additional genotoxic agents to suppress. These assumptions regarding etiology and therapy may be inadequate to answer fundamental questions regarding this disease, such as why only certain individuals exposed to the same chemotherapeutic agents develop MDS/secondary AML, why certain individuals evolve from MDS to secondary AML more rapidly than others, and why treatment with additional genotoxic agents has not proven curative.

It is likely that the understanding of MDS and secondary AML may be promoted by the application of the principles of evolutionary biology, sometimes referred to as "Darwinian Medicine" (Nesse and Williams, 1994). Evolutionary biology seeks to understand human disease by placing the human species within the realm of the rest of the biological world, in which natural selection has shaped the genetic structure of populations, and genetic variation between individuals determines the response to the environment. In this context, human disease may be understood as the biological consequence of the interaction of genes and the environment (Burdon, 1999).

MODERN MEDICINE AND EVOLUTIONARY BIOLOGY

The tradition of modern medicine, since the era of Osler, has been to view the human body as a generic "machine", designed to function in an absolute "normal" state, regardless of genetic background or environment (Childs, 1999). This placed human biology in contradistinction to the remainder of the living world, in which the design of organisms was the result of adaptation to their environment, and the health of those organisms dependent upon the interaction between genes and environment. Human "disease" was viewed by modern medicine, therefore, as simply a "dysfunction" of the bodily machine. Oslerian Medicine managed human disease by primarily addressing its proximate, or immediate cause, with the only goal being to return the machine to its absolute normal state.

Molecular biology and genetics has, however, consistently illuminated the common thread between human biology and that of other organisms, and supported the argument that evolutionary biology was relevant to human health. Although evolution has been the basis of modern biology for 150 years, modern medicine has remained untouched by Darwin, until recently:

" Evolutionary Biology is so firmly integrated with the rest of biology that it is not at all possible to mark a boundary between them. But modern medicine has been a peninsula. It is broadly connected with most regions of biology such as anatomy, physiology, biochemistry, ... but has just a few thin bridges traversing the gulf to evolutionary biology." (Ewald, 1994)

The application of evolutionary biology to the field of medicine has altered the way in which a growing number of physicians explain disease (Nesse and Williams, 1994) (Stearns, 1999). "Darwinian Medicine" views the human body more appropriately as the product of evolution, for which there is no absolute "normal" or "abnormal" state, but rather degrees of adaptation to a particular environment. Many diseases may therefore best be explained as the result of evolutionary factors such as natural selection, genetic variation among individuals, and maladaptation to a particular environment.

APPLYING EVOLUTIONARY BIOLOGY TO ONCOLOGY

The application of the principles of evolutionary biology to oncology promises to be perhaps the most fruitful area of analysis, in view of the many parallels between evolutionary biology and the process of carcinogenesis and malignant progression (Weiss, 1993) (Greaves, 2000). In addition, the enormous amount of genetic variation found in human populations (Cavalli-Sforza, Menozzi, Piazza, 1994), in the form of genetic polymorphisms, is proving, in may cases, to be of functional significance in the complex process involved in carcinogenesis (Caporaso and Rothman, 1998). It is apparent, therefore, that evolutionary biology is an indispensable tool for the understanding of the development of malignancy in the human species, at the level of the cell, the individual, and the population.

Evolutionary Biology on the Cellular Level

On the somatic cellular level, it is clear that the malignant cell population develops as the result of a process of selection and adaptation, much the same as any population of organisms. Weiss (1993) observed that carcinogenesis " reflects processes very similar to those that generate genetic variation among individuals over time. The evolving tissue mosaic may simulate many evolutionary mechanisms in microcosm" (p. 303).

A key mechanism of evolution used by bacteria, arguably the most successful and ubiquitous of all life forms, is the generation of genetic variation in the face of selective pressure (Hoffman and Parsons, 1993). Increased genetic variation in the population is an evolutionary strategy that increases the likelihood of an individual arising with a genetic mutation that confers the ability to tolerate, or even thrive upon, the selective pressures within the environment. Increased genetic variation is generated in bacterial populations by a rise in the rate of endogenous mutations, or hypermutability, which is accomplished by a variety of means. These include the induction of diminished fidelity of replication through the use of variant DNA polymerases, diminished DNA mismatch repair, and increased chromosomal instability.

Adaptive hypermutability via diminished DNA mismatch repair is accomplished in bacteria by the horizontal transfer of defective mismatch repair genes, and is considered a hallmark of adaptive evolution (Denamur, et al, 2000). It is important to note that defective DNA mismatch repair, as evidenced by microsatellite instability, has been implicated as an operative mechanism in a number of human malignancies, as well as MDS (Maeck, et al, 2000). Adaptive amplification, an inducible mechanism for generating chromosomal instability, has also been observed in bacteria, allowing rapid evolution under stress (Hastings, et al, 2000). Again, chromosomal instability, resulting in loss of heterozygosity, deletions and translocations, has been a consistent finding in all malignancies, as well as in hematopoietic stem cells in MDS (Lichtman and Brennan, 2001).

The inducible hypermutability of bacteria directly parallels the observation of a "mutator phenotype" in malignancy, as both provide the mechanism by which genetic diversity may be generated, and evolutionary adaptation accelerated (Hanahan and Weinberg, 2000). The "universal" selective pressures which drive the clonal evolution of solid tumors lead to the development of genetic traits identified as the "Hallmarks of Cancer." The mutations that produce these traits very likely account for nearly all of the recurring genetic changes that appear essential for cancer development. In order for cancer to evolve, a cell and its progeny must acquire mutations that confer at least some of the following traits:

1. Self-Sufficiency of Growth Signals
2. Insensitivity to Anti-Growth Signals
3. Evasion of Apoptosis
4. Limitless Replicative Potential
5. Maintenance of sustained angiogenesis
6. Tissue invasion and metastasis

While this list is derived from analysis of solid tumors, it is clear that the same (or fewer) adaptive genetic traits are acquired in the progression of hematologic malignancies (Ponten, 1998) and MDS (Sullivan and Willis, 1994). The acquisition of these "adaptive" traits is facilitated by the genetic instability of the premalignant clone, and thus anything that enhances genetic instability is likely to accelerate the evolution of malignancy. The use of mutagenic or genotoxic agents for the treatment of incipient or established malignancy would therefore appear to run the risk of promoting the evolutionary progression of the malignant clone, unless all abnormal cells were killed outright by the therapy, or induced to stop proliferating.

Human Genetic Variation and Disease

There is considerable genetic variation between human populations, and between individuals within the same population (Cavalli-Sforza, Menozzi, and Piazza, 1994). Much of this variation, in the form of genetic polymorphisms, is without known biological significance. Variation in allele frequencies in human populations may represent the effect of natural selection, as well as founder effects, and random genetic drift. However, many genes do have functionally variable alleles, which produce measurable differences in gene expression, protein structure and function. These differences involve a number of genes affecting human health, including those encoding metabolic enzymes, DNA repair enzymes, cell surface receptors, cytokines and coagulation factors (Cooper, 1999). It is this functional variation between populations and individuals upon which natural selection acts, although the importance of natural selection in shaping the modern human gene pool is uncertain (Weatherall, 1996). Whatever the cause of human genetic variation, it is clear that many of these polymorphisms greatly affect human health, including the predisposition to malignancy.

Infectious agents have exerted considerable selective pressure on human populations throughout history (Cavalli-Sforza, Menozzi, Piazza, 1994). Much of the best-studied genetic variation seen in modern day human populations is presumed to be due to the past and present effect of infectious agents as a selective force. Examples include the diverse HLA antigen polymorphisms involved in innate immunity to infectious agents in general, and hemoglobin and tumor necrosis factor (TNF) polymorphisms in the case of specific agents such as malaria (Cooper, 1999).

The effect of other types of selection pressure may also be reflected in widespread, functional polymorphisms, which may have arisen as adaptations that were of value in a past environment, but now pose a liability in the current environment. Examples include the heritable traits of avid storage of dietary calories as fat (the "thrifty" genotype), or particularly effective hemostasis (coagulation factor polymorphisms such as Factor V leiden), which may have been important for survival in prior times of famine or high risk of hemorrhage, but are maladaptive in the face of the modern high calorie diet and sedentary lifestyle (Nesse and Williams, 1994) (Stearns, 1999) (Weatherall, 1996). The genetic polymorphisms that form this "signature" of natural selection may be thought of as the underlying cause of a number of modern diseases of "maladaptation" (Neel, 1999), such as diabetes, cardiovascular disease, and predisposition to malignancy. Polymorphic genes producing functional variation in xenobiotic metabolism (Caporaso and Rothman, 1998), and DNA repair (Berwick and Vineis, 2000) are also likely to reflect prior selection pressures, and in the modern environment have been associated with significant predisposition to malignancy (Frame et al., 1998).

Human Genetic Variation and Predisposition to Malignancy

The phylogenetically ancient xenobiotic metabolizing enzymes evolved as a result of the need to detoxify and remove potentially toxic or non-nutritive xenobiotic substances absorbed from the environment (Caporaso and Rothman, 1998). A wide array of enzymes and polymorphic alleles characterize these gene families, which include the cytochrome p450 (CYP) and glutathione-s-transferase (GST) enzyme systems. In humans, over 100 CYP genes have been identified, with subfamilies scattered throughout the genome. The CYP genes encode mono-oxygenases which perform oxidation reactions on a wide variety of xenobiotic as well as endogenous substrates. The GST enzymes conjugate a cofactor, glutathione, to the oxidized substrate, producing enhanced water-solubility, and more efficient excretion of the metabolite. Over many millions of years, these enzyme systems have evolved to deal with environmental, and in the case of human evolution, dietary xenobiotics. In the modern environment, xenobiotics never before encountered in nature, such as drugs and chemicals from human sources, are also metabolized by the same enzyme systems (Lazar, 2000). While human genetic variation in CYP and GST enzymes may have evolved due to past environmental and dietary selective pressures, these variations profoundly affect drug and carcinogen metabolism in the modern environment (Frame et al., 2000). Genetic variants of xenobiotic metabolising enzymes have been associated with an increased risk of MDS and secondary AML, due to the link with exposure to genotoxic agents such as drugs and carcinogens (Willman, 2000).

While metabolism of non-nutritive xenobiotics is clearly of relevance to predisposition to malignancy, variation in metabolism of the dietary micronutrient folate may also be important. Folate is necessary for the maintenance of DNA integrity, and folate deficiency has been associated with increased risk of malignancy by causing altered methylation and disruption of DNA repair (Choi and Mason, 2000). Dietary folate is metabolised by methylenetetrahydrofolate reductase (MTHFR), and functional polymorphisms in this enzyme which confer enhanced sensitivity to folate deficiency have been associated with colorectal cancer (Chen, J, 1996). A number of so-called "fragile sites" within chromosomes are sensitive to folate deficiency, and in myeloid malignancies and MDS, consistent interstitial deletions have been correlated with fragile sites (Hirst, Czepulkowski, and Mufti, 1993). It is therefore likely that genetic variation in folate metabolism may also play a role in the development of MDS and myeloid malignancy, as well as colorectal cancer.

The capacity for repair of DNA damage appears to be extremely variable within human populations, and almost certainly plays a role in predisposition to malignancy (Berwick and Vineis, 2000). Individuals with malignancies of all kinds have been observed to have ineffective repair of a variety of DNA lesions, although the specific genes have, for the most part, not been identified. Germline mutations in DNA mismatch repair genes MSH2 and MLH1 (human homologues of the bacterial mismatch repair genes important in adaptive hypermutability) confer an increased risk for a variety of human cancers, although their role in MDS is unclear.

APPLYING EVOLUTIONARY BIOLOGY TO MDS AND SECONDARY AML

Selective Pressures and Clonal Evolution at the Cellular Level

From the perspective of evolutionary biology, MDS and secondary AML develop through the stepwise acquistion of key somatic mutations, each of which confer a selective advantage to the developing clone (Sullivan and Willis, 1994). The hallmarks of malignancy which comprise the adaptive traits which must be acquired are likely to be similar, if not identical, to those of solid tumors (Hanahan and Weinberg, 2000).

Diminished sensitivity to growth inhibitory signals, for example, may be a critical adaptive trait in the development of MDS and secondary AML. The mechanism by which this occurs may initially be chromosomal deletions which paradoxically confer hypersensitivity to the inhibitory effects of IFNgamma and TNFalpha, leading to strong selective pressure for clonal outgrowths of resistant cells (Lensch, 1999). Other cellular adaptations observed in MDS with progression to secondary AML include loss of apoptosis due to increased bcl-2 expression and p53 mutation (Kurotaki et al., 2000), as well as a variety of recurring allelic losses and chromosomal deletions (Mori et al., 2000). Identification of the genetic pathways involved in these consistent genetic changes will reveal the adaptive traits that are critical for the development of MDS and secondary AML.

Also revealing are the types of genetic lesions that appear in MDS during the evolution of disease, as they provide insight into the degree and nature of genetic instability driving the process. Gene rearrangements, interstitial deletions, loss of heterozygosity and microsatellite instability have all been observed, supporting the notion that generalized genetic instability is an early and critical feature of MDS (Willman, 2000) (Maeck et al., 2000). Microsatellite instability may be acquired somatically through mutation of mismatch repair genes, or transcriptional silencing of the intact gene by promoter methylation. Microsatellite instability has been detected more frequently than expected in secondary breast and lung cancers following chemotherapy and radiation for Hodgkin's Disease (Behrens et al., 2000), suggesting that genotoxic therapy may induce genetic instability. However, the possibility of an inherited germline defect in DNA repair, which led to both the primary Hodgkin's Disease and second cancers, cannot be ruled out, and the same question may be raised in treatment-related MDS and secondary leukemia.

Genetic Variation and Predisposition to MDS and Secondary AML

Why do only certain individuals exposed to genotoxic agents such as chemotherapy and envirnomental carcinogens develop MDS and secondary AML? Although environmental co-factors such as chemicals and infectious agents may be important, genetic predisposition is likely to be of great significance. What are the genetic traits that would predispose an individual to MDS and secondary AML? They are likely to be genetic polymorphisms with high frequency and low penetrance in the human population, which have arisen as the result of selective pressure, genetic drift, or founder effects. Metabolism of genotoxic agents and proficiency of DNA repair are traits that are likely to the affect the risk of MDS and secondary AML.

Epidemiologic studies have identified exposure to benzene and chemotherapeutic agents as risk factors for MDS and secondary AML, and considerable genetic variation exists in the host response to these agents. Variation in the ability to activate or excrete these compounds may lead to variability in the likelihood of genetic damage following exposure. Benzene is metabolized by CYP 2E1, and variation in enzyme activity is seen with certain polymorphic variants (Caporaso and Rothman, 1998). There is also variation in the expression of CYP 2E1 in the bone marrow (Bernauer et al., 2000). Cyclophosphamide, an important chemotherapeutic alkylating agent associated with the risk of MDS and secondary AML, is metabolized by CYP 2B6, which also has shown inter-individual variation. Epipodophyllotoxin is metabolized by CYP 3A4, and a polymorphic variant, CYP 3A4-W has been associated with an increased risk of secondary AML following treatment. The CYP 3A4 variant may generate increased levels of potentially DNA-damaging reactive intermediates (Felix at al., 1998). Other chemotherapeutic agents implicated in secondary AML, such as doxorubicin and mitoxantrone (Chaplain et al., 2000), are also metabolized by these polymorphic enzymes.

Genetic variation in Phase II enzymes such as GST have also been studied in MDS and secondary AML, and an association with deletion of GST-T1 has been observed (Chen et al., 1996), although other studies have found no association (Crump et al., 2000). Because of the complexity of xenobiotic metabolism, it is unlikely that a single polymorphic enzyme will confer significant risks for disease, although studies that have combined analysis of phase I (CYP) and phase II (GST) in smoking-related cancers have detected 40 to 100 fold variation in risk (Caporaso and Rothman, 1998).

Another important aspect of the host-response to genotoxic agents is the capacity for DNA repair. Although genetic instability is a key aspect of MDS, there has been no systematic study to determine whether an inherited defect in DNA repair is present in individuals with MDS and secondary leukemia. It is interesting to speculate that treatment-related MDS and secondary AML may have developed in individuals who have an underlying tendency to genetic instability, which gave rise to the initial malignancy for which chemotherapy was given. In this regard, the observation of microsatellite instability in a subset of MDS (Maeck et al., 2000) , and in secondary solid tumors, raises the question of a genetic predisposition. Variation in human populations in the ability to maintain DNA integrity in the face of environmental challenge will result, in part, from the observed variation in DNA repair (Berwick and Vineis, 2000) and folate metabolism (Choi and Mason, 2000). These areas of human genetic variation may be useful in identifying individuals at increased risk for treatment-related MDS and secondary AML.

CONCLUSION

Evolutionary biology is essential for the understanding of predisposition to malignancy, and malignant progression. MDS and secondary AML represent a disease process in hematopoietic stem cells that may result from the interaction of predisposing genes with certain environmental factors. Epidemiology has identified genotoxic agents such as chemotherapy as a major causative environmental factor, but evolutionary biology suggests that this is only half of the story. Genetically mediated variation in the host response to the environment is equally important in understanding, treating, and perhaps preventing this disease. The host-response to other factors sometimes implicated in MDS, such as infectious agents, is equally dependent on genetic background. Evolutionary biology would suggest that MDS and secondary AML be viewed as resulting from the maladaptation of particular genotypes to the modern environment, and implicates a tendency to genetic instability in the face of environmental challenges. This tendency may be manifest in the host response to xenobiotocs, the capacity for DNA repair, or some as yet undiscovered trait. The outcome of this approach may be to allow identification of susceptible individuals, to prevent MDS and secondary AML, and to employ non-genotoxic methods when treatment is necessary.

REFERENCES

Behrens, C., Travis, L.B., Wistuba, I.I., Davis, S., Maitra, A., Clarke, E.A., Lynch, C.F., Glimelius, B., Wiklund, T., Tarone, R., & Gazdar, A.F. (2000) Molecular Changes in Second Primary Lung and Breast Cancers after Therapy for Hodgkin's Disease. *Cancer Epidemiology, Biomarkers and Prevention* **9:** 1027-1035.

Bernauer, U., Vieth, B., Ellrich, R., Heinrich-Hirsch, B., Janig, G.R., & Gundert-Remy, U.(2000) CYP 2E1 expression in bone marrow and its intra- and interspecies variability. *Archives of Toxicology* **73**: 618-624

Berwick, M. & Vineis, P. (2000) Markers of DNA Repair and Susceptibility to Cancer in Humans: An Epidemiologic Review. *Journal of the National Cancer Institute* **92:** 874-897

Burdon, R. H. (1999) *Genes and the Environment.* Philadelphia. Taylor and Francis, Inc.

Caporaso, N. & Rothman, N. (1998) Genetic Susceptibility and Cancer Risk, in *Human Variability in Response to Chemical Exposures.* Neuman, D. and Kimmel, C., Editors. Boca Raton. CRC Press

Cavalli-Sforza,L.L., Menozzi, P., & Piazza, A. (1994) *The History and Geography of Human Genes.* Princeton. Princeton University Press.

Chaplain, G., Milan, C., Sgro, C., Carli, P.M., & Bonithon-Kopp, C. (2000) Increased Risk of Acute Leukemia After Adjuvant Chemotherapy for Breast Cancer: A Population-Based Study. *Journal of Clinical Oncology* **18:** 2836-2842

Chen, H., Sandler, D.P., Taylor, J.A., Shore, D.L., Liu, E., Bloomfield, C.E., & Bell, D.A. (1996) Increased risk for myelodysplastic syndromes in individuals with glutathione transferase theta 1 (GSTT1) gene defect. *Lancet* **347** : 295-287

Chen, J., Giovannucci, E., Kelsey, K., Rimm, E.B., Stampfer, M.J., Colditz, G.A., Spiegelman, D., Willett, W.C., & Hunter, D.J. (1996) A methylenetetrahydrofolate reductase polymorphism and the risk of colorectal cancer. *Cancer Research* **56 :** 4862 - 4864

Childs, B. (1999) *Genetic Medicine : A Logic of Disease* Baltimore. Johns Hopkins University Press.

Choi, S.W. & Mason, J.B. (2000) Folate and carconigenesis : an integrated scheme. *Journal of Nutrition* **130 :** 129-132

Cooper, D. N. (1999) *Human Gene Evolution.* Oxford. Bios Scientific Publishers

Crump, C., Chen, C., Applebaum, F.R., Kopecky, K.J., Schwartz, S.M., Willman C.L., Slovak, M.L., & Weiss, N.S. (2000) Glutathion S-Transferase Theta 1 gene Deletion and Risk of Acute Myeloid Leukemia. *Cancer Epidemiology, Biomarkers and Prevention* **9:** 457-460

Denamur, E. Lecointre, G., Darlu, P., Tenaillon, O., Acquaviva, C., Sayada, C., Sunjevaric, I., Rothstein, R., Elion, J., Tadderi, F., Radman, M. & Matic, I. (2000). Evolutionary Implications of the Frequent Horizontal Transfer of Mismatch Repair Genes. *Cell* **103:** 711-721

Dobzhansky, T. (1970) *Genetics of the Evolutionary Process* New York. Columbia University Press.

Ewald, P. (1994) *Evolution of Infectious Disease.* New York. Oxford University Press.

Felix, C.A., Walker, A.H., Lange, B.J., Williams, T.M., Winick, N.J., Cheung, N.K., Lovett, B.D., Nowell, P.C., Blair, I.A., & Rebbeck, T.R. (1998) Association of CYP3A4 genotype with treatment-related leukemia. *Proceedings National Academy of Sciences* **95 :** 13176-13181

Frame, L.T., Ambrosone, C.B., Kadlubar, F.F., & Lang, N.P. (1998) Host-Environment Interactions That Affect Variability in Human Cancer Susceptibility, in *Human Variability in Response to Chemical Exposures.* Neuman, D. and Kimmel, C., Editors. Boca Raton. CRC Press.

Greaves, M. (2000) *Cancer : The Evolutionary Legacy.* New York. Oxford University Press

Hanahan, D. & Weinberg, R. (2000) The Hallmarks of Cancer. *Cell* **100**: 57-70

Hastings, P.J., Bull, H.J., Klump, J.R., & Rosenberg, S.M. (2000) Adaptive Amplification : An Inducible Chromosomal Instability Mechanism. *Cell* **103:** 723-731

Hirst, W.J., Czepulkowski, B. & Mufti, G.J. (1993) Consistent interstitial chromosomal deletions in myeloid malignancies and their correltaion with fragile sites. *Cancer Genetics and Cytogenetics.* **65** : 51-57

Hoffman, A.A. & Parsons, P.A. (1993) *Evolutionary Genetics and Environmental Stress* New York. Oxford University Press.

Kurotaki, H., Tsushima, Y., Nagai, K., & Yagihashi, S. (1999) Apoptosis, bcl-2 expression and p53 accumulation in myelodysplastic syndrome, myelodysplastic syndrome-derived acute myelogenous leukemia and de novo acute myelogenous leukemia. *Acta Haematologica*, **102**, 115-123.

Lazar, M. A. (2000) Gene Regulation : One man's food. *Nature* **407:** 852-853

Lensch, M.W., Rathbun, R.K., Olson, S.B., Jones, G.R., & Bagby, G.C. (1999) Selective Pressure as an essential force in molecular evolution of myeloid leukemic clones : a view from the window of Fanconi anemia *Leukemia* **13:** 1784-1789

Lichtman, M. & Brennan, J. K. (2001) Chapter 92: Myelodysplastic Disorders, in *Williams Hematology, 6th Edition.* New York. McGraw-Hill

Maeck, L., Haase, D., Schoch, C., Hiddeman, W., & Alves, F. (2000) Genetic instability in myelodysplastic syndrome : detection of microsatellite instability and loss of heterozygosity in bone marrow samples with karyotype alterations. *British Journal of Hematology* **109:** 842 – 846

Mori, N., Morosetti, R., Hoflehner, E., Lubbert, M., Mizoguchi, H., & Koeffler, H. (2000) Allelic loss in the progression of myelodysplastic syndrome. *Cancer Research* **60:** 3039-3042

Neel, J.V. (1999) When Some Fine Old Genes Meet a "New" Environment, in *Evolutionary Aspects of Nutrition and Health,* Simopoulos, A.P., Editor. Basel. Karger

Nesse, R. & Williams, G. (1994) *Why We Get Sick : The New Science of Darwinian Medicine* New York. Random House.

Ponten, J. (1998) *Cancer Surveys: Precancer : Biology, Importance, and Possible Prevention.* New York. Cold Spring Harbor Laboratory Press.

Stearns, S. C. (1999) *Evolution in Health and Disease.* New York. Oxford University Press

Sullivan, N. F. & Willis, A. E. (1994) Chapter 8: Acquisition of Premalignant Lesions: Myelodysplastic Syndrome, in *The Molecular Mechanisms of Cancer Predisposition.* Austin. R.G.Landis

Thagard, P. (1999) *How Scientists Explain Disease.* Princeton. Princeton University Press

Weatherall, D.J. (1996) The genetics of common diseases: the implications of population variability, in *Variation in the Human Genome.* (Ciba Foundation Symposium 197) Chichester. Wiley

Weiss, K. W. (1993) *Genetic Variation and Human Disease : Principles and Evolutionary Approaches.* New York. Cambridge University Press

Willman, C. (2000) Biologic and Genetic Features of the Myelodysplastic Syndrome. *Hematology 2000* p100-117.

INDEX